Microvascular Decompression Surgery

Shi-Ting Li • Jun Zhong
Marc Sindou • Raymond F. Sekula
Editors

Microvascular Decompression Surgery

Advances and Expansion of Strategy and Techniques

Second Edition

Springer

Editors
Shi-Ting Li
Department of Neurosurgery
XinHua Hospital, Shanghai JiaoTong
University School of Medicine
Shanghai, China

Jun Zhong
Department of Neurosurgery
XinHua Hospital, Shanghai JiaoTong
University School of Medicine
Shanghai, China

Marc Sindou
Department of Neurosurgery
University of Lyon
Lyon, France

Raymond F. Sekula
Department of Neurosurgery
Columbia University Irving
Medical Center
New York, NY, USA

ISBN 978-981-96-0766-2 ISBN 978-981-96-0767-9 (eBook)
https://doi.org/10.1007/978-981-96-0767-9

This Springer imprint is published by the registered company Springer Nature Singapore Pte Ltd.
The registered company address is: 152 Beach Road, #21-01/04 Gateway East, Singapore 189721, Singapore

Preface

Since the publication of the monograph *Microvascular Decompression Surgery* in 2015, the global promotion and popularization of microvascular decompression (MVD) technology has been accelerated, and the number of patients treated has significantly increased, and the surgical efficacy has also been improved. Looking back at the past 8 years, new progress has been made in both the research on the pathogenesis of diseases and clinical diagnosis and treatment techniques. In particular, there have been significant advances in decompression techniques for complex vascular compression, surgical techniques for atypical patients, reoperation techniques for patients who have failed the first MVD operation, perioperative electrophysiological monitoring techniques, and other treatment techniques for common cranial nerve diseases. For example, the improvement of trigeminal nerve balloon compression technology, facial paralysis repair technology, surgical technology of facial paralysis sequelae, minimally invasive treatment of masseter spasm, MVD technology of oculomotor nerve paralysis, and so on. Therefore, we have written this monograph, hoping to help you better carry out the clinical diagnosis and treatment of cranial nerve diseases.

Cranial nerve diseases are very common in clinical practice, except for trigeminal neuralgia, hemifacial spasm and glossopharyngeal nerve pain, and there are quite a few diseases that affect the quality of life of patients, such as vision loss, double vision, oculomotor nerve paralysis, abducent nerve paralysis, facial numbness, masseter spasm, tinnitus, vertigo, intermediate neuralgia, all kinds of facial nerve paralysis, facial paralysis sequelae, hypoglossal nerve damage, and so on. In recent years, there have been a lot of new ideas, new methods, and new surgical techniques surrounding the diagnosis and treatment of cranial nerve diseases. In this monograph, we will summarize the relevant technical progress as far as possible, and also introduce the research hotspots in related fields. We hope that this monograph can be a good teacher and friend for everyone and help popularize and promote the new techniques for the diagnosis and treatment of cranial nerve diseases so that more patients can get better treatment.

In the process of preparing and writing this monograph, we have received great support from famous experts from more than 20 countries around the world, who not only undertook different writing tasks, but also provided many valuable suggestions for the overall arrangement of the monograph publication. Experts involved in the preparation of the monograph were Marc P. Sindou, Raymond F. Sekula, Anthony M. Kaufmann, Takamitsu Fujimaki,

Mojgan Hodaie, Richard S. Zimmerman, Jun Zhong, Fuminari Komatsu, Xuesheng Zheng, Joachim K. Krauss, Mauro Segura, Jin Woo Chang, Ludvic Zrinzo, Jamil Rzaev, Kim Burchiel, Shusaku Noro, Massimiliano Visocchi, Yinda Tang, Baimiao Wang, Tingting Ying, and Shi-Ting Li.

In the preparation of this book, new developments are highlighted, including new theories, new ideas, new methods, new techniques, new models, and so on. Due to the limitations of time and monograph space, there are still many research developments that have not been introduced in this monograph. I hope you can understand. In addition, due to the limitations of personal experience, omissions are inevitable. I hope that the majority of readers put forward valuable suggestions.

Shanghai, China Shi-Ting Li

Contents

History of the Jannetta Procedure

1

Alwyn Gomez and Anthony M. Kaufmann

1.1 Introduction

The Jannetta procedure, now more commonly known as microvascular decompression (MVD), has become a commonly practiced surgery that is a widely accepted and effective treatment for trigeminal neuralgia (TN), hemifacial spasm (HFS) and glossopharyngeal neuralgia (GPN) [1]. While the history of the procedure extends long before its namesake, without the careful refinement of surgical technique, documentation of outcomes and resilience of Peter Jannetta it may not have taken its place as one of the great advancements in neurosurgery and medicine.

1.2 The History of Surgical Management of Trigeminal Neuralgia

To understand the development of the Jannetta procedure the historical context of TN must be reviewed. While descriptions of TN-like ailments date back to the first century AD, the precise characterization of the clinical condition, then known as tic douloureux, was only undertaken in the 17th and eighteenth century by Locke, André and Fothergill [2]. Surgical management of this debilitating disease would only appear in the mid-nineteenth century with the Hartley-Krause technique. This would later be refined into the Spiller-Frazier technique by 1928 and involve an extradural, subtemporal approach to a retrogasserian rhizotomy that targeted only the affected fibers resulting in long-term pain relief [3]. The procedure became the accepted management of TN at the time but was often associated with significant facial sensory loss, keratitis, retraction injury of the temporal lobe and injury of the geniculate ganglion with resultant facial paralysis [4]. Given the debilitating nature of TN, especially at the time, these were considered acceptable complications.

Dr. Walter Dandy was a vocal opponent to the subtemporal approach, instead advocating for a retromastoid craniectomy approach in 1920s and 1930s [5]. The lack of surgical microscope made the technique particularly challenging but provided a more direct approach with less blood loss. Additionally, through selective or partial rhizotomy he was able to preserve some facial sensation and mastication strength. This was made possible through his recognition of the topographic organization of the sensory fibers of portio major and distinction of the portio minor, caring motor fibers [6].

A. Gomez
Section of Neurosurgery, Department of Surgery, University of Manitoba, Winnipeg, MB, Canada

Department of Human Anatomy and Cell Science, University of Manitoba, Winnipeg, MB, Canada

A. M. Kaufmann (✉)
Section of Neurosurgery, Department of Surgery, University of Manitoba, Winnipeg, MB, Canada
e-mail: AKaufmann@hsc.mb.ca

S.-T. Li et al. (eds.), *Microvascular Decompression Surgery*,
https://doi.org/10.1007/978-981-96-0767-9_1

Despite the technically challenging nature of his technique, Dandy was able to perform a relatively large number of these cases and went on to publish a case series of 215 procedures in which there was complete or partial sectioning of the trigeminal root. It was during this seminal work that Dandy first hypothesized a compressive etiology of TN. He additionally noted compression of the nerve root by the superior cerebellar artery (SCA) in 30.7% of cases and by the petrosal vein in 14% of cases. He also acknowledged that other causes of compression might have been present but not observable by the naked eye [7]. He did not, however, hypothesize that there was a difference between static and pulsatile compression and made no note of any potential susceptibility of the proximal nerve root. Of note, he made no claim that treatment of TN could be achieved through translocation of the compressive vessel. This may have been due to the already high degree of scrutiny he was receiving for the operation or the difficulty of attempting this without magnification [8]. In any case, while Dandy was able to achieve excellent outcomes, his novel approach and observations were largely abandoned as others failed to replicate the success of this technically complex procedure with the surgical tools of that era.

In the 1950s the notion of a compressive etiology of TN was brought back into vogue by Taarnhøj, Gardener, and Miklos [9, 10]. Still without the aid of a surgical microscope, they returned to the subtemporal approach, but this time extended it to allow for opening of the dural mater overlying the proximal entry to Meckel's cave. This freed the sensory root of the trigeminal nerve from its dural sleeve. From there Gardner and Miklos described the "non-traumatic manipulation" of the nerve. Believing in the necessity of neurolysis, they described gently brushing with a cotton pledget and vigorous irrigation of the nerve [10].

Gardner also hypothesized an analogous mechanism for HFS and also began treating this condition with "non-traumatic manipulation." In the early 1960s he reported a series of suboccipital approaches that followed failed middle fossa attempts in 18 cases of TN and 19 cases of HFS. Again, despite the lack of magnification, he noted vascular compression in 6 of the TN cases and 7 of the HFS cases; a similar proportion as Dandy had decades earlier. In one such case, he treated the patient through interposing the vessel away from the nerve using a Gelfoam pad, becoming the first neurosurgeon to perform an MVD for HFS. Despite this, Gardner retained his recommendation to treat both TN and HFS with neurolysis [4, 11, 12].

1.3 Developing the Jannetta Procedure

Born in 1932 in Philadelphia, Peter Joseph Jannetta attended medical school at the University of Pennsylvania, graduating in 1957. He went on to undertake his General Surgery residency and was granted a National Institutes of Health (NIH) neurophysiology research fellowship under the supervision of Professor Sol Erulkar [13]. It was there where he gained initial proficiency in the use of a binocular microscope in experiments on the feline spinal cord. Following this, he went on to complete neurosurgical training at the University of California, Los Angeles (UCLA) from 1963 to 1966 under the mentorship of Robert Rand and Theodore Kurze. As both were early adopters of the operating microscope, it was here that Jannetta was first introduced to microneurosurgery [14].

The 1950s and 1960s were also a time of major evolutions in the management of TN. This primarily involved the identification and utilization of phenytoin and carbamazepine as medical treatments for TN. Additionally, during this time period, rhizotomy became further engrained with the refinement of less-invasive percutaneous procedures. The medical community had seemingly settled into its understanding of TN and its treatments. Fortunately, a young Jannetta was primed to challenge these entrenched notions [15].

In a biography of Jannetta by Shelton, three serendipitous events in 1965–66 are described that led to his development of the neurovascular compression theory [16]. The first was in the spring of 1965 when Rand had tasked Jannetta with performing cadaveric dissections of the cranial nerves for dental students to view on closed-circuit television. Through these dissections, Jannetta was able to develop his microsurgical approach to the trigeminal nerve for TN. It also led to his discovery of a small bundle of nerve fibers at the proximal end of the nerve root that lay between the portio major and minor. In discussing these findings with Rand, he was directed to the previous work of Dandy, who had identified these fibers decades earlier and had described preserving them during sectioning of the portio major for TN [17]. Jannetta and Rand continued work on developing a subtemporal transtentorial microsurgical approach to the trigeminal nerve for the purposes of sectioning the portio major, while preserving the portio minor and "portio intermediate," for the treatment of TN [18]. However, despite having performed numerous cadaveric trials of the procedure, they were forbidden from performing this new microneurosurgery procedure at UCLA (Fig. 1.1).

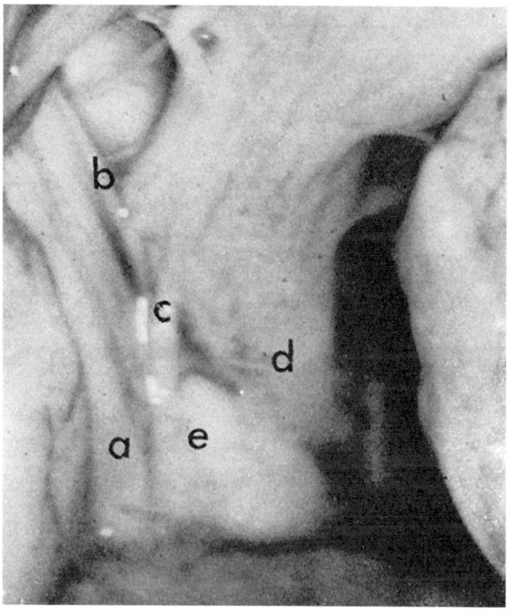

Fig. 1.1 In 1965, as a resident, Jannetta was assigned to prosect cranial nerve specimens for teaching demonstrations to dental students. He identified sensory fiber bundles intermediate to the portio major and minor. This was the basis of his development of a selective or partial trigeminal rhizotomy, which was intended to treat TN while preserving a degree of facial sensation. Seen is the view through a dissecting microscope of the right trigeminal never at 10× magnification: (**a**) motor branches; (**b**) intermediate fibers with motor branches; (**c**) intermediate fibers leaving the portio major and entering the pons between motor and major sensory roots; (**d**) "fibrous cone" region of the portio major; (**e**) pons. Reprinted with permission from Jannetta PJ: Gross (mesoscopic) description of the human trigeminal nerve and ganglion. J Neurosurg 26 (1 Suppl):109–111, 1967

The second serendipitous event would occur during the index case of this new procedure, but to call it luck would discount the perseverance and astute nature of Jannetta. With the procedure barred at UCLA, the first patient would actually be treated at the neighboring Harbor General Hospital. The patient, a 52-year-old man with a 10-year history of TN, had become refractory to conventional management including alcohol injections and medications. He had been admitted under the care of the neurosurgeon John Alksne. Alksne was also an early adopter of microneurosurgery and a supporter of Jannetta's novel ideas [19]. The patient, now suffering from approximately 200 pain attacks per day, consented to undergo selective sensory rhizotomy.

Jannetta, determined to perform the surgery, disassembled the operating microscope, personally purchased by Rand and located at UCLA, and transported it in his 1957 Ford station wagon to Harbor General Hospital, where he reassembled it for the surgery. The procedure was performed by Jannetta with Alksne assisting and Rand observing. Through the subtemporal transtentorial approach, they we able to view of the proximal trigeminal nerve where Jannetta noted a pulsating artery compressing the nerve. Jannetta had an epiphany and quietly exclaimed to Alksne "That's the cause of the tic!" While they went on to section the nerve as planned, the seeds of the neurovascular compression theory had been planted in Jannetta's mind. Jannetta would go on to make similar observations in subsequent procedures. Conversely, in a series of 56 cadaveric dissections of subjects presumed to not have TN, Jannetta reported that no vascular compression of the trigeminal nerve was noted [20]. Jannetta was convinced of the vascular compression etiology of TN and hypothesized that transposition of the vessel would potentially cure the disease (Fig. 1.2).

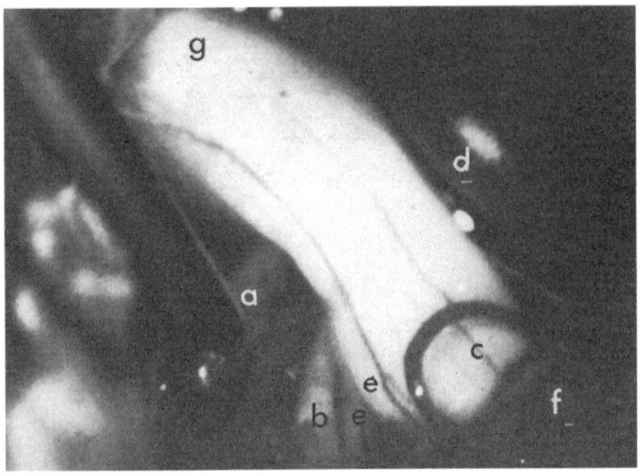

Fig. 1.2 View of the right trigeminal nerve at the pons through a dissecting microscope as would have been seen by Jannetta and Alksne during Jannetta's first selective trigeminal rhizotomy operation for TN: (**a**) small tortuous branches of the SCA compressing nerve at pons; (**b**) motor roots; (**c**) "fibrous cone" region of portio major; (**d**) another arterial branch; (**e**) intermediate fibers; (**f**) cerebellum (retracted); and (**g**) trigeminal nerve entering dural canal. Tortuous arterial branches are supported partly away from the nerve by the instrument. Original magnification ×16. Reprinted with permission from Jannetta PJ: Arterial compression of the trigeminal nerve at the pons in patients with trigeminal neuralgia. J Neurosurg 26:159–162, 1967

The third serendipitous event occurred in May of 1966 during one of Jannetta's clinics. He observed a 41-year-old precision mechanic in the hallway suffering from severe left-sided HFS. It was in that moment that he suddenly recognized that vascular compression could also be the root cause of this condition, just as he hypothesized with TN. He also was convinced this could be cured through mobilization of the offending vessel away from the facial nerve. The patient had been debilitated from this disease, unable to work due to the forceful eye closures. Jannetta presented him with the standard treatment of facial nerve injury through a posterior fossa approach. Somewhat daringly, he also presented his nascent theory on neurovascular compression and proposed that through atraumatic translocation of the offending vessel they could potentially avoid facial weakness and cure the disease for good. The patient consented to the experimental procedure and became the first to undergo Jannetta's MVD procedure [16].

Through coincidence or pure luck, the obstructive senior faculty members were away when the procedure was performed on June 2, 1966, at UCLA. Paul Crandall, the supervising neurosurgeon at the time granted Jannetta permission to perform the surgery. Under the operative microscope, through a retromastoid approach in the seated position, Jannetta observed an anterior inferior cerebellar artery in proximity to the distal facial nerve; however, he was not convinced that this was the causative vessel. Undeterred, he inspected the nerve more carefully to find that its distortion was caused by a vein located on the pons. Committed to his theory, he coagulated and cut the vessel and marveled as the nerve immediately returned to a more typical course [16]. Following the procedure, the patient recovered well, with his spasms resolving in what would turn out to be a durable result. Those well versed in the HFS literature will note the rarity of a venous etiology. The insight and pois that Jannetta demonstrated surely prevented the premature rejection of the neurovascular compression theory.

Two months later, with the first successful MVD treatment of HFS under his belt, Jannetta and Rand would perform the first MVD for TN. Initially consented for a selective rhizotomy, under the surgical microscope they observed that the superior cerebellar artery (SCA) was compressing the trigeminal nerve. Eager to test the neurovascular coupling theory in TN, they obtained consent to perform a vascular decompression of the nerve intraoperatively from the patient's husband. They mobilized the SCA and maintained the separation with a piece of Ivalon sponge. The procedure was a success with the patient experiencing lifelong relief from TN [21].

1.4 The Early Years of the Jannetta Procedure

As their experience grew, Rand and Jannetta began presenting their neurovascular compression hypothesis for TN and HFS at neurosurgical conferences in 1967. However, much resistance

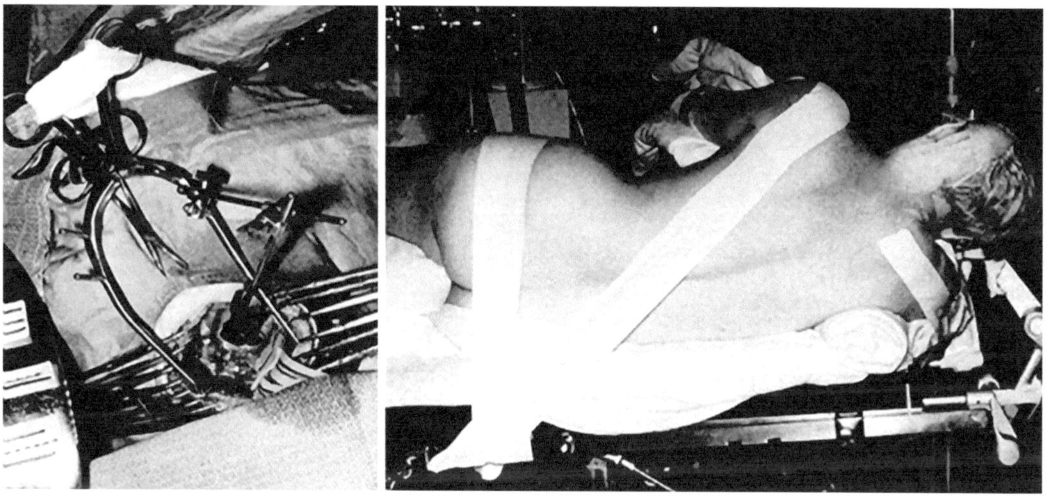

Fig. 1.3 Jannetta moved away from utilizing the subtemporal approach for TN and instead adopted a lateral position and retromastoid craniectomy to access the cranial nerves of the posterior fossa, much like Dandy decades earlier. Reprinted with permission from Jannetta PJ, Abbasy M, Maroon JC, Ramos FM, Albin MS: Etiology and definitive microsurgical treatment of hemifacial spasm. Operative techniques and results in 47 patients. J Neuorsurg 47:321–328, 1977

was met to this hypothesis and further to the notion of a nondestructive approach to the treatment of these conditions [20]. Even those that agreed with the neurovascular etiology of TN and HFS, such as Gardner, felt that at the very least, neurolytic interventions were still most appropriate [12].

Following residency, Jannetta accepted a faculty position at Louisiana State University Medical Center in the Department of Neurosurgery. Jannetta continued there his development of the MVD procedure and came to abandon the subtemporal approach to the trigeminal nerve in favor of the more contemporary retrosigmoid approach. This transition was driven, in part, through the temporal lobe injuries that occurred without the expert assistance of Rand [22]. Further, the subtemporal approach was developed with the section of the nerve in mind and not the translocation of causative vessel. Jannetta recognized that the retrosigmoid approach was much better suited to this new objective [23] (Fig. 1.3).

Following a move to the University of Pittsburg Medical Center in 1971, Jannetta continued to refine the MVD procedure and kept diligent records about his cases and the outcomes of his patients [24]. Through the 1970s Jannetta actively published his results in the neurosurgical literature and presented at numerous neurosurgical meetings [25, 26]. Beyond this, he began training others in the procedure, thereby allowing the impact of his advancements to extend far beyond his own institution. Through these dedicated and honest efforts, the neurosurgical community slowly began to accept the neurovascular compression theory of TN and HFS as well as the utility and safety of the MVD procedure. However, it would take until the mid-1990s until safely and efficacy of MVD for TN would be accepted by the larger medical community after the publication of the long-term results of the procedure in the New England Journal of medicine [27], together with similar papers regarding HFS and GPN [28, 29] (Fig. 1.4).

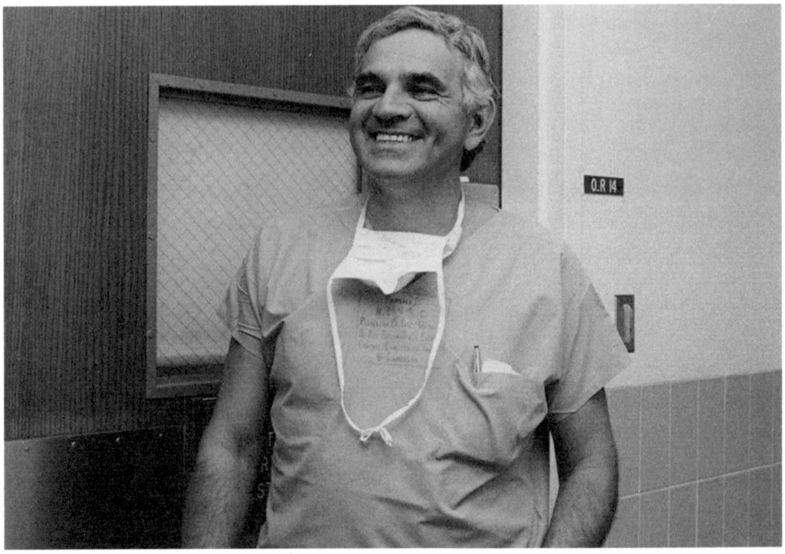

Fig. 1.4 Through his early career Jannetta faced much skepticism regarding his neurovascular compression theory and his proposed surgery for these conditions. Despite this he persevered through meticulous self-evaluation, driven by the desire to do the best for the patients he cared for. Copyright Raymond F. Sekula Jr. Published with permission from World Neurosurgery (https://doi.org/10.1016/j.wneu.2016.06.068)

1.5 Conclusion

As time has passed, the MVD procedure has continued to be proven a safe, effective, and durable treatment for TN, HFS, and GPN. It is now widely considered the gold-standard treatment for these conditions. Further, the notion of a neurovascular compressive etiology of these conditions is now generally accepted. While the roots of the surgical management of these pathologies extend far before Jannetta, there is no doubt that without his dedication and conviction, the medical community would be without this great discovery.

References

1. Kaufmann AM, Price AV. A history of the Jannetta procedure. J Neurosurg. 2020;132:639–46.
2. Stookey B, Ransohoff J. Trigeminal neuralgia: its history and treatment. Springfield, IL: Charles C Thomas; 1959.
3. Pinkus RL. Innovation in neurosurgery: Walter Dandy in his day. Neurosurgery. 1984;14:623.
4. Patel SK, Liu JK. Overview and history of trigeminal neuralgia. Neurosurg Clin N Am. 2016;27:265–76.
5. Dandy WE. An operation for the cure of tic Douloureaux: partial section of the sensory root at the pons. Arch Surg. 1929;18:687.
6. Sweet WH, Wepsic JG. Controlled thermocoagulation of trigeminal ganglion and rootlets for differential destruction of pain fibers: part 1: trigeminal neuralgia. J Neurosurg. 1974;40:143–56.
7. Dandy WE. Concerning the cause of trigeminal neuralgia. Am J Surg. 1934;24:447–55.
8. Van Wagenen WP. Some indications for section of the trigeminal nerve through the posterior fossa. Ann Surg. 1931;94:1013–7.
9. Taarnhøj P. Decompression of the trigeminal root and the posterior part of the ganglion as treatment in trigeminal neuralgia: preliminary communication. J Neurosurg. 1952;9:288–90.
10. Gardner WJ. Response of trigeminal neuralgia to decompression of sensory root; discussion of cause of trigeminal neuralgia. JAMA. 1959;170:1773.
11. Gardner WJ, Sava GA. Hemifacial spasm—a reversible pathophysiologic state. J Neurosurg. 1962;19:240–7.
12. Gardner WJ. Concerning the mechanism of trigeminal neuralgia and Hemifacial spasm. J Neurosurg. 1962;19:947–58.
13. Erulkar SD, Sprague JM, Whitsel BL, Dogan S, Jannetta PJ. Organization of the vestibular projection to the spinal cord of the cat. J Neurophysiol. 1966;29:626–64.
14. Rand RW, Kurze TL. Facial nerve preservation by posterior fossa transmeatal microdissection in total removal of acoustic tumors. J Neurol Neurosurg Psychiatry. 1965;28:311–6.
15. Jannetta PJ. Preface. In: Trigeminal Neuralgia. New York: Oxford University Press; 2011. p. ix–xi.
16. Shelton M. Working in a very small place: the making of a neurosurgeon. New York: First Vintage Books Edition; 1990.
17. Jannetta PJ. Gross (mesoscopic) description of the human trigeminal nerve and ganglion. J Neurosurg. 1967;26:109–11.

18. Jannetta PJ, Rand RW. Transtentorial retrogasserian rhizotomy in trigeminal neuralgia by microneurosurgical technique. Bull Los Angel Neurol Soc. 1966;31:93–9.
19. Alksne JF. Microsurgical vascular decompression of cranial nerves. Am J Surg. 1980;140:156–7.
20. Jannetta PJ. Arterial compression of the trigeminal nerve at the pons in patients with trigeminal neuralgia. J Neurosurg. 1967;26:159–62.
21. Rand RW. Gardner neurovascular decompression of the trigeminal and facial nerves for tic douloureux and hemifacial spasm. Surg Neurol. 1981;16:329–32.
22. Jannetta PJ. Letter: complications from microsurgical treatment of tic douloureux. J Neurosurg. 1974;40:675.
23. Jannetta PJ, McLaughlin MR, Sekula RF, Jannetta PJ. Microvascular decompression. New York: Oxford University Press; 2011. p. 213.
24. Jannetta PJ. Microsurgery of cranial nerve cross-compression. Clin Neurosurg. 1979;26:607–15.
25. Jannetta PJ, Skinner DB, Ebert PA. Microsurgical exploration and decompression of the facial nerve in hemifacial spasm, vol. 2. Cham: Springer; 1970. p. 220.
26. Jannetta PJ. The cause of hemifacial spasm: definitive microsurgical treatment at the brainstem in 31 patients. Trans Sect Otolaryngol Am Acad Ophthalmol Otolaryngol. 1975;80:319–22.
27. Barker FG, Jannetta PJ, Bissonette DJ, Larkins MV, Jho HD. The long-term outcome of microvascular decompression for trigeminal neuralgia. N Engl J Med. 1996;334:1077–83.
28. Barker FG, Jannetta PJ, Bissonette DJ, Shields PT, Larkins MV, Jho HD. Microvascular decompression for hemifacial spasm. J Neurosurg. 1995;82:201–10.
29. Resnick DK, Jannetta PJ, Bissonnette D, Jho HD, Lanzino G. Microvascular decompression for glossopharyngeal neuralgia. Neurosurgery. 1995;36:64–9.

2 The Mechanism Underlying Trigeminal Neuralgia

Jun Zhong

Trigeminal neuralgia (TN) is a prevalent form of cranial nerve rhizophathy characterized by hyperexcitability, which also involves hemifacial spasm (HFS), glossopharyngeal neuralgia, masticatory spasm, intermediate neuralgia and some sort of tinnitus or vertigo, etc. [1–5]. Although limited relevant research has been reported in the literature [6, 7], two main schools of thought exist to address this puzzle: the central [8–10] and peripheral theories [11–13]. The former primarily focused on the brain stem structures, specifically the trigeminal nucleus. It was hypothesized that paroxysm represented a form of epileptic seizures, supported by evidence indicating that TN may exhibit response to specific anticonvulsant drugs, notably carbamazepine [14, 15]. The latter primarily focused on the compressed site of the cranial nerve root, as adjacent arterial loops or occasionally tumors, cysts, arteriovenous malformations, or aneurysms can exert compressive force on the nerve in these patients [16–18]. However, the underlying mechanism responsible for the development of hyperfunction rather than hypofunction in compressed nerves remains poorly elucidated.

J. Zhong (✉)
Department of Neurosurgery, XinHua Hospital, Shanghai JiaoTong University School of Medicine, Shanghai, China
e-mail: ZhongJun@Xinhuamed.com.cn

2.1 Compression of Nerve Root

The pathogenesis of these disorders can be attributed to neurovascular conflict or vascular compression of the cranial nerve root, a phenomenon that has been substantiated by successful microvascular decompression surgery [19–21]. The provided etiological explanation may facilitate comprehension of the heightened susceptibility observed in individuals of elder Oriental ancestry [22]. Due to inherent anatomical disparities, individuals with Eastern heritage manifest a more condensed cerebellopontine angle (CPA) relative to other ethnic groups. The aging process can cause cerebral atrophy and vascular sclerosis, bringing them closer together in a limited space. The findings from our previous study indicate that 86.4% of patients with primary HFS exhibit a shifted vertebrobasilar complex deviating towards the symptomatic side [23]. Nevertheless, numerous contradictions persist. Firstly, it is worth noting that similar neurovascular relationships are commonly observed outside the cranium, such as in the femoral sheath or carotid where nerves and vessels are closely arranged; however, no corresponding symptoms have been reported. Secondly, based on Rhoton's cadaver anatomy findings [24–26], the anterior inferior cerebellar artery traverses the space between the acoustic and facial nerves with an approximate occurrence rate of 70%, yet the incidence of HFS is significantly

S.-T. Li et al. (eds.), *Microvascular Decompression Surgery*,
https://doi.org/10.1007/978-981-96-0767-9_2

lower than that. Additionally, magnetic resonance imaging (MRI) scans often reveal a close neurovascular relationship in asymptomatic individuals. Thirdly, why do these cranial nerves exhibit hyperactivity in response to compression? Shouldn't they exhibit reduced excitability when the nerve is damaged? Additionally, why does this symptom manifest in a sudden and intermittent manner with periods of silence, often triggered by emotional stimuli? Consequently, it can be inferred that neurovascular conflict may give rise to neuralgia, while the reverse causality is unlikely. Considering the prompt resolution of symptoms subsequent to a successful microvascular decompression (MVD) in the majority of cases, we hypothesize that the underlying pathogenesis primarily resides at the site of nerve compression. However, the development of the symptom still necessitates various preconditions. In other words, the symptom may only be generated and triggered by a compression that is precisely "calibrated."

2.2 Demyelination

The initial documentation of demyelination associated with TN was originally reported by Hilton and colleagues [27, 28], who discovered degraded central myelin at the location of arterial compression. This observation was subsequently replicated by Rappaport et al [29, 30] analyzed biopsy samples from the compressed site in 12 TN patients undergoing MVD. Interestingly, both demyelination and axonopathy were observed in 11 patients, despite only 7 having confirmed arterial compression during surgery. After years of relevant research, we have come to the realization that establishing the TN or HFS animal model is a more complex task than initially anticipated. In fact, our success rate has been found to be below 60%. Nevertheless, it is important to highlight that demyelination has been consistently observed in all TN or HFS rats [7, 31]. The implication suggests that a certain degree of demyelination, neither excessively severe nor too mild, serves as the essential pathological prerequisite. The effective explanation for why symptoms arise exclusively from intracranial neurovascular contact lies in the distinctive characteristics of these nerves compared to their extracranial counterparts. Unlike extracranial nerves that are encased in protective sheaths and immobile relative to arteries, akin to concealed wires embedded within a wall, intracranial nerves resemble exposed wires, especially in segments positioned medially towards the root entry/exit zone (REZ) where Schwann's cells offer comparatively weaker shielding. It also explains the phenomenon that while the culprit can arise anywhere along the intracranial trigeminal root in TN cases, it is typically limited to the REZ of facial root in most HFS cases [5, 6, 32]. The cranial nerve consists of segments from both the central (CNS) and peripheral nervous (PNS) systems, separated by the REZ. The histological differences suggest that the PNS segment exhibits a higher resistance to compression [13]. According to Moller and De Ridder's findings [33], the PNS segment of the VII root is significantly longer compared to that of the V root. A study by Burchiel and colleagues supported a link between demyelination and TN-like changes in animals [34–36], who observed additional action potentials in the trigeminal root after iatrogenic demyelination due to stimulation. Jannetta hypothesized that compression-induced demyelination facilitated ephaptic impulse transmission at these specific sites [37, 38]. It was postulated that damage to the REZ triggers the development of autorhythmicity in certain regions of the trigeminal ganglion, a phenomenon referred to as the "ignition hypothesis" [11]. The ignition process, however, does not appear to be as simple as a mere "short circuit" in electric wires with worn insulating covers. Nevertheless, these studies have convincingly demonstrated that demyelination serves as the fundamental structural basis required for generating aberrant impulses.

2.3 Ectopic Action Potentials

Based on these findings, it is evident that the neurovascular conflict site assumes a crucial role in this context. The pathogenesis, in fact, can be explained by an impulse or heightened excitability that specifically originates from the axon (cranial nerve root), which is distinct from those originating from neuronal soma or algesiroreceptor. Upon propagation of such deviant impulses towards the central cortex, they engender a perceptual illusion characterized by profound pain sensation. This particular form of atypical impulse may aptly be termed as an ectopic action potential.

2.4 Ion Channels

2.4.1 Voltage-Gated Channels

Considering the efficacy of use-dependent Na^+ channel blockers, such as carbamazepine, in the pharmacological treatment of TN or HFS, it is crucial to acknowledge the significance of targeting sodium channels. In fact, it is the primary molecular entity responsible for generating the propagatable action potential. In the embryonic promyelinating stage, a diffuse distribution of various isoforms ($Na_v1.1$–1.9) was observed along the axon. During the myelination process, Schwann cells extend and wrap around the nerve, resulting in exclusive presence of $Na_v1.6$ at the Ranvier nodes, which is responsible for propagating rather than generating action potentials [39, 40]. The presence of amorphous and enlarged channel clusters on the demyelinated axons has been observed to significantly increase in cases of chronic demyelination or developmental failure of myelin formation, as demonstrated by several studies [41–43]. Among these clusters, certain isoforms with lower thresholds may exert a particularly significant influence on the inherent excitability of nerve fiber. The expression of $Na_v1.3$ mRNA in the dorsal root ganglion (DRG) has been extensively documented to be high during embryonic stages, but significantly lower in adult rats. However, it undergoes upregulation subsequent to axotomy or peripheral nerve injury [44–47]. Additionally, administering a specific Nav1.3 antisense construct directly into the spinal cord effectively reduced hyperexcitability in dorsal horn neurons and improved pain-related behaviors associated with both spinal cord injury and chronic constriction injury of the peripheral nerve [48, 49]. The expression of $Na_v1.3$ in the infraorbital nerve and trigeminal ganglion, rather than the brain stem, has been demonstrated in our previous study on rat models of trigeminal neuralgia [50].

2.4.2 Mechanosensitive Channels

Based on the aforementioned evidence and analysis, it appears that certain isoforms of Na^+ channels play a pivotal role in generating ectopic action potentials. However, being voltage-gated channels, their activation is contingent upon membrane potential. Consequently, the presence of a threshold potential becomes imperative for initiating Na^+ channel opening.

Recently, the potential involvement of mechanotransduction ion channels in the pathogenesis of TN has garnered attention [51–55]. The TREK-1 potassium channel plays a crucial role in regulating cell excitability by maintaining a hyperpolarized resting membrane potential through mediating K^+-selective leak currents [55]. Piezos are Ca^{2+}-permeable nonselective cation channels that have now been shown to participate in a number of processes, ranging from arterial modeling to sensing muscle stretch [56–58]. In a preclinical investigation, Piezos were observed to be expressed in the axonal membrane subsequent to nerve injury, exhibiting responsiveness towards mechanical stimuli [59–62]. Specifically, the deficiency of Piezo2 may lead to impaired mechanical nociception [63]. However, being a low-threshold channel, Piezos exhibit activation in response to a wide range of mechanical stimuli [51, 54, 58].

TRP (transient receptor potential) ion channels are Ca^{2+}-permeable nonselective cation channels that have now been shown to locate in nociceptive nerve fiber Aδ and C. When external physicochemical stimuli are received, these channels induce neuronal depolarization by facilitating the transmembrane influx of cations along their electrochemical gradients, thereby initiating the generation of pain sensation [64]. TRPA1, TRPV1, TRPV4, and TRPM8 have been identified in the trigeminal nerve under normal conditions and play significant roles in the pathogenesis of orofacial pain, including trigeminal neuralgia [65]. The upregulation of these channels has been observed in rats with trigeminal nerve injury, along with the alleviation of pain following channel blockade [66–68]. The TRPA1 and TRPM8 channels have been reported to exhibit responsiveness to mechanical stimulation, while the activation of TRPA1 is up-regulated under low temperatures, which aligns with the characteristic features observed in TN. The unique mechanical ring structure of TRPA1 enables it to exhibit sensitivity towards physical stimulation, albeit with a relatively high threshold. This leads to membrane depolarization and the generation of a baseline voltage for downstream voltage-gated channels [64, 69]. Therefore, TRPA1 may function as a trigger for converting compression of a certain degree into voltage, thereby eliciting action potential generation in the nerve.

2.5 Inflammation

Given the apparent establishment of the structural foundation, it remains intriguing how these transmembrane ion channels are formed subsequent to nerve lesion (demyelination). As an inherent response to tissue damage, inflammation may contribute to the signaling pathway associated with the development of transmembrane ion channels. The expression of TNF-α mRNA was observed to exhibit a significant increase 6 h following chronic constriction injury of the nerve [70, 71]. The initial transient signal of TNF-α triggers a series of events involving other proinflammatory cytokines, which contribute to the persistence of painful symptoms in neuropathy and promote axonal damage. However, inhibiting TNF-α did not completely eliminate this neuropathic pain effect. IL-6 synthesis in the dorsal root ganglia (DRG) was observed following nerve injury, and administration of an IL-6 neutralizing antibody resulted in a reduction in allodynia [72, 73]. Clinically, tocilizumab, an anti-IL-6 receptor antibody, has demonstrated efficacy in the treatment of sciatica [74]. Our clinical study has demonstrated that the serum levels of TNF-α, IL-1β, IL-6, and IL-8 were significantly elevated in both patients with HFS or TN compared to healthy volunteers. Notably, the concentration of IL-6 exhibited a significant correlation with the severity of HFS or TN [75]. Additionally, our study has demonstrated the upregulation of $Na_v1.3$ in a rodent model of trigeminal neuralgia [50]. Furthermore, there is compelling evidence indicating that the activity of the Piezo2 channel is potentiated in sensory neurons through diverse inflammatory signaling pathways [59, 76]. However, further investigation is warranted to ascertain whether IL-6 exerts a direct influence on the expression of ion channels.

2.6 Hypothesis

According to the evidence and analysis mentioned above, we conclude that TN involves the generation of ectopic action potentials due to nerve root compression. The molecular basis of this phenomenon involves the emergence of transmembrane proteins, such as voltage-gated and mechanosensitive ion channels. This process starts with demyelination and is facilitated by inflammation following nerve damage. During pulsatile compressions, mechanosensitive channels activate and cause a depolarizing shift in the resting potential, resulting in subthreshold membrane potential oscillations. The unstable state can be triggered by an appropriate stimulus to surpass the threshold and subsequently activate voltage-gated channels, thereby eliciting conductible ectopic action potentials (Fig. 2.1).

This hypothesis potentially elucidates the characteristic symptoms of paroxysmal attacks precipitated by emotional stimuli. When experiencing nervousness or excitement, the corresponding changes in blood pressure and heart beat rate may lead to a precise compression with a specific frequency and amplitude that impacts the involved nerve root, reaching the threshold for initiating impulses. After a successful MVD, symptoms are

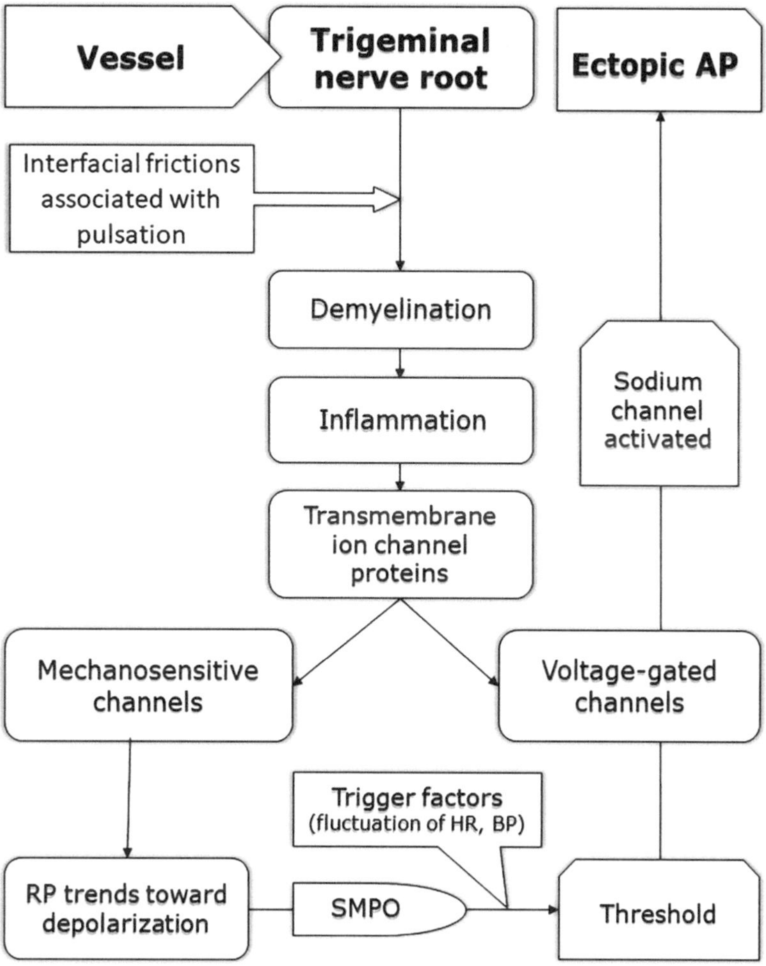

Fig. 2.1 A diagram elucidating the mechanism of trigeminal neuralgia. In individuals with a crowded cerebellopontine angle, the proximity of the trigeminal nerve root and surrounding vessel increases with age, ultimately resulting in neurovascular conflict. Due to the presence of interfacial friction caused by brain pulsations, demyelination of the nerve occurs. Upon reaching a certain pathological stage, the activation of inflammatory cytokine-mediated signaling pathways leads to the emergence of specific transmembrane proteins from the nerve. The transmembrane proteins include voltage-gated and mechanosensitive ion channels. With pulsatile compressions, the mechanosensitive channel induces a state of subthreshold membrane potential oscillation (SMPO) by driving the resting potential (RP) towards depolarization. During this state of instability, if the amplitude (BP) and/or frequency (HR) of compression fluctuates beyond a certain level, it can cause the membrane potential to surpass its activation threshold for voltage-gated sodium channels. Consequently, an action potential (AP) will be generated in the axon.

immediately relieved by repositioning the artery away from the nerve. However, excessive placement of Teflon felt between the nerve and the artery may result in gradual development of Teflon granuloma over time, leading to recompression of the vulnerable nerve root and subsequent recurrence [77]. Additionally, it may help clarify the clinical observation that secondary trigeminal neuralgia cases are predominantly associated with cholesteatoma or meningioma rather than schwannoma, as the latter provides nerve insulation through its proliferative sheath [17, 78].

References

1. Zhong J, Zhu J, Li ST, Li XY, Wang XH, Yang M, et al. An analysis of failed microvascular decompression in patients with hemifacial spasm: focused on the early reoperative findings. Acta Neurochir. 2010;152(12):2119–23.
2. Zhong J, Zhu J, Li ST, Guan HX. Microvascular decompressions in patients with coexistent hemifacial spasm and trigeminal neuralgia. Neurosurgery. 2011;68(4):916–20. discussion 20
3. Wang YN, Dou NN, Zhou QM, Jiao W, Zhu J, Zhong J, et al. Treatment of hemimasticatory spasm with microvascular decompression. J Craniofac Surg. 2013;24(5):1753–5.
4. Wang YN, Zhong J, Zhu J, Dou NN, Xia L, Visocchi M, et al. Microvascular decompression in patients with coexistent trigeminal neuralgia, hemifacial spasm and glossopharyngeal neuralgia. Acta Neurochir. 2014;156(6):1167–71.
5. Xia L, Li YS, Liu MX, Zhong J, Dou NN, Li B, et al. Microvascular decompression for glossopharyngeal neuralgia: a retrospective analysis of 228 cases. Acta Neurochir. 2018;160(1):117–23.
6. Dou NN, Zhong J, Zhou QM, Zhu J, Wang YN, Xia L, et al. The mechanism of hemifacial spasm: a new understanding of the offending artery. Neurol Res. 2015;37(2):184–8.
7. Zhou QM, Zhong J, Jiao W, Zhu J, Yang XS, Ying TT, et al. The role of autonomic nervous system in the pathophysiology of hemifacial spasm. Neurol Res. 2012;34(7):643–8.
8. Wang Y, Yang Q, Cao D, Seminowicz D, Remeniuk B, Gao L, et al. Correlation between nerve atrophy, brain grey matter volume and pain severity in patients with primary trigeminal neuralgia. Cephalalgia. 2018;333102418793643:515.
9. Peker S, Sirin A. Primary trigeminal neuralgia and the role of pars oralis of the spinal trigeminal nucleus. Med Hypotheses. 2017;100:15–8.
10. May A, Büchel C, Bahra A, Goadsby PJ, Frackowiak RS. Intracranial vessels in trigeminal transmitted pain: a PET study. NeuroImage. 1999;9(5):453–60.
11. Devor M, Amir R, Rappaport ZH. Pathophysiology of trigeminal neuralgia: the ignition hypothesis. Clin J Pain. 2002;18(1):4–13.
12. Lefaucheur JP. New insights into the pathophysiology of primary hemifacial spasm. Neurochirurgie. 2018;64(2):87–93.
13. Li ST, Zhong J, Sekula JR. Microvascular decompression surgery. Cham: Springer; 2016.
14. Liang YC, Huang CC, Hsu KS. Therapeutic potential of cannabinoids in trigeminal neuralgia. Curr Drug Targets CNS Neurol Disord. 2004;3(6):507–14.
15. Obermann M, Katsarava Z. Update on trigeminal neuralgia. Expert Rev Neurother. 2009;9(3):323–9.
16. Yang XS, Li ST, Zhong J, Zhu J, Du Q, Zhou QM, et al. Microvascular decompression on patients with trigeminal neuralgia caused by ectatic vertebrobasilar artery complex: technique notes. Acta Neurochir. 2012;154(5):793–7; discussion 7.
17. Liu MX, Zhong J, Dou NN, Xia L, Li B, Li ST. Management of symptomatic hemifacial spasm or trigeminal neuralgia. Neurosurg Rev. 2016;39(3):411–8.
18. Wang C, Wang YN, Sun K, Yin J, Xiao HS, Zhong J. A successful treatment of coexistent trigeminal neuralgia and ipsilateral superior cerebellar artery aneurysm. J Craniofac Surg. 2015;26(4):1270–2.
19. Zhong J, Zhu J, Sun H, Dou NN, Wang YN, Ying TT, et al. Microvascular decompression surgery: surgical principles and technical nuances based on 4000 cases. Neurol Res. 2014;36(10):882–93.
20. Zhong J, Xia L, Dou NN, Ying TT, Zhu J, Liu MX, et al. Delayed relief of hemifacial spasm after microvascular decompression: can it be avoided? Acta Neurochir. 2015;157(1):93–8; discussion 8–9.
21. Zhong J. An ideal microvascular decompression technique should be simple and safe. Neurosurg Rev. 2012;35(1):137–40. author reply 40
22. Dao Trong P, Beynon C, Unterberg A, Schneider T, Jesser J. Racial differences in the anatomy of the posterior fossa: neurosurgical considerations. World Neurosurg. 2018;117:e571–e4.
23. Guan HX, Zhu J, Zhong J. Correlation between idiopathic hemifacial spasm and the MRI characteristics of the vertebral artery. J Clin Neurosci. 2011;18(4):528–30.
24. Matsushima K, Yagmurlu K, Kohno M, Rhoton AL Jr. Anatomy and approaches along the cerebellar-brainstem fissures. J Neurosurg. 2016;124(1):248–63.
25. Martin RG, Grant JL, Peace D, Theiss C, Rhoton AL Jr. Microsurgical relationships of the anterior inferior cerebellar artery and the facial-vestibulocochlear nerve complex. Neurosurgery. 1980;6(5):483–507.
26. Lister JR, Rhoton AL Jr, Matsushima T, Peace DA. Microsurgical anatomy of the posterior inferior cerebellar artery. Neurosurgery. 1982;10(2):170–99.
27. Love S, Hilton DA, Coakham HB. Central demyelination of the Vth nerve root in trigeminal neuralgia associated with vascular compression. Brain Pathol. 1998;8(1):1–11; discussion −2, 1.
28. Hilton DA, Love S, Gradidge T, Coakham HB. Pathological findings associated with trigeminal neuralgia caused by vascular compression. Neurosurgery. 1994;35(2):299–303; discussion.
29. Rappaport ZH. Microvascular decompression in trigeminal neuralgia. Harefuah. 1996;130(8):515–6, 84.
30. Devor M, Govrin-Lippmann R, Rappaport ZH. Mechanism of trigeminal neuralgia: an ultrastructural analysis of trigeminal root specimens obtained during microvascular decompression surgery. J Neurosurg. 2002;96(3):532–43.
31. Xia L, Liu MX, Zhong J, Dou NN. Pain threshold monitoring during chronic constriction injury of the infraorbital nerve in rats. Br J Neurosurg. 2019;33(4):409–12.

32. Zhong J, Dou N. A novel hypothesis on the mechanism of Hemifacial spasm. In: Li S, Zhong J, Sekula R, editors. Microvascular decompression surgery. Cham: Springer; 2016. p. 51–8.
33. De Ridder D, Møller A, Verlooy J, Cornelissen M, De Ridder L. Is the root entry/exit zone important in microvascular compression syndromes? Neurosurgery. 2002;51(2):427–33; discussion 33–4.
34. Burchiel KJ. Trigeminal neuropathic pain. Acta Neurochir Suppl (Wien). 1993;58:145–9.
35. Burchiel KJ. Ectopic impulse generation in focally demyelinated trigeminal nerve. Exp Neurol. 1980;69(2):423–9.
36. Burchiel KJ. Abnormal impulse generation in focally demyelinated trigeminal roots. J Neurosurg. 1980;53(5):674–83.
37. Sekula RF Jr, Marchan EM, Baghai P, Jannetta PJ, Quigley MR. Central brain herniation secondary to fulminant acute disseminated encephalomyelitis: implications for neurosurgical management. Case report. J Neurosurg. 2006;105(3):472–4.
38. Resnick DK, Jannetta PJ, Lunsford LD, Bissonette DJ. Microvascular decompression for trigeminal neuralgia in patients with multiple sclerosis. Surg Neurol. 1996;46(4):358–61; discussion 61–2.
39. Suzuki A, Hoshi T, Ishibashi T, Hayashi A, Yamaguchi Y, Baba H. Paranodal axoglial junction is required for the maintenance of the Nav1.6-type sodium channel in the node of Ranvier in the optic nerves but not in peripheral nerve fibers in the sulfatide-deficient mice. Glia. 2004;46(3):274–83.
40. Luo S, Jaegle M, Li R, Ehring GR, Meijer D, Levinson SR. The sodium channel isoform transition at developing nodes of Ranvier in the peripheral nervous system: dependence on a genetic program and myelination-induced cluster formation. J Comp Neurol. 2014;522(18):4057–73.
41. Rasband MN, Kagawa T, Park EW, Ikenaka K, Trimmer JS. Dysregulation of axonal sodium channel isoforms after adult-onset chronic demyelination. J Neurosci Res. 2003;73(4):465–70.
42. Hamada MS, Kole MH. Myelin loss and axonal ion channel adaptations associated with gray matter neuronal hyperexcitability. J Neurosci. 2015;35(18):7272–86.
43. Freeman SA, Desmazières A, Fricker D, Lubetzki C, Sol-Foulon N. Mechanisms of sodium channel clustering and its influence on axonal impulse conduction. Cell Mol Life Sci. 2016;73(4):723–35.
44. Xu W, Zhang J, Wang Y, Wang L, Wang X. Changes in the expression of voltage-gated sodium channels Nav1.3, Nav1.7, Nav1.8, and Nav1.9 in rat trigeminal ganglia following chronic constriction injury. Neuroreport. 2016;27(12):929–34.
45. Siqueira SR, Alves B, Malpartida HM, Teixeira MJ, Siqueira JT. Abnormal expression of voltage-gated sodium channels Nav1.7, Nav1.3 and Nav1.8 in trigeminal neuralgia. Neuroscience. 2009;164(2):573–7.
46. Nassar MA, Baker MD, Levato A, Ingram R, Mallucci G, McMahon SB, et al. Nerve injury induces robust allodynia and ectopic discharges in Nav1.3 null mutant mice. Mol Pain. 2006;2:33.
47. He XH, Zang Y, Chen X, Pang RP, Xu JT, Zhou X, et al. TNF-alpha contributes to up-regulation of Nav1.3 and Nav1.8 in DRG neurons following motor fiber injury. Pain. 2010;151(2):266–79.
48. Lindia JA, Köhler MG, Martin WJ, Abbadie C. Relationship between sodium channel NaV1.3 expression and neuropathic pain behavior in rats. Pain. 2005;117(1–2):145–53.
49. Hains BC, Saab CY, Waxman SG. Changes in electrophysiological properties and sodium channel Nav1.3 expression in thalamic neurons after spinal cord injury. Brain. 2005;128(Pt 10):2359–71.
50. Liu M, Zhong J, Xia L, Dou N, Li S. The expression of voltage-gated sodium channels in trigeminal nerve following chronic constriction injury in rats. Int J Neurosci. 2019;1-12:955.
51. Giniatullin R. Ion channels of nociception. Int J Mol Sci. 2020;21(10):835.
52. Mikhailov N, Leskinen J, Fagerlund I, Poguzhelskaya E, Giniatullina R, Gafurov O, et al. Mechanosensitive meningeal nociception via piezo channels: implications for pulsatile pain in migraine? Neuropharmacology. 2019;149:113–23.
53. Kim SE, Coste B, Chadha A, Cook B, Patapoutian A. The role of drosophila piezo in mechanical nociception. Nature. 2012;483(7388):209–12.
54. Earley S, Santana LF, Lederer WJ. The physiological sensor channels TRP and piezo: Nobel prize in physiology or medicine 2021. Physiol Rev. 2022;102(2):1153–8.
55. Honoré E. The neuronal background K2P channels: focus on TREK1. Nat Rev Neurosci. 2007;8(4):251–61.
56. Wu J, Lewis AH, Grandl J. Touch, tension, and transduction—the function and regulation of piezo ion channels. Trends Biochem Sci. 2017;42(1):57–71.
57. Murthy SE, Dubin AE, Patapoutian A. Piezos thrive under pressure: mechanically activated ion channels in health and disease. Nat Rev Mol Cell Biol. 2017;18(12):771–83.
58. Coste B, Mathur J, Schmidt M, Earley TJ, Ranade S, Petrus MJ, et al. Piezo1 and Piezo2 are essential components of distinct mechanically activated cation channels. Science. 2010;330(6000):55–60.
59. Murthy SE, Loud MC, Daou I, Marshall KL, Schwaller F, Kuhnemund J, et al. The mechanosensitive ion channel Piezo2 mediates sensitivity to mechanical pain in mice. Sci Transl Med. 2018;10(462):eaat9897.
60. Malet M, Leiguarda C, Gastón G, McCarthy C, Brumovsky P. Spinal activation of the NPY Y1 receptor reduces mechanical and cold allodynia in rats with chronic constriction injury. Peptides. 2017;92:38–45.
61. Hulse RP. Identification of mechano-sensitive C fibre sensitization and contribution to nerve injury-induced mechanical hyperalgesia. Eur J Pain. 2016;20(4):615–25.
62. Boada MD, Gutierrez S, Aschenbrenner CA, Houle TT, Hayashida K, Ririe DG, et al. Nerve injury induces a new profile of tactile and mechanical noci-

ceptor input from undamaged peripheral afferents. J Neurophysiol. 2015;113(1):100–9.
63. Murthy SE, Loud MC, Daou I, Marshall KL, Schwaller F, Kühnemund J, et al. The mechanosensitive ion channel Piezo2 mediates sensitivity to mechanical pain in mice. Sci Transl Med. 2018;10(462):eaat9897.
64. Ramsey IS, Delling M, Clapham DE. An introduction to TRP channels. Annu Rev Physiol. 2006;68:619–47.
65. Luo Y, Suttle A, Zhang Q, Wang P, Chen Y. Transient receptor potential (TRP) ion channels in orofacial pain. Mol Neurobiol. 2021;58(6):2836–50.
66. Demartini C, Greco R, Zanaboni AM, Francesconi O, Nativi C, Tassorelli C, et al. Antagonism of transient receptor potential Ankyrin Type-1 channels as a potential target for the treatment of trigeminal neuropathic pain: study in an animal model. Int J Mol Sci. 2018;19(11):3320.
67. Trevisan G, Benemei S, Materazzi S, De Logu F, De Siena G, Fusi C, et al. TRPA1 mediates trigeminal neuropathic pain in mice downstream of monocytes/macrophages and oxidative stress. Brain. 2016;139(Pt 5):1361–77.
68. Kim YS, Chu Y, Han L, Li M, Li Z, LaVinka PC, et al. Central terminal sensitization of TRPV1 by descending serotonergic facilitation modulates chronic pain. Neuron. 2014;81(4):873–87.
69. Talavera K, Startek JB, Alvarez-Collazo J, Boonen B, Alpizar YA, Sanchez A, et al. Mammalian transient receptor potential TRPA1 channels: from structure to disease. Physiol Rev. 2020;100(2):725–803.
70. Zhang H, Zhang H, Dougherty PM. Dynamic effects of TNF-alpha on synaptic transmission in mice over time following sciatic nerve chronic constriction injury. J Neurophysiol. 2013;110(7):1663–71.
71. Onodera Y, Kanao-Kanda M, Kanda H, Sasakawa T, Iwasaki H, Kunisawa T. Pregnancy suppresses neuropathic pain induced by chronic constriction injury in rats through the inhibition of TNF-alpha. J Pain Res. 2017;10:567–74.
72. Wei XH, Na XD, Liao GJ, Chen QY, Cui Y, Chen FY, et al. The up-regulation of IL-6 in DRG and spinal dorsal horn contributes to neuropathic pain following L5 ventral root transection. Exp Neurol. 2013;241:159–68.
73. Thier M, März P, Otten U, Weis J, Rose-John S. Interleukin-6 (IL-6) and its soluble receptor support survival of sensory neurons. J Neurosci Res. 1999;55(4):411–22.
74. Ohtori S, Miyagi M, Eguchi Y, Inoue G, Orita S, Ochiai N, et al. Efficacy of epidural administration of anti-interleukin-6 receptor antibody onto spinal nerve for treatment of sciatica. Eur Spine J. 2012;21(10):2079–84.
75. Liu MX, Zhong J, Xia L, Dou NN, Li ST. A correlative analysis between inflammatory cytokines and trigeminal neuralgia or hemifacial spasm. Neurol Res. 2019;1-6:335.
76. Dubin AE, Schmidt M, Mathur J, Petrus MJ, Xiao B, Coste B, et al. Inflammatory signals enhance piezo2-mediated mechanosensitive currents. Cell Rep. 2012;2(3):511–7.
77. Dou NN, Zhong J, Liu MX, Xia L, Sun H, Li B, et al. Teflon might be a factor accounting for a failed microvascular decompression in Hemifacial spasm: a technical note. Stereotact Funct Neurosurg. 2016;94(3):154–8.
78. Xia L, Zhong J, Zhu J, Wang YN, Dou NN, Liu MX, et al. Cholesteatoma of cerebellopontine angle presented as trigeminal neuralgia. J Craniofac Surg. 2014;25(4):1540–2.

3 Hypothesis of Hemifacial Spasm

Xuesheng Zheng

Hemifacial spasm (HFS) is a common disease in functional neurosurgery, which is featured by uncontrollable contractions of facial muscles, strictly limited in one side. This can cause physical discomfort, emotional distress, and impair quality of life. While the exact cause remains unknown [1], the leading theory attributes HFS to compression of the cranial nerve VII at its root exit zone (REZ) [2, 3]. This compression, typically by arteries like the anterior inferior cerebellar, posterior inferior cerebellar or vertebral, disrupts nerve signals, leading to the involuntary muscle contractions. Interestingly, close neighboring between the arteries and the facial nerve is actually quite frequent, occurring in over half the population with no symptoms [4]. It suggests that additional factors beyond compression, still under investigation, contribute to the development of HFS.

During operation, surgeons often find obvious indentation and sometimes even color change (Fig. 3.1) on the facial nerve root at the site of vessel–nerve conflict [5, 6]. What are the microscopic changes in the compressed facial nerve root and the motor nucleus? There is very limited pathologic evidence as to the pathologic changes in the nerve root from human cases of primary hemifacial spasm [7, 8], which revealed that demyelination and even degeneration of axons take place at the neurovascular conflict. To our knowledge, there is no report as to the pathologic changes in the facial motonucleus up till now. This scarcity arises from several factors. Firstly, the nonfatal nature of the disease limits opportunities for postmortem examination. Secondly, microvascular decompression surgery, the primary treatment, doesn't involve tissue sampling of the nerve root or the motonucleus. Consequently, understanding the pathogenesis of hemifacial spasm relies heavily on indirect methods like intraoperative electrophysiology, clinical observations, and animal models.

As for the normal people, there is no cross-transmission among the facial nerve branches (Fig. 3.2a). Nonetheless, in individuals afflicted with hemifacial spasm, electrical stimulation of a single facial nerve branch on the affected side triggers a delayed muscular response from regions innervated by alternate branches. For instance, the temporal or zygomatic branches is stimulated and then waveforms are recorded in the mentalis muscle. This phenomenon, termed an "abnormal muscle response" (AMR) or alternatively "lateral spread response" (LSR), exhibits an initial latency of roughly 10 milliseconds. The occurrence of AMR is exclusive to HFS, rendering it a pivotal diagnostic tool and invaluable for intraoperative monitoring during microvascular decompression surgery [9]. The AMR indicates the presence of abnormal cross-talk among

X. Zheng (✉)
Neurosurgery, Xinhua Hospital, Affiliated to Shanghai Jiao Tong University School of Medicine, Shanghai, China

S.-T. Li et al. (eds.), *Microvascular Decompression Surgery*,
https://doi.org/10.1007/978-981-96-0767-9_3

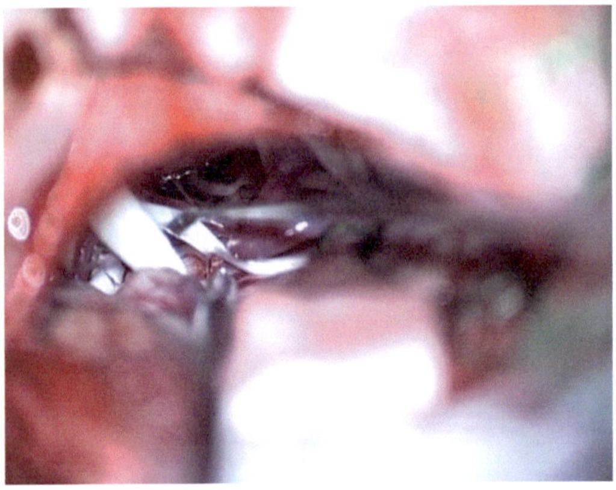

Fig. 3.1 Clear indentation and color change on the cranial nerve VII at the vessel–nerve conflict

facial nerve branches, which is hypothesized to underlie the primary pathogenesis of HFS [9]. Nevertheless, the precise location of this cross-transmission remains a subject of ongoing debate.

Two prevailing hypotheses have emerged to explain the underlying mechanisms. The first hypothesis, known as the "ephaptic transmission hypothesis" (depicted in Fig. 3.2b), posits that neurovascular compression leads to demyelination of nerve fibers [7, 8], and pushes bare axons into close proximity [10], thereby facilitating abnormal electrical signals between them. The second hypothesis, termed the "nucleus hyperexcitability hypothesis" (depicted in Fig. 3.2c), asserts that chronic injury to the facial nerve triggers hyperexcitability within the facial motor nucleus. The constant striking is believed to lead to the opening of dormant synapses, ultimately causing cross-transmission within the motor nucleus [9]. Both hypotheses offer insights into the complex etiology of HFS, though the precise mechanisms remain an active area of research.

The ephaptic transmission hypothesis [11] postulates that cross-communication arises among facial nerve fibers subjected to vascular compression. This hypothesis posits that ephaptic transmission, or "cross talk," occurs between adjacent nerve axons when they come into close contact, leading to ectopic excitation that could account for the manifestations of hemifacial spasm [11]. This concept finds support in pathological studies revealing histological alterations at compression sites on facial nerves, including demyelination, vacuolation of the myelin sheath, and partial axonal degeneration [7, 8]. Ephaptic transmission thus emerges as a plausible explanation for various symptoms, notably synkinesis in HFS. Nevertheless, critics contend that the restricted number of nerve fibers in contact is insufficient to explain the extensive facial muscle contractions observed in HFS [12].

The ephaptic transmission hypothesis predicts that the abnormal muscle response (AMR) latency should precisely match the combined conduction times along the facial nerve pathways involved in cross-transmission at the neurovascular conflict site. However, studies have consistently shown a discrepancy: the AMR latency is roughly 2 milliseconds longer than expected [9]. This suggests that the neural activity triggered by stimulation actually travels further, potentially reaching the facial motonucleus before activating descending facial structures. Furthermore, blocking neural conduction in the facial nerve proximal to the point of vascular compression eliminates the abnormal muscle contractions, thereby suggesting that the anatomical site of cross-transmission is proximal to the vascular compression. [13].

Recent investigations have underscored the pivotal role of facial motor nucleus hyperexcitability in the manifestation of hemifacial spasm. Wilkinson and colleagues corroborated this finding by assessing facial motor evoked potentials during microvascular decompression (MVD) surgery. Notably, their study revealed that desflurane, a commonly administered general anesthetic, exerted a lesser inhibitory effect on the affected side, thus lending credence to the hypothesis of a central pathophysiological mechanism underlying HFS [14]. Ishikawa and his team examined F waves, which provide insights into antidromically activated neurons within the facial motor nucleus, both prior to and following MVD. Intriguingly, they observed that elevated F waves and abnormal muscle responses lingered for several months post-surgery in some patients, despite a successful MVD procedure. These abnormal responses normalized only after a decrease in F waves, suggesting a potential link

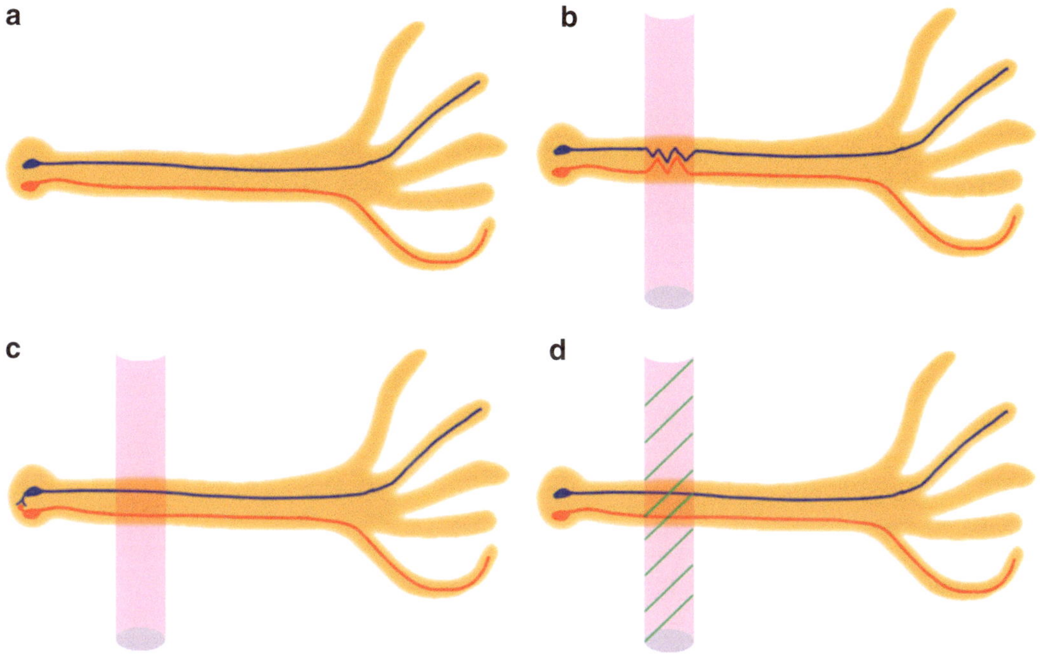

Fig. 3.2 Three hypotheses for cross-transmission in hemifacial spasm: (**a**) Normal facial nerve scenario: In the illustration, the blue and red lines represent the healthy facial nerve fibers belonging to the temporal and marginal mandibular branches, respectively. Under normal physiological conditions, these fibers function independently without any cross-transmission occurring between them. (**b**) Ephaptic transmission hypothesis: This hypothesis postulates that ephaptic transmission arises specifically at the site of neurovascular compression, where individual facial nerve fibers come into close proximity. (**c**) Nucleus hyperexcitability hypothesis: According to this hypothesis, chronic injury to the facial nerve triggers a state of hyperexcitability within the facial motor nucleus. This constant striking is thought to lead to the activation of dormant synapses, resulting in cross-transmission within the motor nucleus. (**d**) Sympathetic bridge hypothesis: This hypothesis proposes that at the site of neurovascular compression, cross-transmission between facial nerve fibers is facilitated by sympathetic nerve fibers (depicted as green lines) located on the offending artery wall. These sympathetic fibers serve as a bridge, enabling abnormal communication between the facial nerve fibers and contributing to the development of hemifacial spasm

between hyperexcitability and the persistence of symptoms [15, 16]. Early on, Møller and Jannetta posited the hyperexcitable nucleus hypothesis, postulating that cross-transmission within the facial motor nucleus might underlie this condition [9].

The facial motor nucleus, although not directly compressed by vessels, can become hyperexcitable as a result of vascular irritation to the facial nerve. This abnormal neural activity triggers the opening of dormant synapses within the facial motor nucleus, leading to cross-transmission and potentially exacerbating symptoms. A mechanism akin to the kindling phenomenon observed in epilepsy may contribute to the hyperactivation of the facial motonucleus [9]. Experimental evidence supports this hypothesis, as electrical stimulation of the facial nerve in rats using a specific “kindling” protocol has been shown to induce HFS-like symptoms. In these studies, the facial nerve was subjected to repeated electrical stimulations twice daily for several weeks at its entry point into the skull. Following 4–6 weeks of this regimen, the rats exhibited manifestations resembling human HFS [17, 18]. These findings suggest that the alterations in facial motonucleus function are a consequence of plastic changes within the nucleus itself. It is further postulated that the activation of neuroplasticity stems from the irritation of the facial nerve due to its proximity to blood vessels [12].

In individuals afflicted with HFS, additional indicators suggest hyperactivity within the facial motonucleus. Notably, despite the general suppression of the blink reflex by electrical stimulation under anesthesia, HFS patients exhibit a remarkable persistence of this reflex (specifically, the R1 component) on the affected side when the supraorbital nerve is stimulated [19]. This unexpected response underscores the abnormal excitability of the facial motonucleus in HFS. Moreover, when the offending vessel is successfully decompressed from the facial nerve, resulting in the disappearance of abnormal muscle response (AMR), the blink reflex becomes unprovokable under anesthesia, further confirming the vessel's role in modulating facial motonucleus activity. In addition, studies have reported an enhanced F-response in HFS patients compared to healthy controls [20]. The F-response, which is a reflection of the motonucleus's excitability in response to antidromic activity within its motor nerve, serves as a direct measure of motonucleus hyperexcitability.

However, the nucleus hyperexcitability hypothesis faces some challenges. Yamashita et al. conducted a study involving double stimulation in 12 HFS patients to investigate the nature of abnormal muscle responses (AMRs). Their findings revealed that the second response (R2) emerged after a consistent refractory period, exhibiting neither facilitation nor depression in the latency and amplitude recovery curve [21]. This observation lends support to the notion that the AMR may not solely originate from facial motor neurons, thereby posing a potential limitation to the nucleus hyperexcitability hypothesis as the sole explanatory mechanism for HFS.

In clinical practice, we frequently observe that upon detachment of the offending vessel from the facial nerve, the AMR promptly disappears, resulting in immediate relief of spasms for patients. This observation aligns well with the existing literature [22]. Nonetheless, both the ephaptic transmission hypothesis and the nucleus hyperexcitability hypothesis fall short in fully explaining this prevalent and pivotal clinical manifestation. It appears counterintuitive that facial motor neuron hyperexcitability would diminish instantaneously following vessel detachment. Likewise, it is implausible for histological alterations at the compression sites, including demyelination, myelin sheath vacuolization, and partial axonal degeneration [7, 8], to swiftly recover post-decompression. These findings underscore the complexity of HFS and the need for further exploration of its underlying mechanisms. The observed abnormal cross-transmission appears to be contingent upon the intimate proximity between the facial nerve and the offending vessel, postulating that the offending vessel itself might constitute an integral part of the cross-transmission circuitry. Consequently, when the vessel is detached from the facial nerve, the circuit is disrupted, resulting in an immediate cessation of the abnormal transmission. Given that nerve impulses, or action potentials, propagate through nerve fibers, and considering the abundance of sympathetic nerve fibers on the arterial wall [23], we further advanced the hypothesis that these sympathetic nerve fibers, situated on the offending artery, may act as a "bridge" between demyelinated facial nerve fibers. This hypothetical mechanism, which we term the "sympathetic bridge hypothesis," posits that these sympathetic fibers facilitate the abnormal cross-transmission (Fig. 3.2d).

The sympathetic bridge hypothesis leads to three logical deductions: Firstly, if the sympathetic nerve fibers on the offending artery wall are electrically stimulated, the resulting action potentials would propagate to the facial nerve fibers, potentially eliciting a novel facial muscle response that could be recorded. Secondly, if these sympathetic nerve fibers are blocked with lidocaine, the cross-transmission circuit would be disrupted, leading to the elimination of AMR, while preserving the integrity of facial nerve conduction. Lastly, if the sympathetic ganglion responsible for innervating the offending artery is resected, the cross-transmission circuit would be permanently severed.

In a rat model of HFS, electrical stimulation of the offending artery wall elicited a novel facial muscle response, termed the Z-L response (ZLR), thereby validating the first deduction of the sympathetic bridge hypothesis [24, 25]. It could be argued that the electrical stimulation on the offending artery may have directly propagated to the facial nerve via physical current flow. However, the fact that ZLR was exclusively observed in the HFS group and not in the control group suggests that the slight impulse (1 mA × 0.1 ms) delivered to the offending artery wall was conducted to the facial nerve through nerve conduction, rather than as a result of physical current flow. This conclusion is further supported by the close proximity of the temporal artery to the facial nerve in both groups.

Upon blocking the nerve fibers on the offending artery wall with lidocaine, AMR was abolished, while facial nerve conduction remained unaffected. Additionally, the complete elimination of AMR following resection of the sympathetic ganglion innervating the offending artery further validated the second and third deductions of the sympathetic bridge hypothesis [24, 25]. In conclusion, these findings underscore the indispensable role of sympathetic nerve fibers on the offending artery wall in the abnormal cross-transmission circuit underlying hemifacial spasm.

Anatomic studies conducted by Chen [23] revealed the extensive distribution of sympathetic fibers on the surface of arteries, residing beneath the tunica adventitia vasorum. Prolonged irritation from arterial pulsations (in humans) or chromic gut ligatures (in animal models) may compromise the integrity of both the tunica adventitia vasorum and epineurium, resulting in the exposure of naked sympathetic nerve fibers that subsequently come into close proximity with demyelinated facial nerve fibers. This proximity facilitates the spread of action potentials from one facial nerve fiber to many others via the "bridge" formed by the sympathetic fibers. The sympathetic bridge hypothesis incorporates Moller and Jannetta's "2-ms difference" observation [9], acknowledging that sympathetic nerve fibers, being grade C fibers, conduct at a much slower velocity than grade A facial nerve fibers. Thus, the additional 2 ms conduction time is attributed to the sympathetic bridge. Furthermore, this hypothesis aligns with the findings of Yamashita et al. [21], as it does not implicate the facial nucleus in the underlying mechanism.

During microvascular decompression procedures, a pivotal observation has been made. When the offending vessel is meticulously detached from the nerve, AMR disappears, only to reappear upon the vessel's inadvertent re-contact with the nerve [26]. This pivotal evidence appears to lend greater credence to the "sympathetic bridge hypothesis" over the "nucleus hyperexcitability hypothesis," as it underscores the role of the vessel–nerve interaction and the intervening sympathetic fibers in mediating AMR.

The sympathetic bridge hypothesis underscores the potential for treating hemifacial spasm by targeting the sympathetic nerves. For patients who have experienced unsuccessful MVD surgery, alternative approaches such as stellate ganglion block or selective resection of vertebral plexus sympathetic nerves may offer therapeutic benefits. While these sympathetic nerve-targeted therapies may carry risks of complications including Horner's syndrome, seizures, locked-in syndrome, and pneumothorax [27], they are considerably less invasive than posterior cranial fossa operations and can often be performed under local anesthesia. Consequently, they may serve as viable alternatives for those who have failed MVD surgery or who are hesitant or unable to undergo the more extensive cranial surgery.

ZLR, which is based on the anticipation of sympathetic bridge hypothesis, has been applied in clinical practice, which is very helpful in the cases of multiple compressing vessels [24, 25, 28–30]. However, the sympathetic bridge hypothesis is also under debate currently [28].

In summary, the study on the pathophysiology of hemifacial spasm is very important. Due to the lack of direct pathologic evidence from human specimens, the current available knowledge, however, is mainly based on such secondary evidence as intraoperative electrophysiological monitoring, clinical observations, and animal experiments, and thus not overwhelmingly convincing. In order to completely solve this problem, we strongly advocate for body donation and autopsy research of patients with hemifacial spasm.

References

1. Yaltho TC, Jankovic J. The many faces of hemifacial spasm: differential diagnosis of unilateral facial spasms. Mov Disord. 2011;26(9):1582–92. https://doi.org/10.1002/mds.23692.
2. Campos-Benitez M, Kaufmann AM. Neurovascular compression findings in hemifacial spasm. J Neurosurg. 2008;109(3):416–20. https://doi.org/10.3171/JNS/2008/109/9/0416.
3. Jannetta PJ. Neurovascular compression in cranial nerve and systemic disease. Ann Surg. 1980;192(4):518–25. https://doi.org/10.1097/00000658-198010000-00010.
4. Sunderland S. Neurovascular relations and anomalies at the base of the brain. J Neurol Neurosurg Psychiatry. 1948;11(4):243–57. https://doi.org/10.1136/jnnp.11.4.243.
5. Lee JA, Park K. Short-term versus long-term outcomes of microvascular decompression for hemifacial spasm. Acta Neurochir. 2019;161(10):2027–33. https://doi.org/10.1007/s00701-019-04032-x.
6. Li S, Feng B, Xie C, You C, Wei X, Zheng X. Good surgical outcomes of Hemifacial spasm patients with obvious facial nerve indentation and color change. World Neurosurg. 2016;92:218–22. https://doi.org/10.1016/j.wneu.2016.05.012.
7. Ruby JR, Jannetta PJ. Hemifacial spasm: ultrastructural changes in the facial nerve induced by neurovascular compression. Surg Neurol. 1975;4(4):369–70.
8. Wang H. Ultrastructural changes in the facial nerve root in patients with hemifacial spasm. Zhonghua Er Bi Yan Hou Ke Za Zhi. 1991;26(5):262–4, 316. [In Chinese].
9. Møller AR, Jannetta PJ. On the origin of synkinesis in hemifacial spasm: results of intracranial recordings. J Neurosurg. 1984;61(3):569–76. https://doi.org/10.3171/jns.1984.61.3.0569.
10. Gardner WJ. Concerning the mechanism of trigeminal neuralgia and hemifacial spasm. J Neurosurg. 1962;19:947–58. https://doi.org/10.3171/jns.1962.19.11.0947.
11. Nielsen VK. Electrophysiology of the facial nerve in hemifacial spasm: ectopic/ephaptic excitation. Muscle Nerve. 1985;8(7):545–55. https://doi.org/10.1002/mus.880080702.
12. Møller AR. Vascular compression of cranial nerves: II: pathophysiology. Neurol Res. 1999;21(5):439–43.
13. Kuroki A, Møller AR. Facial nerve demyelination and vascular compression are both needed to induce facial hyperactivity: a study in rats. Acta Neurochir. 1994;126(2–4):149–57. https://doi.org/10.1007/BF01476426.
14. Wilkinson MF, Chowdhury T, Mutch WA, Kaufmann AM. Analysis of facial motor evoked potentials for assessing a central mechanism in hemifacial spasm. J Neurosurg. 2017;126(2):379–85. https://doi.org/10.3171/2016.2.JNS151384.
15. Ishikawa M, Ohira T, Namiki J, Ajimi Y, Takase M, Toya S. Abnormal muscle response (lateral spread) and F-wave in patients with hemifacial spasm. J Neurol Sci. 1996;137(2):109–16. https://doi.org/10.1016/0022-510x(95)00308-o.
16. Ishikawa M, Ohira T, Namiki J, Kobayashi M, Takase M, Kawase T, Toya S. Electrophysiological investigation of hemifacial spasm after microvascular decompression: F waves of the facial muscles, blink reflexes, and abnormal muscle responses. J Neurosurg. 1997 Apr;86(4):654–61. https://doi.org/10.3171/jns.1997.86.4.0654.
17. Saito S, Møller AR. Chronic electrical stimulation of the facial nerve causes signs of facial nucleus hyperactivity. Neurol Res. 1993;15(4):225–31. https://doi.org/10.1080/01616412.1993.11740141.
18. Sen CN, Møller AR. Signs of hemifacial spasm created by chronic periodic stimulation of the facial nerve in the rat. Exp Neurol. 1987;98(2):336–49. https://doi.org/10.1016/0014-4886(87)90246-9.
19. Møller AR, Jannetta PJ. Blink reflex in patients with hemifacial spasm. Observations during microvascular decompression operations. J Neurol Sci. 1986;72(2–3):171–82. https://doi.org/10.1016/0022-510x(86)90005-5.
20. Hai J, Pan QG. Experimental study on the correlation between abnormal muscle responses and F waves in hemifacial spasm. Neurol Res. 2007;29(6):553–6. https://doi.org/10.1179/016164107X166263.
21. Yamashita S, Kawaguchi T, Fukuda M, Suzuki K, Watanabe M, Tanaka R, Kameyama S. Lateral spread response elicited by double stimulation in patients with hemifacial spasm. Muscle Nerve. 2002;25(6):845–9. https://doi.org/10.1002/mus.10123.
22. Møller AR, Jannetta PJ. Monitoring facial EMG responses during microvascular decompression operations for hemifacial spasm. J Neurosurg. 1987;66(5):681–5. https://doi.org/10.3171/jns.1987.66.5.0681.
23. Chen XQ, Bo S, Zhong SZ. Nerves accompanying the vertebral artery and their clinical relevance. Spine (Phila Pa 1976). 1988;13(12):1360–4. https://doi.org/10.1097/00007632-198812000-00006.
24. Zheng X, Hong W, Tang Y, Ying T, Wu Z, Shang M, Feng B, Zhang W, Hua X, Zhong J, Li S. Discovery of a new waveform for intraoperative monitoring of hemifacial spasms. Acta Neurochir. 2012a;154(5):799–805. https://doi.org/10.1007/s00701-012-1304-6.
25. Zheng X, Hong W, Tang Y, Wu Z, Shang M, Zhang W, Zhong J, Li S. Sympathetic nerves bridge the cross-transmission in hemifacial spasm. Neurosci Lett. 2012b;517(1):52–5. https://doi.org/10.1016/j.neulet.2012.04.023.
26. Møller AR, Jannetta PJ. Microvascular decompression in hemifacial spasm: intraoperative electrophysiological observations. Neurosurgery. 1985;16(5):612–8. https://doi.org/10.1227/00006123-198505000-00005.

27. Jadon A. Revalidation of a modified and safe approach of stellate ganglion block. Indian J Anaesth. 2011;55(1):52–6. https://doi.org/10.4103/0019-5049.76601.
28. Son BC, Ko HC, Choi JG. Intraoperative monitoring of Z-L response (ZLR) and abnormal muscle response (AMR) during microvascular decompression for hemifacial spasm. Interpreting the role of ZLR. Acta Neurochir. 2018;160(5):963–70. https://doi.org/10.1007/s00701-017-3462-z. Epub 2018 Jan 17.
29. Yang M, Zheng X, Ying T, Zhu J, Zhang W, Yang X, Li S. Combined intraoperative monitoring of abnormal muscle response and Z-L response for hemifacial spasm with tandem compression type. Acta Neurochir. 2014;156(6):1161–6; discussion 1166. https://doi.org/10.1007/s00701-014-2015-y.
30. Zhang X, Zhao H, Tang YD, Zhu J, Zhou P, Yuan Y, Li ST. The effects of combined intraoperative monitoring of abnormal muscle response and Z-L response for Hemifacial spasm. World Neurosurg. 2017;108:367–73. https://doi.org/10.1016/j.wneu.2017.08.160.

4 Tips for Opening and Closure to Ensure Successful Microvascular Decompression Surgery and Prevention of Complications

Takamitsu Fujimaki

4.1 Introduction

For treatment of trigeminal neuralgia (TN) and hemifacial spasm (HFS), there have been many descriptions of intracranial procedures for microvascular decompression (MVD) [1–10], but relatively few articles have provided step by step descriptions of skin incision, craniotomy, or cranial closure [1, 2, 5, 9]. If appropriate extradural manipulations are not performed, intradural surgical procedures become difficult, and if the head closure process is inappropriate, there is a risk of complications such as subcutaneous accumulation of cerebrospinal fluid or cerebrospinal fluid leakage and infections [11–13]. Complications due to metal plates used for bone fixation have also been reported [14]. Fibrin glue, which is often used in MVD, is a blood product, and therefore carries a theoretical risk of infection [15, 16], albeit very rare.

The authors perform MVD using a keyhole approach via a 6–7 cm skin incision and a small craniotomy 2.8–3 cm in diameter. Closure is performed without using any metal materials or fibrin glue. (Fibrin glue is also not used for any intracranial procedures.) The procedures we employ have yielded good surgical results with minimal complications.

T. Fujimaki (✉)
Department of Neurosurgery, Saitama Medical University, Saitama, Japan
e-mail: tfujimak@saitama-med.ac.jp

4.2 Surgical Procedures Leading to Craniotomy

When performing MVD surgery with a keyhole approach, the first important consideration is to decide the appropriate location of the craniotomy. For TN, the craniotomy should be placed at the corner of the transverse-sigmoid junction, and for HFS, it should be behind the sigmoid sinus and slightly below that for TN. The skin incisions are made as shown in the figure, directly above the planned craniotomy location for TN, and about 1 cm behind the craniotomy for HFS (Fig. 4.1). For HFS, this positioning ensures that the muscle layer posterior to the craniotomy does not impede the view of the microscope.

Once the fascia is reached after the skin incision and subcutaneous incision, some fibrous tissue from the fascia of the superficial muscles is collected and stored during craniotomy to be used as a patch graft when closing the dura. For this, after incision, the connective tissue layer under the skin is dissected subcutaneously (leaving a thin layer of connective tissue on the skin side), and the layer underneath is harvested for grafting (Fig. 4.2). Also, the fibrous layer on the muscle side should be left intact in order to facilitate suturing when closing the wound. If the lesser occipital nerve is identified at this time, it should be preserved as far as possible, as described previously [17, 18]. The fibrous tissue

S.-T. Li et al. (eds.), *Microvascular Decompression Surgery*,
https://doi.org/10.1007/978-981-96-0767-9_4

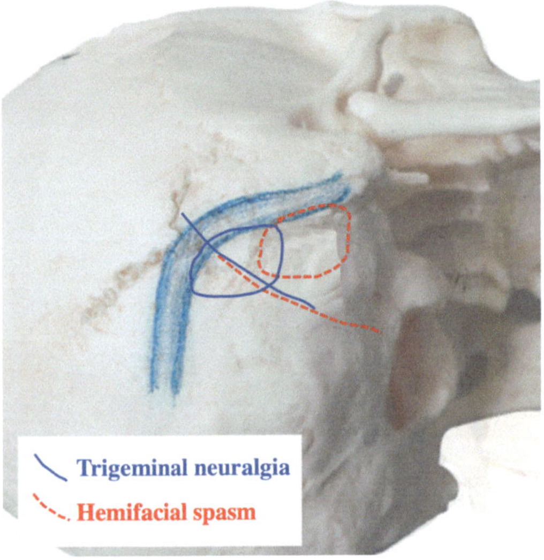

Fig. 4.1 Skin incision and craniotomy for trigeminal neuralgia (solid line) and hemifacial spasm (dashed line). For trigeminal neuralgia, place the craniotomy so that it touches the corner of the transverse sinus and sigmoid sinus, and for hemifacial spasm, place it so that it touches the sigmoid sinus. For trigeminal neuralgia, the skin incision is placed directly above the craniotomy, and for hemifacial spasm, the skin incision is placed posteriorly

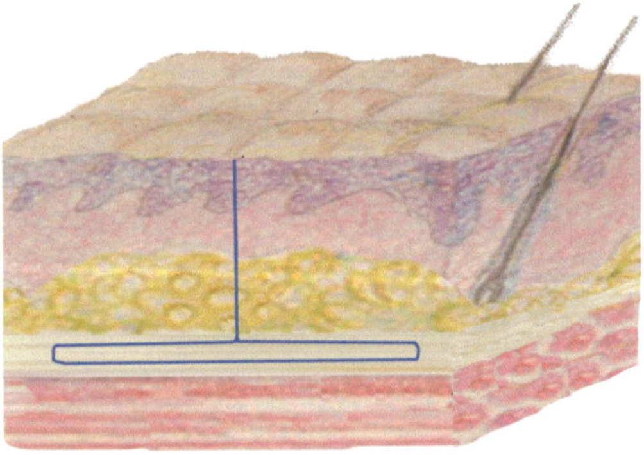

Fig. 4.2 Harvesting the fascia for dural plasty. When the skin incision reaches the superficial fascial layer of the superficial muscle group, this layer is peeled off, leaving some fibrous tissue on the subcutaneous side and on the muscle side, and the central layer is harvested as a graft

collected from the fascia is soaked in physiological saline.

The layers of muscle, i.e. the sternocleidomastoideus, the splenius capitis, the longissimus capitis, the obliquus capitis superior, the semispinalis capitis, and the rectus capitis posterior major are classified into two groups. Incision of the superficial muscles (sternocleidomastoideus and splenius capitis) reveals a layer of fibrous tissue, the so-called deep fascia, through which the occipital artery runs. This artery should be thoroughly cauterized and incised.

In the deepest layer, peeling of the rectus capitis posterior major muscle away from the occipital bone in a caudal direction reveals a loose layer of connective tissue. In TN there is no need to expose this loose connective tissue region. In HFS, posterior condylar emissary vein(s) and venous plexuses are evident at the craniocervical junction deeper to this connective tissue, and vertebral arteries run further back. Although it is not necessary to fully expose this area, it is recommended to dissect it to some extent so that the venous plexus can be observed up to the very edge. When peeling muscles to this point, the tip of the digastric muscle between the superficial and deep muscle groups is peeled away from the tip of the mastoid process, exposing the digastric groove. It is important to perform craniotomy to the point where the edge of the venous sinus (transverse and/or sigmoid) can be seen. Since the dural incision cannot extend above the venous sinus, further craniotomy is meaningless, although it is important to obtain a sufficient view above and lateral to the cerebellum. To obtain a better view, the dura should be incised as widely as possible on the lateral sigmoid sinus side. On the other hand, if the craniotomy is wide, the mastoid air cells may be opened, leading to leakage of cerebrospinal fluid from the dura. As this can lead to rhinorrhea, it is better to avoid opening the mastoid air cells if at all possible.

The mastoid emissary vein is often a useful guide for craniotomy positioning (Fig. 4.3). Although the size and location of this vein vary among individuals, the range of craniotomy is planned based on the relationship between the location of this vein and the sigmoid. One burr hole is placed at a position where the sigmoid is slightly exposed, and then the craniotomy is performed. First, it is better to avoid opening the mastoid air cells. The craniotomy is then extended laterally using a drill, rongeur, or Kerrison punch

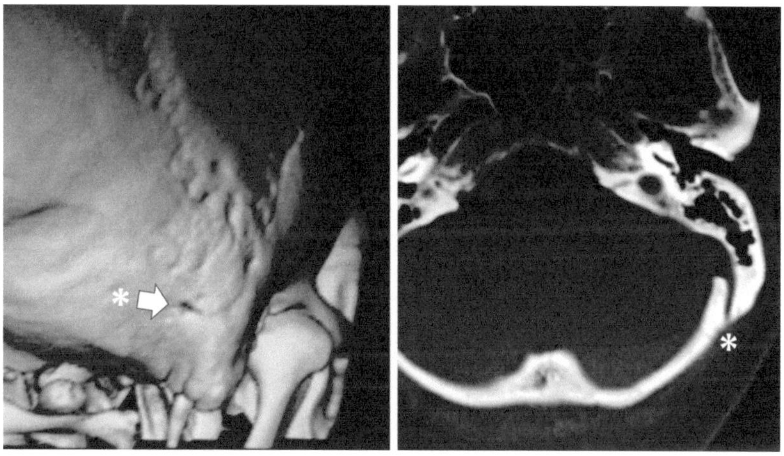

Fig. 4.3 Emissary vein(s) (*) are useful as indicators for craniotomy. Modified from Fujimaki et al. [9]

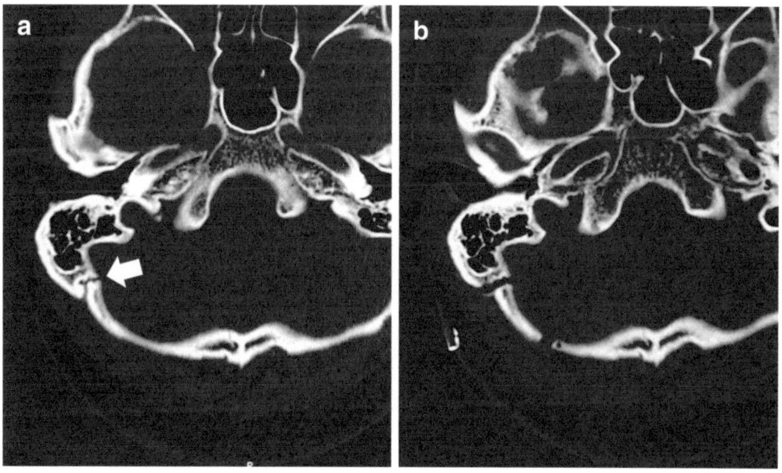

Fig. 4.4 A patient with right hemifacial spasm. Preoperative CT (**a**) and postoperative CT (**b**). A craniotomy was performed using the occipitotemporal suture (white arrow) as a landmark. The mastoid air cells are not opened

to expose the sigmoid sinus. At this point, the occipitotemporal suture is a good landmark. It is often possible to remove the bone fragments at the suture using a rongeur or Kerrison punch (Fig. 4.4).

With these procedures there is no possibility of the mastoid air cells being opened unless the temporal bone is opened through craniotomy. If this does not sufficiently expose the sigmoid, further bone removal is necessary while giving due consideration to the possibility of mastoid air cell opening. If some mastoid air cells are opened, they should be filled with small bone fragments to create "new mastoid air cell walls" (Fig. 4.5). For this, sufficient bone wax should be applied to the lateral side of the bone edge including the opened mastoid. As will be described later, in order to use a clamp system to fix the bone flap when the head is closed, a gelatin sponge is initially inserted between the dura mater and the bone at this stage, and then one dural tenting is placed (Fig. 4.6).

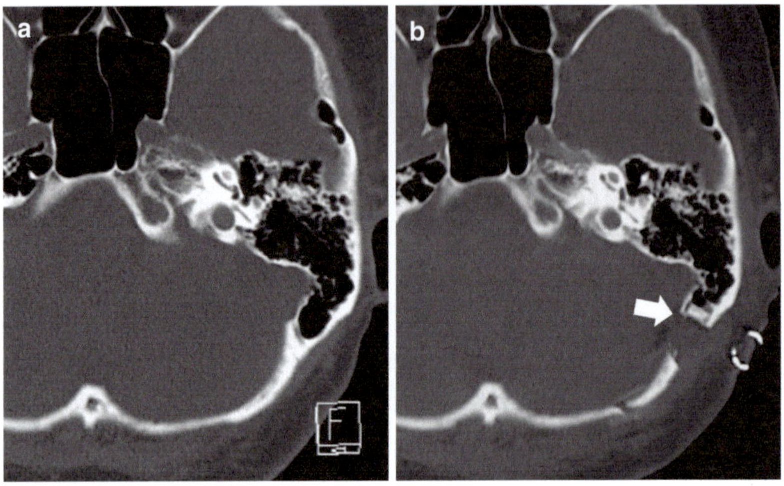

Fig. 4.5 A patient with right hemifacial spasm. Preoperative CT (**a**) and postoperative CT (**b**). A new wall (white arrow) was formed to close the opened mastoid air cells using bone fragments

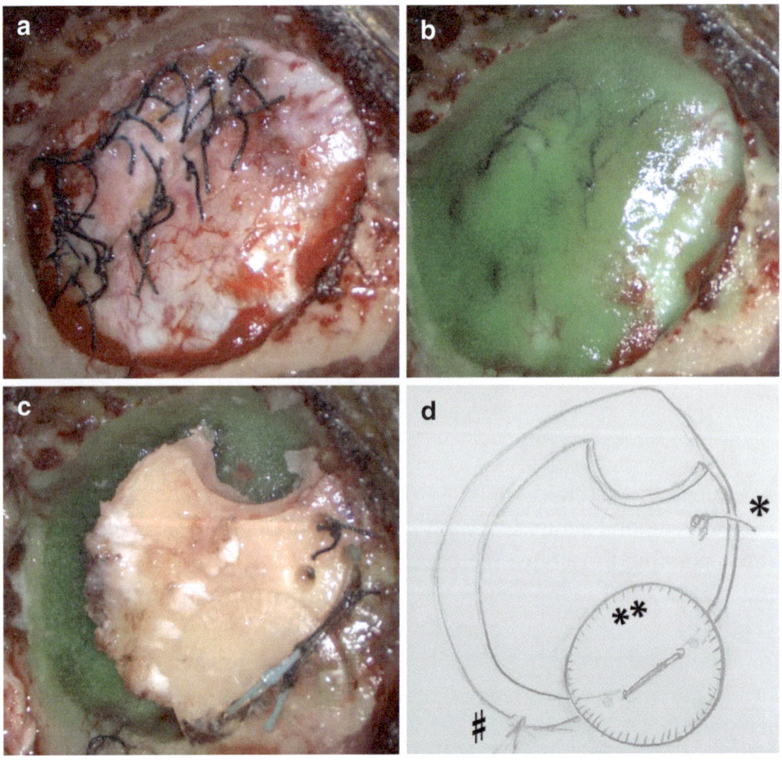

Fig. 4.6 Intraoperative photographs (**a**–**c**) and a sketch of dural closure and bone fixation (**d**). (**a**) Dural plasty was done with fascia and sutures. (**b**) Polyethylene glycol glue was sprayed. (**c**–**d**) The bone flap was fixed with nonabsorbable thread (*) and an absorbable plastic clamp (**). Dural tenting (♯)

4.3 Closure of the Dura and Fixation of the Bone Flap

Using interrupted sutures, dural closure is performed with the fascia graft collected during opening. The epidural area is sprayed with polyethylene glycol glue (Adherus®, Stryker, Tokyo, Japan). The bone flap is then fixed at one point with one or two nonabsorbable suture(s) and further fixed with an absorbable plastic clamp (CranioFix® absorbable, B.Brown, Tokyo, Japan). Clamps can cause bleeding between the dura and bone at the site where they are inserted epidurally, but if a gelatin sponge is inserted in advance at the beginning of surgery, as described earlier, no bleeding will occur (Fig. 4.6). After confirming that the bone is well fixed, each muscle layer is sutured, followed by the subcutaneous layer, and finally the skin. Since the craniotomy is small, no drain is usually required.

We have performed more than 750 microvascular decompression procedures with dural closure using auto-fascial grafts, and experienced only 2 instances of subcutaneous cerebrospinal fluid accumulation and 2 instances of subcutaneous infection, which is a far lower frequency than reported elsewhere. On the basis of our experience, we conclude that dural closure with an auto-fascial graft is an effective strategy for MVD surgery with a keyhole approach.

References

1. McLaughlin MR, Jannetta PJ, Clyde BL, et al. Microvascular decompression of cranial nerves: lessons leaarned after 4400 operations. J Neurosurg. 1999;90:1–8.
2. Fujimaki T. Microvascular decompression surgery for trigeminal neuralgia: technical review based on surgical anatomy. No Shinkei Geka. 2008;36:593–9.
3. Park JS, Kong D-S, Lee J-A, et al. Hemifacial spasm: neurovascular compressive patterns and surgical significance. Acta Neurochir. 2008;150:235–41.
4. Hyun S-J, Kong D-S, Park K. Microvascular decompression for treating hemifacial spasm : lessons learned from a prospective study of 1174 operations. Neurosurg Rev. 2010;33:325–54.
5. Zhong J, Li S-T. Zhou J, et al is entire nerve root decompression necessary for hemifacial spasm? Int J Surg. 2011;9:254–7.
6. Yang X-S, Li S-T, Zhong J, et al. Microvascular decompression on patients with trigeninal neuralgia caused by ectatic vertebrobasilar artery complex : technique notes. Acta Neurochir. 2012;154:793–7.
7. Zhong J, Li S-T. Zhou J, et al. Is entire nerve root decompression necessary for hemifacial spasm? Int J Surg. 2011;9:254–7.
8. Lee S, Joo KM, Park K. Challenging microvascular decompression surgery for hemifacial spasm. World Neurosurg. 2021;151:e94–9.
9. Fujimaki T, Ujihara M, Hirata S, et al. Technique of microvascular decompression for hemifacial spasm based on surgical anatomy. No Shinkei Geka. 2022;50:467–79.
10. Nagahiro S, Mizobuchi Y, Nakajima K, et al. A novel approach to microvascular decompression for hemifacial spasm: method description and associated outcomes. Oper Neurosurg (Hagerstown). 2022;23:e16–22.
11. Sindou M, Mercier P. Microvascular decompression for hemifacial spasm: outcome on spasm and complications. A review. Neurochirurgie. 2018;64:106–16.
12. Lee H-S, Cho K-R, Park K, et al. Management of cerebrospinal fluid leakage after microvascular decompression surgery: clinical strategy. Life. 2023;13:1771.
13. Menabbawy AA, Rafaee EE, Elwy RE, et al. Preemptive strategies and lessons learned from complications encountered with microvascular decompression for hemifacial spasm. J Neurosurg. 2024;140:248–59.
14. Gupta R, Adeeb N, Griessenuer GJ, et al. Removal of symptomatic titanium fixation plates after craniotomy. Acta Neurochir. 2016;158:1845–484.
15. Jackson MR. Fibrin sealants in surgical practice: an overview. Am J Surg. 2001;182:15–75.
16. Horowitz B, Busch M. Estimating the pathogen safety of manufactured human plasma products: application to fibrin sealants and to thrombin. Transfusion. 2008;48:1739–53.
17. Fujimaki T, Son JH, Takanashi S, et al. Preservation of the lesser occipital nerve during microvascular decompression for hemifacial spasm. Technical note. J Neurosurg. 2007;107:1235–7.
18. Hirata S, Kobayashi M, Wakiya K, et al. Preservation of the lesser occipital nerve prevents occipital sensory disturbance after microvascular decompression: long-term results. World Neurosurg. 2020;136:e126–31.

Development of MVD Technology 5

Shi-Ting Li

Since the establishment of MVD technology in the 1960s, MVD surgery has become an effective method for the treatment of cranial nerve hyperexcitability diseases such as trigeminal neuralgia, hemifacial spasm, and glossopharyngeal neuralgia, and has been promoted and popularized worldwide. After more than 70 years of development, MVD technology has made a lot of progress, involving MVD surgical principles, surgical approaches, decompression range, decompression methods, decompression materials, electrophysiological monitoring technology, anti-adhesion technology, complex blood vessels Decompression techniques during compression, anesthesia techniques, and treatment techniques for relapsed patients will be introduced separately below.

5.1 The Surgical Principle of MVD

Compression of cranial nerves by blood vessels may lead to dysfunction of cranial nerves, which is the theoretical basis for the formation of MVD technology. The principle of MVD surgery is to separate and relocate the blood vessels that compress the cranial nerves, so that the blood vessels and cranial nerves are completely separated. However, it is not easy to determine what kind of blood vessels are the real offending vessels, or there is no generally accepted judgment standard so far. In fact, any blood vessels that have anatomical contact with cranial nerves may become responsible blood vessels, including large vertebral artery, basilar artery, anterior inferior cerebellar artery, posterior inferior cerebellar artery, large petrosal veins, and even small perforating arteries may also be responsible vessels. Therefore, all vessels that have anatomical contact with cranial nerves need to be removed during MVD surgery. Separation and isolation include both current responsible vessels and vessels that may become pathogenic factors in the future. Completing the above-mentioned operating skills ensures the efficiency of MVD surgery and can also significantly reduce the recurrence rate of the disease.

5.2 Indications for MVD Surgery

All cranial nerve diseases caused by vascular compression should undergo MVD surgery. Therefore, before choosing MVD surgery, patients need to undergo detailed imaging examinations to exclude any possible secondary causes, such as cholesteatoma, schwannoma, meningiomas, aneurysms, and cavernous hemangiomas. At the same time, all patients need to undergo MRTA examination before surgery to clarify the anatomical relationship between cranial nerves and surrounding vessels.

S.-T. Li (✉)
Department of Neurosurgery, XinHua Hospital, Shanghai JiaoTong University School of Medicine, Shanghai, China

S.-T. Li et al. (eds.), *Microvascular Decompression Surgery*,
https://doi.org/10.1007/978-981-96-0767-9_5

For a long time, people have believed that primary trigeminal neuralgia, hemifacial spasm, and glossopharyngeal neuralgia are the best indications for MVD surgery, and a large number of clinical applications have also confirmed the effectiveness of MVD surgery. In medical centers with mature technology, The cure rate of MVD surgery is greater than 95%, even close to 100% [1, 2]. It is particularly important to point out that the indications for MVD surgery have been significantly expanded in recent years, and satisfactory results have been obtained after clinical application. This is worthy of further research and improvement, such as unexplained ptosis, abducens nerve palsy, Masseter spasm, intermediary neuralgia, some refractory neurogenic tinnitus, spasmodic torticollis, and neurogenic hypertension. Although MVD treatment of these diseases lacks support from RCT research results, the actual effects observed in clinical practice provide new hope for MVD treatment of these diseases.

5.3 The Value of MRTA Examination

All patients with cranial nerve disease must undergo imaging evaluation before undergoing vascular decompression surgery. Magnetic resonance MRI is the best option. Patients who cannot undergo magnetic resonance imaging should undergo a head CT scan. The significance of MRI examination is to rule out intracranial lesions that may cause cranial nerve diseases, such as tumors, cavernous hemangiomas, cerebral arteriovenous malformations (AVMs), posterior circulation aneurysms, cysts, skull base malformations, etc. The importance of MRI examination is also to clarify the vessels that have anatomical contact with the cranial nerve even show the type, thickness, and degree of compression to the cranial nerve (Fig. 5.1). In particular, three-dimensional time-of-flight magnetic resonance angiography (3D-TOF-MRA) has become a routine examination before MVD surgery. MRI imaging technology based on this has continued to develop and can now display 360 degrees of all anatomical relationships between cranial nerves and offending vessels. However, it must be pointed out that the vessels displayed by MRI examination are not necessarily the real responsible vessels. At the same time, a negative 3D-TOF-MRA examination is not an absolute contraindication for MVD surgery [3], but for 3D-TOF-MRA examination, Negative patients need to be more cautious when choosing MVD. At the same time, MRI examination can also observe the width of the subarachnoid space

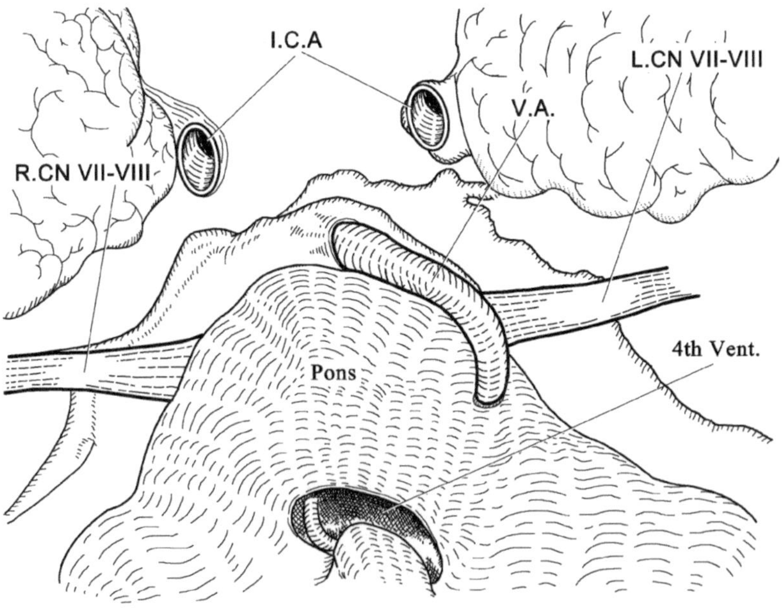

Fig. 5.1 MRI can show the anatomical relationship between cranial nerves and blood vessels

in the posterior fossa and the anatomical relationship between the sigmoid sinus, mastoid, and cerebellum, which helps to improve the safety and accuracy of vascular decompression surgery.

5.4 Surgical Approach of MVD

The selection of surgical approach for vascular decompression is based on the type of cranial nerve disease, and the selection of surgical approach is based on improving surgical safety and adequate exposure. For example, MVD surgery for trigeminal neuralgia advocates the use of the suboccipital sigmoid sinus transcerebellar fissure approach (Fig. 5.2) [4], and vascular decompression surgery for hemifacial spasm and glossopharyngeal neuralgia advocates the use of the suboccipital sigmoid sinus. Posterior subcerebellar flocculent approach (Fig. 5.3) [5, 6], for MVD surgery on the abducens nerve, you can choose a subcerebellar flocculent surgical approach that combines the head and tail ends of the vagus nerve. There are two optional surgical approaches for oculomotor nerve vascular decompression surgery, including the transsylvian paratemporal sulcal surgical approach and the suboccipital retrosigmoid sinus transsuperior cerebellar surgical approach. In practical application, it is necessary to select the appropriate surgical approach according to the type and location of the responsible vessels. No matter which surgical approach is adopted, it is necessary to use the natural anatomical gap in the skull for surgery, and at the same time, use sharp incision to fully separate the arachnoid membrane in the surgical field, especially the arachnoid membrane between the cranial nerves and the cerebellum. The key to fully separating and evaluating the quality of the surgical approach is whether the cranial nerves can be fully exposed without increasing the traction on the cranial nerves. This is also the technical key to reducing surgical complications [7].

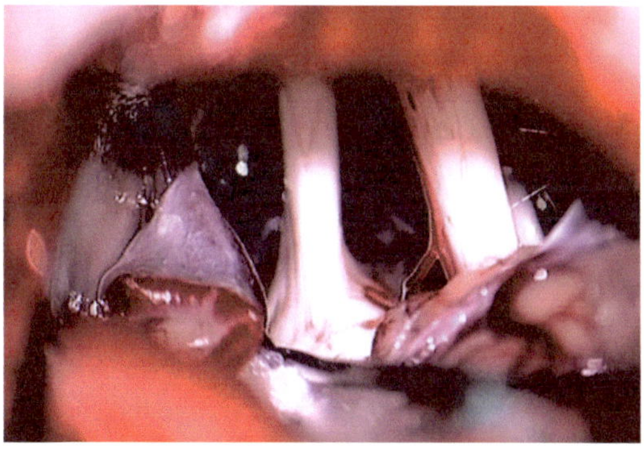

Fig. 5.2 The trigeminal nerve is exposed via cerebellar fissure approach

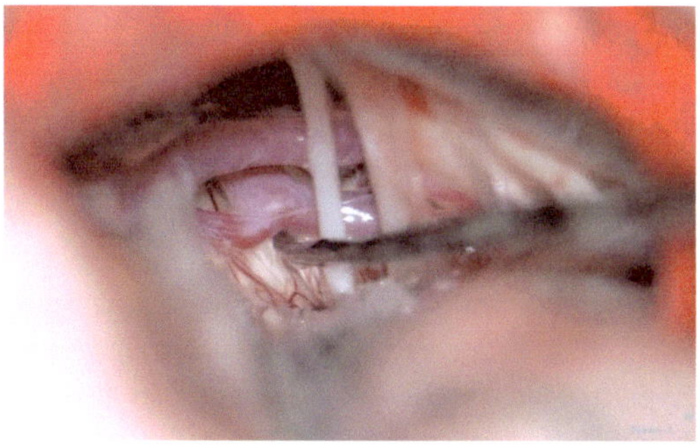

Fig. 5.3 The facial nerve was shown by a subcerebellar floccular approach

There are two main surgical approaches for treating hemifacial spasm with vascular decompression: the lateral cerebellar approach and the posterolateral cerebellar approach. The lateral cerebellar approach means to directly pull the cerebellar hemisphere medially after incising the dura mater to expose the facial auditory nerve trunk and gradually separate and cut the arachnoid membrane around it with spring scissors to expose the facial nerve area II and its nearby blood vessels, and then perform separation and decompression (Fig. 5.4). The advantage of this surgical approach is that it directly faces the auditory nerve trunk and can expose facial nerve zone II and nearby blood vessels earlier. If the responsible vessel is located in zone II, the operation time can be shortened. However, this approach also has obvious shortcomings. It often requires excessive pulling of the cerebellar hemisphere, and this pulling is done before the arachnoid is completely released, which is likely to damage the vestibulocochlear nerve, glossopharyngeal nerve, and vagus nerve, and may also cause cerebellar contusion, when the petrosal vein passes through the dorsal side of the vagus nerve, blind traction may also lead to venous bleeding or even petrosal vein tearing. Moreover, this surgical

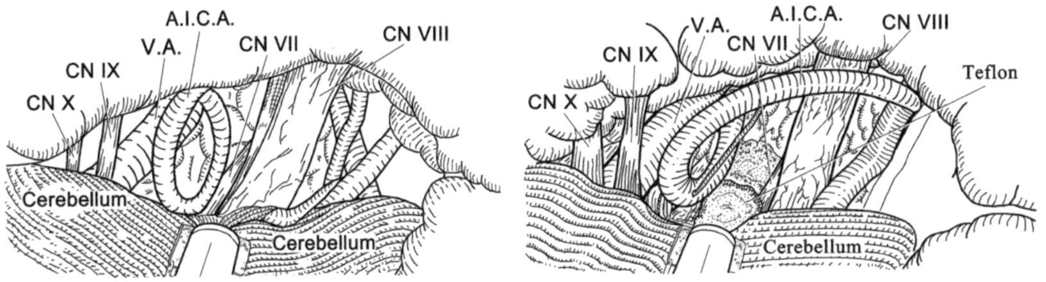

Fig. 5.4 (**a**) Left facial spasm during MVD surgery; AICA compression of the facial nerve was observed. (**b**) Teflon is placed between the AICA and the facial nerve

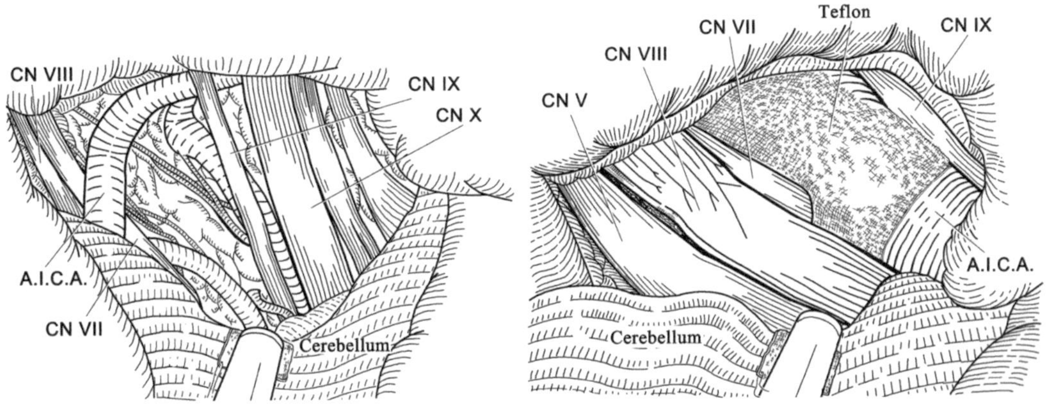

Fig. 5.5 (**a**) AICA passes between the facial nerve and the auditory nerve and compresses the facial nerve. (**b**) A thin layer of Teflon cotton is placed between the AICA and the facial nerve

approach can not only better expose the facial nerve zone II, but it is also difficult to fully expose the facial nerve zones I, III, and IV. Especially when the responsible vessels are located between the facial and auditory nerves, it will be very difficult to complete vascular decompression, so this surgical approach is rarely used now. The currently recommended surgical approach is the posterolateral cerebellar approach (Fig. 5.5). The key points of this approach are to first pull the cerebellum anteromedially after incising the dura mater to expose the arachnoid mater at the lower end of the cerebellomedullary fissure, first use a pointed blade to incise the arachnoid membrane here to slowly release cerebrospinal fluid, and then use spring scissors to gradually separate and incise the arachnoid membrane from the tail end to the head end until the vagus nerve, glossopharyngeal nerve, and vestibulocochlear nerve are completely released. In some patients, there is a petrosal vein passing through on the dorsal side of the vagus nerve. It is not allowed to easily electrocoagulate and cut off the petrosal vein here. It is recommended to carefully separate the adhesions around the petrosal vein to the cerebellomedullary fissure. If the posterior inferior cerebellar artery or the anterior inferior cerebellar artery also passes through the dorsal side of the posterior cranial nerve, it is recommended to use the same method to separate them. In some patients, the cerebellar flocculus will be abnormally proliferated and hypertrophied. It is difficult to fully expose the entire facial nerve by simply releasing the arachnoid membrane. In such cases, it is not recommended to forcibly pull the cerebellar flocculus to obtain exposure. Instead, it is recommended to first remove the hypertrophic cerebellum. Pompon, so that the facial nerve and its responsible vessels can be fully exposed without excessive stretching of the cerebellum, and vascular decompression can be safely performed.

5.5 MVD Decompression Range

REZ is an internationally recognized decompression range for MVD surgery. For a long period of time, MVD surgery in the REZ zone was considered the gold standard for MVD surgery for all cranial nerve diseases. Even today, many experts still adhere to this view. It should be pointed out that the effective rate of MVD surgery using the REZ zone remains at about 85% and cannot reach 100%, and more and more experts have found that any part of the cranial nerve compressed by vessels may cause the disease, or offending vessels may be present in any part of the cranial nerves in the posterior fossa, and our clinical practice has long found this rule [8, 9]. Therefore, we have focused on observing the distribution of responsible vessels since 2000. Represented by trigeminal neuralgia and hemifacial spasm, the probability that the responsible vessels are located in the REZ zone is about 85%, while the probability that the responsible vessels are located in areas outside the REZ zone is about 15%, so we believe that MVD surgery should explore the entire cranial nerve in the posterior fossa and separate and isolate all vessels that have anatomical contact with the cranial nerves. In order to better grasp and promote the above MVD principles, we divide the posterior root of the trigeminal nerve and the facial nerve into five zones. The definition of the five zones of the trigeminal nerve is (Fig. 5.6): Zone I: the inner 1/3 of the head, Zone II: The caudal end of the inner 1/3, area III: the ventral inner 1/3, area IV: the dorsal inner 1/3, area V: the middle and outer 2/3 of the root of the trigeminal nerve. The definition of the five zones of the facial nerve is (Fig. 5.7): Zone I: the pontine sulcus segment, Zone II: the pontine segment, Zone III: the transition zone where the facial nerve leaves the pons and enters the subarachnoid space, Zone IV: the cisternal segment, and V Area: inner auditorium section. It is currently believed that MVD surgeries for trigeminal neuralgia and hemifacial spasm should adhere to the principle of five-zone exploration and decompression, and that MVD surgeries for other cranial nerve diseases should also adhere to the same principles.

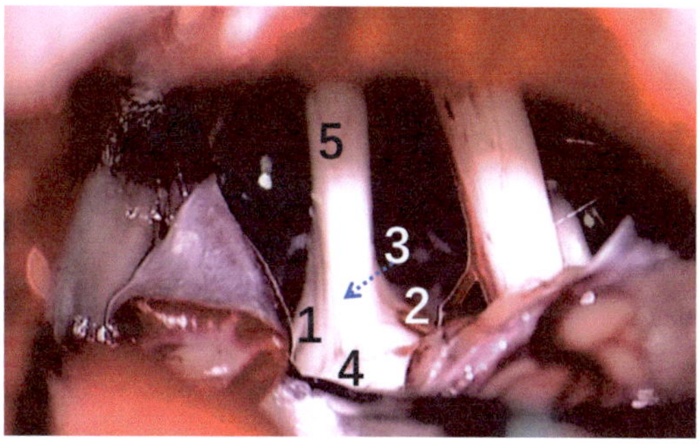

Fig. 5.6 Five areas to explore in MVD operation for trigeminal neuralgia

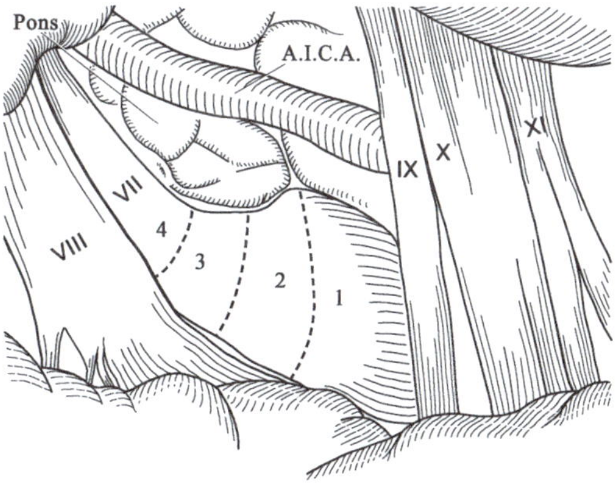

Fig. 5.7 Five areas need to be explored in MVD surgery for hemifacial spasm

5.6 MVD Decompression Method

The decompression principle of MVD is to separate and shift the offending vessels to achieve complete isolation from the cranial nerves. Therefore, the main decompression methods of MVD include the following: (1) Separate the responsible vessels and suspend them on the lateral wall of the posterior fossa, keeping the vessels completely away from the cranial nerves, and there is no need to place Teflon pads [10–14]; (2) Separate the responsible vessels and adhere them to the lateral wall of the posterior cranial fossa with biological glue. In order to prevent the blood vessels from resetting, it is recommended to place padding around the vessels [15]; (3) Separate the responsible vessels and push them away from cranial nerves, and use padding to fix them away from the cranial nerves; (4) After the responsible vessels are separated, if they cannot be displaced due to various reasons, place an appropriate amount of padding between the blood vessels and the cranial nerves; (5) For compression of the sclerotic and large vertebrobasilar arteries, it is first necessary to fully release the arachnoid at the caudally end, and then place a sufficient amount of gelatin sponge between the posterior cranial nerves-brainstem and the vertebrobasilar artery to move the vertebrobasilar artery caudally and dorsally. At this time, space can often be obtained between the vertebrobasilar artery and the facial nerve or trigeminal nerve, and finally an appropriate amount of cotton padding is placed between the blood vessel and the vertebrobasilar artery; (6) Compression of the petrosal vein needs to be treated in a classified manner. If the vein is small (less than 2 mm in diameter) and the vein passes through the trigeminal nerve, it is recommended to cut the vein directly after electrocoagulation. On the contrary, if the vein is large, it needs to be preserved. At this time, the adhesion between the vein and the cranial nerve needs to be slowly and carefully separated, and then a thin layer of cotton padding is placed; (7) For compression of small perforating arteries, only a small amount of cotton padding needs to be placed around the vessels to avoid compression and occlusion of the perforating arteries caused by large amounts of cotton padding. Of course, for some patients with complex vascular compression, the above technologies can be integrated [16–18].

Taking the common MVD surgery for primary hemifacial spasm as an example, the method of decompression is further explained. Since the anatomical contact between vessels and facial nerve is a necessary condition for hemifacial spasm to occur, the core task of vascular decompression is to separate, shift and properly fix the responsible vessels from the facial nerve to avoid resetting of the vessels and causing recurrence of the condition. The corresponding decompression method can be selected according to the thickness, elasticity and tortuous length of the responsible vessels. There are three most common methods of stress reduction: isolation, suspension, and bioadhesive adhesion. The so-called isolation is to separate the responsible vessels from the facial nerve and then implant an appropriate amount of Teflon padding between them to ensure that the vessels no longer contact the facial nerve. This is also the most commonly used decompression method at present. The advantage of this method is that the surgical operation is relatively simple, the surgical effect is accurate, and it is suitable for the vast majority of patients. However, its biggest disadvantage is that the implanted Teflon pads will form adhesions with offending vessels and facial nerves, which is the main cause of disease recurrence [19–21]. The so-called suspension is to use muscles, fascia, or artificial cords to wrap and fix the responsible blood vessels to the lateral wall of the posterior cranial fossa or the tentorium after the responsible vessels are anatomically separated from the facial nerve. This type of surgery does not require the implantation of pads around the facial nerve. Cotton. Therefore, the biggest advantage of this type of surgery is that it is suitable for cases where the offending vessels are tortuous and elongated, and there will be no adhesion around the facial nerve, making it easier to operate again. However, this type of surgery also has disadvantages, that is, the operation is very difficult and the risk of the operation itself is significantly increased, so most clinicians are unwilling to use it. In the same way, fibrin glue adhesion is to adhere the separated offending vessels to the lateral wall of the posterior fossa or the tentorium through bioglue. There is no need to implant Teflon pads between the facial nerve and vessels. Therefore, the method of fibrin glue adhesion is mainly to use tortuous and long blood vessels to decompress or as an auxiliary measure to decompress large vessels. The advantages of this method are similar to suspension, but its disadvantage is that it is very difficult to perform another operation due to the adhesion of the glue.

In some individuals, the instability of the glue adhesion becomes the cause of disease recurrence. In addition, the glue itself may also damage the exposed skull. Nerve, in fact, is similar to suspension, and the glue adhesion method is rarely used clinically.

5.7 Decompression Material in MVD

Currently, there are only two types of decompression pads widely used clinically: Teflon pads and polyester pads. Although both types of decompression pads are inert materials, there is still a risk of adhesion to the cranial nerves after operation, which is also the main cause of disease recurrence. Therefore, the location, quantity, and physical properties of the pad implant should meet the needs of non-adhesion as much as possible. Clinically, it has been found that Teflon pads will harden after operation. If the disease recurs, another MVD surgery is required. The hardened Teflon pads are difficult to separate, cut, and shift. These shortcomings have led to the gradual reduction of the application of Teflon pads. Polyester pads are softer than Teflon pads and are easy to shape. They are more suitable for isolating small offending vessels and veins. They are also easy to separate from cranial nerves during reoperation in patients with recurrence. Therefore, the application of polyester pads is increasing day by day. It should be pointed out that both Teflon cotton and polyester cotton still have their own shortcomings, and we look forward to the emergence of materials with better performance.

5.8 Anti-Adhesion Technology

Adhesions between decompression pads and cranial nerves are the main cause of disease recurrence. Reducing the risk of adhesions during MVD surgery is an important measure to reduce disease recurrence. It is the best choice not to use pads or to keep pads away from cranial nerves during MVD surgery. However, most MVD surgeries still require pads between responsible vessels and cranial nerves. At this time, we recommend placing gelatin sponge between pads and cranial nerves. Clinical studies have proven that this method can effectively reduce the risk of adhesions and is a technology worthy of widespread promotion and application [22, 23]. In MVD surgery for different cranial nerve diseases, the application methods are different. If it is MVD surgery for trigeminal neuralgia, after fully exposing the responsible vessels and the posterior root of the trigeminal nerve, pads needs to be placed first, and the pads is used to push the responsible vessels away from trigeminal nerve, and finally place a sufficient amount of gelatin sponge around the trigeminal nerve root. If it is MVD surgery for hemifacial spasm, first the responsible vessel needs to be fully released, then an appropriate amount of gelatin sponge is placed between the blood vessel and the facial nerve, and finally some pads are placed between the gelfoam sponge and the responsible vessels to ensure that the facial nerve is in contact with the pads. Cotton does not come into direct contact.

5.9 Anesthesia Technique for MVD

MVD surgery for cranial nerve diseases needs to be performed under general anesthesia. Before surgery, the anesthesiologist should learn in detail whether the patient has respiratory diseases and surgical history, and whether there is a history of allergies to anesthetic drugs. In order to cooperate with effective electrophysiological monitoring during the surgery, a reasonable anesthesia plan should be formulated, such as the selection, use time, and dosage of muscle relaxants. In order to use beta-blockers (such as esmolol) during surgery to control cerebrospinal fluid fluctuations and facilitate surgical operations, the patient's history of heart disease and experience with beta-blockers should be known in detail before surgery. In particular, surgery for hemifacial spasm and the sequelae of spastic facial paralysis requires the use of muscle relaxants as little as possible to ensure that typical AMR waves can be monitored. During the operation, it is necessary to strictly control intracranial pressure and cerebral pulsation. Use 250 mL of mannitol for dehydration, control the total volume and speed of fluid replacement, and hyperventilate to maintain the partial pressure of carbon dioxide at about 26 mmHg. When cerebrospinal fluid fluctuations seriously affect the surgical operation, beta-blockers can be used appropriately. Usually 40–100 mg of esmolol is injected intravenously, and changes in the patient's heart rate and blood pressure should be closely observed.

5.10 Electrophysiology Monitoring Technology

Electrophysiological monitoring plays a very important role in surgery for cranial nerve diseases, not only making the surgery safer but also making the surgery more effective. The electrophysiological monitoring mentioned here includes brainstem function monitoring and cranial nerve function monitoring. Specific monitoring methods include somatosensory evoked potential SEP, brainstem auditory evoked potential BAEP, motor nerve electromyography EMG, and disease-related abnormal muscle response potentials AMR, LSR, ZLR, etc. [24–26]. Specific monitoring methods should be selected for different cranial nerve diseases. For example, SEP, BAEP, facial and abducens nerve EMG, AMR, and ZLR monitoring should be performed simultaneously during vascular decompression surgery for hemifacial spasm, while vascular decompression surgery for trigeminal neuralgia should be monitored simultaneously. SEP, BAEP, oculomotor nerve EMG, trochlear nerve EMG, and trigeminal nerve BTEP should be monitored simultaneously during compression surgery. In all such surgeries, it is necessary to monitor the function of the brachial plexus on the surgical side to avoid damage to the brachial plexus caused by excessive traction. It should be noted that the monitoring doctor's detailed observation and identification of various monitoring waveforms and close cooperation with the operating surgeon can give full play to the value of monitoring. Generally, a decrease in amplitude of more than 20% and a delay in latency of more than 1 millisecond are considered signs of nerve damage, and changes within this range can be completely restored in most cases. Practical application requires discussion and cooperation between the monitoring physician and the operating physician.

In MVD surgery for hemifacial spasm, the complete disappearance of AMR is an important sign of the end of the operation. For patients whose AMR never disappears, ZLR monitoring can be combined. If the facial nerve has been fully explored and decompressed, and the ZLR has completely disappeared, it can be try to end the surgery. In the above situation, the surgical assistant can also ask the surgical assistant to observe whether the eyelids, cheek muscles and mouth corners are twitching. If there is no twitching, it is recommended to end the surgery. Otherwise, exploration should be continued until the AMR disappears completely. Recognizing the diversity of AMR and the pathophysiological mechanisms of AMR formation is helpful for the scientific application of AMR monitoring. For example, a patient exhibits facial muscle spasm on one side combined with mouth and eye synkinesis, and preoperative electrophysiological testing indicates that the AMR wave is multimodal. This often indicates that there are multiple abnormal conduction pathways in the formation mechanism of the AMR wave. During MVD surgery, it is not only necessary to the offending vessels are separated and displaced, and the compressed and degenerated facial nerve fibers may also need to be combed, otherwise the AMR wave may partially disappear.

Release surgery for sequelae of spastic facial paralysis also requires the assistance of electrophysiological monitoring technology. Typical AMR waves need to be detected before starting the surgery. After the facial nerve is completely exposed from the stylomastoid foramen to the bifurcation area of the upper and lower trunks in the parotid gland, EMG technology needs to be used for detection. Areas with obvious facial nerve degeneration are also an effective method to determine the scope of release surgery. During the operation, the method of membranous release and layered progression should be adhered to. Once the AMR wave completely disappears, it is recommended to terminate the surgical operation.

During masseter spasm surgery, it is not only necessary to separate and relocate the blood vessels that compress the motor roots of the trigeminal nerve, but also to use EMG technology to detect hyperactive motor root fibers. This is also a key step to ensure the effectiveness of the surgery.

5.11 Decompression Techniques for Complex Vascular Compression

Although the vascular decompression operation in typical cases may be very simple, complex cases are often encountered clinically, making the decompression operation extremely difficult, such as compression of large blood vessels, patients with facial nerve compression degeneration, and offending vessels crossing between the facial and auditory nerves, offending vessels across the motor fibers of the facial nerve, treatment of patients whose AMR waves never disappear, and patients whose intraoperative exploration does not reveal obvious vascular compression. Here is a brief description based on the author's clinical experience. Compression from large, sclerotic vertebral artery, when the vertebral artery serves as a direct or indirect responsible blood vessel, it is often accompanied by narrowing of the posterior cranial fossa and narrowing of the ipsilateral cerebellomedullary cistern. At this time, it is very difficult to separate or displace the vertebral artery. If forced implanting pads between the vertebral artery and the facial nerve only increases the compression to the facial nerve and cannot achieve satisfactory surgical results. Even if suspension or fibrin glue adhesion is used, it is difficult to truly decompress the facial nerve [15]. For this kind of situation, the decompression method we adopt is to first open the lower end of the cerebellomedullary cistern, separate the adhesions between the vertebral artery and surrounding tissues from the tail end to the head end, and then pull the vertebral artery toward the tail end. An appropriate amount of gelatin sponge is implanted between the vertebral artery and the medulla oblongata. This step often causes the vertebral artery to move away from the surface of the facial nerve, creating conditions for the eventual implantation of pads between the vertebral artery and the facial nerve (Fig. 5.8). In some patients with facial nerve compression degeneration, due to severe blood vessel compression, obvious indentations appear on the surface of the facial nerve, and the facial nerve even becomes thinner, pigmented, and nerve fibers degenerate (Fig. 5.9). Although

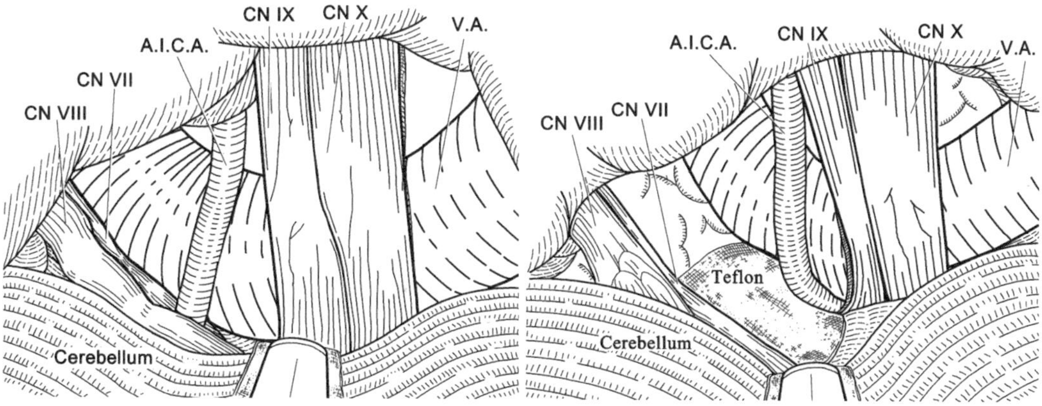

Fig. 5.8 (**a**) VA and AICA compress the facial nerve simultaneously. (**b**) A sufficient amount of Teflon cotton was placed between VA, AICA, and facial nerve

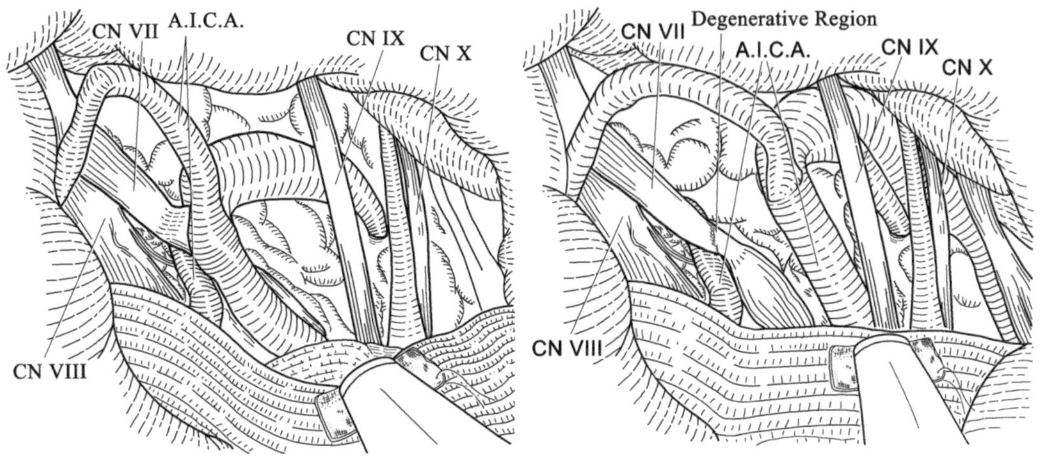

Fig. 5.9 (**a**) AICA compresses the facial nerve at both the cephalic and caudal ends. (**b**) The area showing compression and degeneration of the facial nerve after AICA displacement

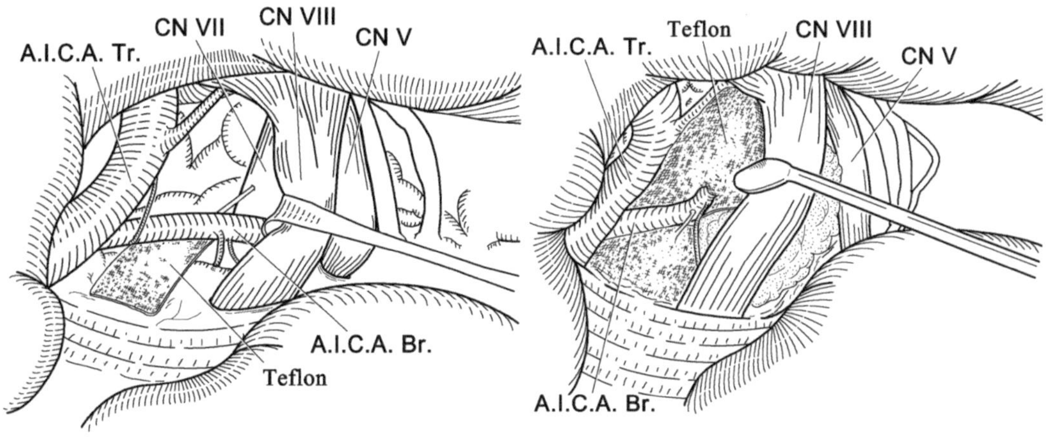

Fig. 5.10 (**a**) MVD for left facial spasm; AICA was seen passing between the facial nerve and the auditory nerve. (**b**) Appropriate amount of Teflon cotton was inserted between AICA and facial nerve and auditory nerve, respectively

it is easier to separate and displace the compressed blood vessels from the facial nerve, simply placing pads between the facial nerve and the offending vessels will not only cause severe adhesion between the blood vessels, pads, and facial nerves but also affect the function of the facial nerve. Functional repair is a common cause of symptom recurrence. To deal with this type of compression, we often implant a certain amount of gelatin sponge between the pads and the facial nerve, which may well solve the above problems. In about 8% of patients, the anterior inferior cerebellar artery that passes between the facial and auditory nerves is the responsible blood vessel that causes hemifacial spasm. Because such an anterior inferior cerebellar artery cannot be completely displaced and it is often difficult to fully decompress blood vessels if there is no sufficient space for decompression. The currently feasible method is to use a "sandwich" decompression [16] (Fig. 5.10). First, the anterior inferior cerebellar artery is safely separated from the facial nerve and vestibular nerve on both sides, and then an appropriate amount of pads are implanted between the anterior inferior cerebellar artery and facial nerve and between the anterior inferior cerebellar artery and vestibular nerve. Finally, an appropriate amount of gelatin sponge is implanted between the pads and the facial nerve and between the pads and the vestibular nerve, which

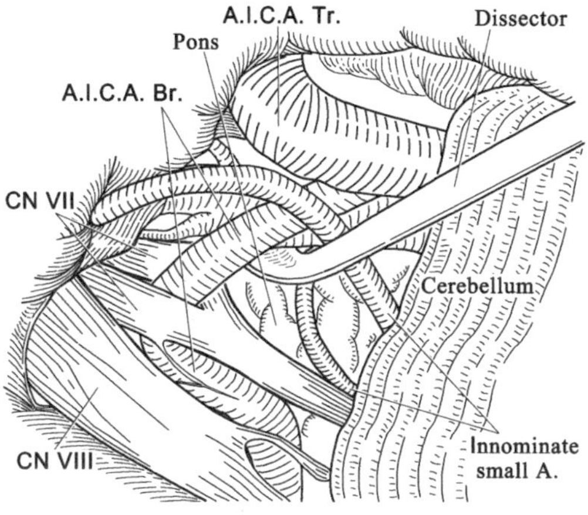

Fig. 5.11 MVD for right facial spasm; AICA was seen passing through the facial nerve

can not only achieve effective isolation but also avoid adhesion between the pads and the cranial nerves. Blood vessels crossing between the motor fibers of the facial nerve are very rare (Fig. 5.11), but once they occur, it is difficult to perform decompression operations, mainly due to ensuring that the facial nerve is not damaged and performing adequate decompression. The "sandwich" decompression method is still used for such responsible blood vessels. However, because the gap between the two facial nerve fibers is much smaller than the gap between the facial nerve and the vestibular nerve, great care should be taken during separation and decompression operations. First, the blood vessels passing through need to be shifted to the end of the facial nerve with a larger gap, and then the gap is appropriately and suddenly separated to expand the gap. Finally, a small amount of pads are implanted around the blood vessels and the surgery is completed. Treatment of patients whose AMR wave never disappears. AMR wave is an abnormal electromyographic response unique to typical hemifacial spasm. A positive AMR wave often indicates the existence of compression of the responsible blood vessel, and the disappearance of AMR wave during surgery often indicates that decompression has been sufficient. However, the biggest disadvantage of AMR waves is that they are not stable enough and are easily affected by many factors, which will reduce the value of AMR wave monitoring. In some patients, AMR waves may always exist no matter how the operation is performed. At this time, it is difficult for the surgeon to decide whether to end the operation or continue exploration. We believe that if the position of the monitoring electrode is correct, a positive AMR wave may indicate that the real responsible blood vessel has not been found or the decompression is not sufficient. It is recommended to use ZLR wave and EMG for joint monitoring, which can often find the small responsible blood vessel that was previously missed and separate and shift it again. After the AMR wave can disappear, the postoperative curative effect will be relatively satisfactory. It needs to be reminded that blindly ending the operation while the AMR wave persists is not encouraged. No obvious vascular compression was found during intraoperative exploration. If no obvious vascular compression of the facial nerve was found during intraoperative exploration, the patient's diagnosis of hemifacial spasm should be rechecked first, and a comprehensive judgment should be made based on the results of preoperative MRTA and intraoperative electrophysiological monitoring. The first possibility is that during the process of separating the arachnoid membrane, the original responsible blood vessel has automatically left the facial nerve; the second possibility is that the thickened arachnoid membrane itself is the cause of hemifacial spasm; the third possibility is that the responsible blood vessel is a small perforating artery and needs to be identified and judged in conjunction with ZLR wave monitoring; it should be pointed out that do not easily judge that there is no vascular compression, but should be comprehensively judged based on the above-mentioned factors to ensure the effectiveness of the surgery. For the treatment of bilateral facial spasm, it is recommended to select the side with severe symptoms for surgery first. After surgery, the other side will be selectively operated based on the degree of symptom relief on the operated side and the patient's physical condition. It is not recommended to perform bilateral vascular decompression surgery at one time. However, there is currently no particular limit on the interval between the two surgeries.

5.12 MVD Surgical Techniques for Recurrent Patients

The management of patients with recurrence of cranial nerve disease after MVD is still challenging, and the management principles vary in different diseases. For oculomotor nerve palsy and abducens nerve palsy, it is not recommended to perform MVD surgery again regardless of whether the disease recurs after MVD. For patients with typical primary trigeminal neuralgia, hemifacial spasm, and glossopharyngeal neuralgia, if the disease recurs after MVD, they can still choose to undergo re-MVD surgery, and the effective rate of re-MVD surgery is still greater than 95% [27–32]. In order to ensure that the surgery is effective and does not increase the risk of cranial nerve dysfunction, the second MVD should adhere to the following principles: (1) continuous electrophysiological monitoring, including AMR, BAEP, SEP, EMG, ZLR, and BTEP., electrophysiological monitoring physician, anesthesiologists, and operating surgeons should cooperate closely; (2) The principle of limited dissection. Adhesion between tissues is the main factor affecting the efficacy of the second MVD surgery. Separation of adhesions is also a key part of the surgery. Of course, the process of separation of adhesions can also easily lead to accidental damage to cranial nerves and surgical complications. Therefore, we recommend a second MVD surgery. The principle of limited dissection should be adhered to, and the trigeminal nerve, facial nerve or glossopharyngeal nerve should be exposed directly without expanding the exposure range; (3) The adhesion between the pads and the cranial nerves should be sharply incised. It is not necessary to completely remove the pads. Exploring along the cranial nerves to see if there are any missing blood vessels and performing corresponding isolation treatment. For trigeminal neuralgia, special attention needs to be paid to whether any motor roots are missed or pushed to the head or ventrally. For hemifacial spasm, attention should be paid to whether there is a gap between the facial and auditory nerves. If a blood vessel is missing, attention should be paid to whether there is a missing perforating artery under the pads. For glossopharyngeal neuralgia, the focus should be on checking whether there is a missing blood vessel in the sulcus; (4) Use gelatin sponge skillfully. After the pad is completely separated from the cranial nerves, it is not recommended to insert a new pad again. Instead, it is encouraged to place a sufficient amount of gelfoam between the original pad and the cranial nerve. Preventing the formation of new adhesions is the goal of re-MVD surgery. Of course, an appropriate amount of padding needs to be inserted into the missing blood vessels for isolation. Whether it is the original padding or a newly inserted padding, the key is to maintain no direct contact with the cranial nerves; (5) For trigeminal neuralgia, if no missing vessels were found during the operation, it is generally recommended to perform grooming of the superficial 1/3 of the trigeminal nerve at the same time to ensure that the patient's postoperative pain can completely disappear. For hemifacial spasm, complete disappearance of AMR is still a prerequisite for ending the operation. If AMR never disappears, full exploration and decompression as well as the combined application of ZLR and EMG will improve the effectiveness and safety of the operation.

5.13 Management Techniques for Patients with Ineffective Treatment After First MVD Surgery

There is no unified academic standard for the treatment principles of patients with ineffective treatment after the first MVD surgery. Many countries also lack guidelines or expert consensus. We read the literature and summarized based on the clinical data of a single center. Here we introduce the treatment principles of cranial nerve Disease Diagnosis and Treatment Center of Shanghai Jiao Tong University. For trigeminal neuralgia, if there is still pain after the first MVD, the degree of pain needs to be assessed first. If the pain reduction is greater than 50%, it is recommended to provide auxiliary drug treatment and follow-up observation. Commonly used drugs include oxcarbazepine, carbamazepine, and Gabapentin capsules. If the degree of pain relief is less than 50%, active surgical intervention is recommended. Possible treatment options include repeat MVD surgery, balloon compression therapy, radiofrequency thermocoagulation therapy, and gamma knife radiosurgery. For cases without any pain relief, Most advocate repeat MVD surgery. For cases with partial pain relief, the application of routine auxiliary balloon compression therapy, radiofrequency thermocoagulation therapy, and gamma knife radiosurgery has a tendency to gradually decrease [30, 33]. If you choose to undergo another MVD surgery, you must perform five-zone exploration and full decompression, and use trigeminal nerve sensory root coming if necessary. If the symptoms of hemifacial spasm are not relieved after MVD surgery, the next treatment plan needs to be decided based on the results of the electrophysiological examination. If the AMR reexamination is positive, it indicates that decompression is insufficient. It is recommended to perform a second MVD surgery as soon as possible, as long as the five days can be maintained. With area exploration and full decompression, surgery can still achieve ideal results. On the contrary, if the AMR reexamination is negative, follow-up observation and drug treatment are recommended. The observation needs to be at least 1 year. If the symptoms still do not improve, you can choose to perform another MVD surgery [34, 35]. If the symptoms of glossopharyngeal neuralgia are not relieved after MVD surgery, it may indicate that the decompression is not sufficient. Since these patients lack other effective treatments, it is recommended to choose another MVD surgery, but careful exploration must be done during the second MVD surgery, ensuring that any blood vessels in anatomical contact with the posterior cranial nerves are isolated and fully decompressed [36]. For other cranial nerve diseases such as oculomotor nerve palsy, abducens nerve palsy, intractable tinnitus, and spasmodic torticollis, if the symptom relief after MVD is not satisfactory, it is generally not recommended to choose MVD treatment again. It needs to be particularly emphasized that whenever you choose to perform another MVD surgery, you need to be particularly cautious. Not only do you need to repeatedly check the surgical video of the first MVD, but you also need to communicate in detail with the patient and their families, because no one can guarantee that the second MVD surgery will be successful. The second MVD surgery will definitely be successful.

5.14 Trigeminal Nerve Grooming

Trigeminal nerve combing is a method of using a combing knife to comb the pain fibers of the trigeminal nerve to relieve pain. In order to better apply this technology, it is necessary to fully understand the anatomical characteristics of the posterior root of the trigeminal nerve. The posterior root of the trigeminal nerve contains pain fibers and general tactile fibers. In the posterior root close to the brainstem, the pain fibers are located in the superficial area, while the tactile fibers are located in the middle. As they extend from the brainstem to Meckel's capsule, the pain fibers gradually spread out, and mixed distribution with tactile fibers. In the posterior root close to Meckel's capsule, tactile fibers are already distributed in superficial parts. According to the above histological characteristics, when combing the posterior root of the trigeminal nerve, it needs to be carried out on the inner 1/3 of the posterior root. And only the superficial area needs to be combed, including the dorsal, cranial, and caudal 1/3 of the posterior root of the trigeminal nerve as much as possible. Using the above combing method can not only effectively relieve pain, but also will not cause facial numbness after surgery. We usually use the combing knife produced by Qimai Medical Co., Ltd. in Suzhou City, Jiangsu Province. The quality of the combing knife will directly affect the surgical effect. It is best not to use ordinary strippers for combing [29, 37].

Grooming of the posterior trigeminal nerve root is a very safe and effective treatment technique that can effectively relieve pain without sacrificing the sensory function of the trigeminal nerve. The main indications of this technique are as follows: (1) In MVD surgery for trigeminal neuralgia, no obvious vascular compression is found; (2) In MVD surgery for trigeminal neuralgia, the responsible blood vessels are veins, and there are large veins that cannot achieve full displacement; (3) In order to ensure the effectiveness of the operation during MVD surgery for recurrent trigeminal neuralgia; (4) Primary trigeminal neuralgia is ineffective after Gamma Knife treatment. During MVD surgery, degeneration of the posterior root of the trigeminal nerve was found. After completing routine blood vessel separation and translocation and inserting some pads, it is often recommended to comb the degenerated posterior roots; (5) Postherpetic secondary trigeminal neuralgia, trigeminal posterior root combing is a very good treatment option .

References

1. Zhong J, Zhu J, Sun H, Dou NN, Wang YN, Ying TT, Xia L, Liu MX, Tao BB, Li ST. Microvascular decompression surgery: surgical principles and technical nuances based on 4000 cases. Neurol Res. 2014;36(10):882–93.
2. Zhong J, Li ST, Zhu J, Guan HX, Zhou QM, Jiao W, Ying TT, Yang XS, Zhan WC, Hua XM. A clinical analysis on microvascular decompression surgery in a series of 3000 cases. Clin Neurol Neurosurg. 2012 Sep;114(7):846–51.
3. Jeon C, Kim M, Lee H-S, Park K. Outcomes after microvascular decompression for Hemifacial spasm without definite radiological neurovascular compression at the root exit zone. Life (Basel). 2023;13(10):2064.
4. Zhu J, Zhong J, Jiao W, Li S-T. Via-cerebellar-fissures approach for microvascular decompression of trigeminal nerve. J Craniofac Surg. 2014;25(4):1438–40.
5. Miller LE, Miller VM. Safety and effectiveness of microvascular decompression for treatment of hemifacial spasm: a systematic review. Br J Neurosurg. 2012;26(4):438–44.
6. Hyun SJ, Kong DS, Park K. Microvascular decompression for treating hemifacial spasm: lessons learned from a prospective study of 1,174 operations. Neurosurg Rev. 2010;33(3):325–34; discussion 334.
7. Lee MH, Lee HS, Jee TK, Jo KI, Kong DS, Lee JA, Park K. Cerebellar retraction and hearing loss after microvascular decompression for hemifacial spasm. Acta Neurochir. 2015 Feb;157(2):337–43.
8. Li Y, Zheng X, Hua X, Li S. Surgical treatment of hemifacial spasm with zone-4 offending vessel. Acta Neurochir. 2013;155(5):849–53.
9. Liang Q, Shi X, Wang Y, Sun Y, Wang R, Li S. Microvascular decompression for hemifacial spasm: technical notes on pontomedullary sulcus decompression. Acta Neurochir. 2012;154(9):1621–6.
10. Sinha Ajit K, Shrey J, Vyas Medha A, Muralikrishnan K. "PTFE sleeve graft" technique to remove neurovascular conflict in micro vascular decompression for trigeminal neuralgia. Neurol India. 2022;70(4):1412–6.
11. Patra Devi P, Turcotte Evelyn L, Chandan K, Bendok Bernard R. Microvascular decompression technique for trigeminal neuralgia using a vascular clip. World Neurosurg. 2021;154:1.
12. Steinberg Jeffrey A, Jayson S, Bayard W, Alksne J. Tentorial sling for microvascular decompression in patients with trigeminal neuralgia: a description of operative technique and clinical outcome. J Neurosurg. 2018;130(4):1315–20.
13. Swiątnicki W, Heleniak M, Komuński P. Hemifacial spasm caused by the cross-compression of the vertebral artery loop—a case-centered report of a stitched sling retraction technique. Bull Soc Sci Med Grand Duche Luxemb. 2014;3:73–82.
14. Khoo HM, Yoshimine T, Taki T. A "sling swing transposition" technique with pedicled dural flap for microvascular decompression in hemifacial spasm. Neurosurgery. 2012;71(1 Suppl Operative):25–30; discussion 30–1.
15. Kurokawa Y, Maeda Y, Toyooka T, Inaba K. Microvascular decompression for hemifacial spasm caused by the vertebral artery: a simple and effective transposition method using surgical glue. Surg Neurol. 2004;61(4):398–403.
16. Ichikawa T, Agari T, Kurozumi K, Maruo T, Satoh T, Date I. "Double-stick tape" technique for transposition of an offending vessel in microvascular decompression: technical case report. Neurosurgery. 2011;68(2 Suppl Operative):377–82; discussion 382.
17. Wang YN, Zhong J, Zhu J, Dou NN, Xia L, Visocchi M, Li ST. Microvascular decompression in patients with coexistent trigeminal neuralgia, hemifacial spasm and glossopharyngeal neuralgia. Acta Neurochir. 2014 Jun;156(6):1167–71.
18. Zhong J, Zhu J, Li S-T, Guan H-X. Microvascular decompressions in patients with coexistent Hemifacial spasm and trigeminal neuralgia. Neurosurgery. 2011;68:916–20.
19. Zheng XS, Feng BH, Zhang WC, Ying TT, Li ST. Hemifacial spasm caused by cross type vascular compression. Neurol Res. 2011;33(9):965–8.
20. Lee H-S, Park K. Penetrating offenders in Hemifacial spasm: surgical tactics and prognosis. Life (Basel). 2023;13(10):2021.
21. Inoue T, Goto Y, Inoue Y, Fukushima T. Potential reasons for failure and recurrence in microvascular decompression for hemifacial spasm. Acta Neurochir. 2023;165:3845.
22. Chang B, Tang Y, Wei X, Li S. A new application of gelatin sponge in the treatment of Hemifacial spasm by microvascular decompression: a technical note. J Neurol Surg Part A. 2022;83(2):183–6.
23. Liu Ming Xing. e900.

24. Rae CK, Hyun-Seok L, Kim M, Kwan P. Optimal method for reliable lateral spread response monitoring during microvascular decompression surgery for hemifacial spasm. Sci Rep. 2023;13(1):21672.
25. Ying TT, Li ST, Zhong J, Li XY, Wang XH, Zhu J. The value of abnormal muscle response monitoring during microvascular decompression surgery for hemifacial spasm. Int J Surg. 2011;9(4):347–51.
26. Yang M, Zheng X, Ying T, Zhu J, Zhang W, Yang X, Li S. Combined intraoperative monitoring of abnormal muscle response and ZL response for hemifacial spasm with tandem compression type. Acta Neurochir. 2014;156(6):1161–6.
27. Zhang X, Zhao H, Tang Y, Li S. Comparison of the efficacy of reoperation, percutaneous radiofrequency Thermocoagulation when microvascular decompression of trigeminal neuralgia is invalid. J Craniofac Surg. 2016;27(7):e688–90.
28. Zhao H, Zhang X, Tang Y-d, Li S. Factors promoting a good outcome in a second microvascular decompression operation when Hemifacial spasm is not relieved after the initial operation. World Neurosurg. 2017;98(872):e11–872.e19.
29. Zhang X, Xu L, Zhao H, Li S-T. Long-term efficacy of nerve combing for patients with trigeminal neuralgia and failed prior microvascular decompression. World Neurosurg. 2017;108:711–5.
30. Nascimento RFV, Pipek LZ, de Aguiar PHP. Is percutaneous balloon compression better than microvascular decompression to treat trigeminal neuralgia? A systematic review and meta-analysis. J Clin Neurosci. 2023;109:11–20.
31. Kureshi SA, Wilkins RH. Posterior fossa reexploration for persistent or recurrent trigeminal neuralgia or hemifacial spasm: surgical findings and therapeutic implications. Neurosurgery. 1998;43(5):1111–7.
32. Payner TD, Tew JM. Recurrence of hemifacial spasm after microvascular decompression. Neurosurgery. 1996;38(4):686–90.
33. Gökce HM, Filipe WF, Shadi A-A, Krauss Joachim K. Microsurgical posterior fossa re-exploration for recurrent trigeminal neuralgia after previous microvascular decompression: common grounds-scarring, deformation, and the "piston effect". Acta Neurochir. 2023;165:3877.
34. Li S, Hong W, Tang Y, Ying T, Zhang W, Li X, Zhu J, Zhong J, Hua X, Shunqing X, Wan L, Wang X, Yang M, Li Y, Zheng X. Re-operation for persistent. Hemifacial spasm after microvascular decompression with the aid of intraoperative monitoring of abnormal muscle response. Acta Neurochir. 2010;152:2113–8.
35. Zhong J, Zhu J, Li S-T, Li X-Y, Wang X-H, Yang M, Wan L, Guan H-X. An analysis of failed microvascular decompression in patients with hemifacial spasm: focused on the early reoperative findings. Acta Neurochir. 2010;152:2119–23.
36. Xia L, Li Y-S, Liu M-X, Li S-T. Microvascular decompression for glossopharyngeal neuralgia: a retrospective analysis of 228 cases. Acta Neurochir. 2018;160(1):117–23.
37. Zhao H, Zhang X, Tang D, Li S. Nerve combing for trigeminal neuralgia without vascular compression. J Craniofac Surg. 2017;28(1):e15–6.

6 The Easier the Better: A Personal Philosophy of MVD

Jun Zhong

The microvascular decompression (MVD) procedure has gained widespread acceptance as the most efficacious treatment modality for hyperactive cranial rhizopathies, including hemifacial spasm and trigeminal neuralgia [1–7]. With the widespread adoption of this surgical procedure, numerous neurosurgeons have shared their expert opinions on operative techniques. For example, it has been deemed essential to expose the entire intracranial course of the nerve root and release any attached vessels [8–13]. As it adheres to the principle of neurovascular conflict resolution instead of using Teflon, the "sling technique" has become increasingly popular in recent years [14–18]. Despite the utilization of diverse methodologies, ensuring safety remains a paramount concern within the realm of functional neurosurgery. Achieving spasm or pain relief at the expense of facial palsy or hearing loss is generally considered unacceptable. The more intricate the surgical technique, the greater number of instruments or foreign objects introduced into the operative field, and the longer the duration of the process, the higher chance of postoperative complications occurring. Actually, this procedure could be simplified and made more straightforward. The accomplishment of over 10,000 MVDs in our center has given us valuable experience in optimizing the procedure to minimize time and effort [19, 20].

6.1 The Simpler the Better

The literature has recently witnessed a prevailing inclination towards the adoption of the sling technique [16, 18, 21–24]. It was designed to separate the neurovascular conflict without any physical intervention between the artery and the nerve. However, due to its numerous limitations, it is not suitable for widespread adoption. In such a confined surgical field, the adjacent delicate anatomical structures such as the facial and vestibulocochlear nerves as well as petrosal veins are at risk of damage while the surgeon focuses on suturing and knotting around the artery. Specifically, there is a potentially significant risk at the moment when an abrupt rupture occurs during needle puncture of the petrous dura or tentorium [25]. Lately, some authors have made advancements in the technique, for instance, by substituting the thread with alternative materials and eliminating the need for stitching or knotting through the adoption of glue or clips [26–29]. However, the inclusion of these additional procedures requires a longer duration and the use of a spatula for cerebellum retraction to optimize the

J. Zhong (✉)
Department of Neurosurgery, XinHua Hospital,
Shanghai JiaoTong University School of Medicine,
Shanghai, China
e-mail: ZhongMDPhD@sjtu.edu.cn

S.-T. Li et al. (eds.), *Microvascular Decompression Surgery*,
https://doi.org/10.1007/978-981-96-0767-9_6

surgical field. Actually, a satisfactory exposure could have achieved by efficient dissection instead of retraction. Based on our experience, even a dolichoectatic vertebrobasilar complex can be repositioned without the need for slinging. By fully dissecting the arachnoid membrane, an enhanced elevation of the cerebellar hemisphere can be achieved to facilitate a precise medial exposure. Once a broader exposure is achieved, gelfoams or Teflon felts can be sequentially inserted between the vertebral artery and the medulla, starting from cranial nerve XI towards VII. Once reaching the rostral facial nerve root, it would be observed that the offending artery has already been mobilized laterally and proximally without any tension. Compared to a distal pull (sling), this proximal push offers greater ease in maintaining arterial transposition [9, 30–33]. Therefore, it is worthwhile to invest time in dissecting the caudal nerves medially rather than focusing on lateral slinging of a tortuous vertebral artery. The decompression is mainly carried out by manipulating the artery, with a special focus on reducing any disruption to the nerve. The key is to identify the pivotal (leveraged) point along the offending artery, where the culprit can be easily pushed away in line with its natural inclination and sustain its position without rebound. Eventually, the prioritization of technical simplification is of utmost importance in this context (Fig. 6.1).

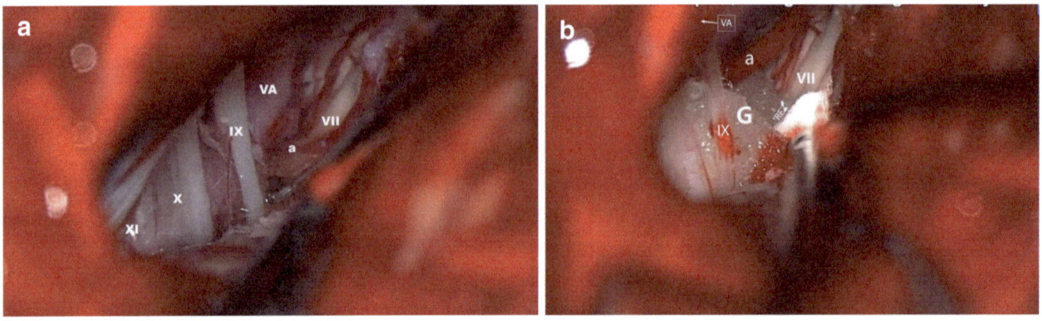

Fig. 6.1 A caudal-to-rostral approach achieves more with less. (a) This is a typical hemifacial spasm case caused by a twisted vertebral artery (VA) pushing a small artery (**a**) towards the root exit zone of the facial nerve (VII). (b) Instead of inserting Teflon felts between the offending artery and facial nerve, geofoams (G) are used to gradually displace the VA in a proximal and lateral direction from caudal (XI) to rostral (IX), achieving effective decompression of the facial root while maintaining a clear neurovascular conflict site (REZ) without dissecting the rostral structures (the acoustic nerve was not exposed in this case)

6.2 The Lesser the Better

The complete decompression procedure can be effortlessly executed by the operator through concurrent manipulation of a microdissector and a microsuction. The use of forceps for arterial manipulation should be avoided to mitigate the risk of vasospasm [19]. Even in the absence of forceps, Teflon felt can coat on the tip of a microdissector for delivery. The placement should be gradually conducted using small fragments, as a substantial quantity of Teflon may obstruct the operator's line of sight and inadvertently displace the vessel towards the nerve instead. The emplacement should be managed to avoid the conflict site, as a granuloma may develop later and contribute to its recurrence [34–36]. Therefore, if the offending artery can be effectively separated from the nerve through careful dissection, the utilization of Teflon may not be deemed imperative.

The use of retracting blades is unnecessary because a narrow suction tip on a padding cottonoid offers better maneuverability for dissecting a specific area compared to using a wider spatula at any given moment. A satisfactory operative field is attained through meticulous arachnoid dissection rather than relying on blind cerebellar retraction.

Therefore, it is advisable to minimize the presence of surgical instruments or foreign objects within the operative field to the greatest possible extent (Fig. 6.1).

6.3 The Shorter the Better

While the procedure is encouraged to conduct in a short time as possible to minimize the chances of complications increasing over time, it remains crucial to execute each step meticulously and efficiently in a routine manner without rushing or redundance [19]. If the principle of commencing from a lower level had not been implemented until encountering an obstructed flocculus, additional time would have been expended due to the redundant manipulation at that juncture. In the majority of hemifacial spasm cases, caudal dissection alone can identify the conflict, thereby obviating the need for additional rostral exposure [10, 12, 37, 38]. Conversely, in most trigeminal cases, instead of dissecting from the tentorium, a viable alternative is to perform dissection at the level of the VIII root in order to circumvent these troublesome petrosal veins [39]. If a favorable angle remains unattainable using this approach, it is recommended to optimize exposure by opening the cerebellar fissures while preserving the veins as much as possible [40]. Moreover, it is crucial to acknowledge the significance of pre-microscopic procedures such as positioning, incision, craniectomy, and duratomy. Neglecting these procedures can result in situations where the patient's shoulder obstructs the operator's arm access or the craniectomy restricts lateral exposure during surgery, necessitating adjustments in positioning or the use of a rongeur for additional bone removal. The extra time consumed in these repeated manipulations may gradually exhaust your mood, judgment, and accuracy, resulting in an increase in risks. In fact, a standardized routine manipulation can effectively reduce the overall operation time. Hence, as emphasized by a Chinese proverb: "*sharpening an axe does not impede cutting firewood*."

6.3.1 Cure Vs. Safety

Operative safety should always be prioritized, particularly in the context of functional neurosurgery. Considering the infrequent occurrence of conflicts in the cisternal segment among hemifacial spasm cases, it is recommended to cease the procedure once a clearly identifiable offending artery has been detected at the axilla (caudal REZ) of the VII root, particularly when a nerve imprint is also observed and intraoperative electrophysiology indicates a negative abnormal muscle response (AMR) upon removal of the artery [5, 41]. The anterior inferior cerebellar artery (AICA) passing between the VIII and VII roots is often observed if the dissection extends rostrally, but it is not considered the primary cause. Prolonged time spent in this area may increase the risk of postoperative facial palsy or hearing loss. Hence, we propose a guiding principle: "*adequate exposure of those essential and no manipulation of those unnecessary*" (Fig. 6.1).

Although rare, this phenomenon may occur in certain patients with an inaccessible neurovascular conflict due to anatomical variations, such as an artery adhering to the petrous bone and preventing retraction of the cerebellum. Real-time electrophysiological assistance can be used to manage this situation instead of forcibly elevating the cerebellum. If a portion of the VII root is visible, gradually inserting small pieces of geofoam waddings between the nerve and artery can move them medially alongside the nerve while simultaneously pushing the artery away until disappearance of AMR wave. The concept can be illustrated by a Chinese proverb: "*follow the vine to get the melon*." Even if the exact location of the conflict cannot be visualized, it is still possible to separate the offending artery from the nerve.

Reoperative cases of trigeminal neuralgia often present challenging adhesions or Teflon granulomas that hinder surgical exposure, posing a significant obstacle. In situations where achieving complete V root exposure proves excessively difficult, an alternative approach involving combing or low-power thermocautery on the trigeminal nerve can be considered. Prioritizing safety over cure and avoiding prolonged struggle is the wise choice.

6.4 Conclusion

A successful MVD depends on promptly and accurately discovering the neurovascular conflict through sufficient exposure. Attaining an optimal surgical field necessitates proper patient positioning, appropriate craniectomy, and a caudal-to-rostral approach. By dissecting arachnoids carefully, the cerebellum can be elevated medially to access the REZ on the brainstem without using a retractor, thus facilitating detachment of the offending artery from the nerve. When *a leverage point* along the artery is identified, preserving neurovascular separation can be achieved by repositioning the artery instead of Teflon insertion in the conflict region. Ultimately, prioritizing safety remains the paramount concern. To strike a harmonious balance between efficacy and safety, the process should be expedited with a rational approach while minimizing potential disruption to the brain as much as possible. In this regard, Confucius's *doctrine of the mean* holds significant relevance.

References

1. Sekula RF Jr, Frederickson AM, Jannetta PJ, Quigley MR, Aziz KM, Arnone GD. Microvascular decompression for elderly patients with trigeminal neuralgia: a prospective study and systematic review with meta-analysis. J Neurosurg. 2011;114(1):172–9.
2. Jannetta PJ, McLaughlin MR, Casey KF. Technique of microvascular decompression. Technical note. Neurosurg Focus. 2005;18(5):E5.
3. McLaughlin MR, Jannetta PJ, Clyde BL, Subach BR, Comey CH, Resnick DK. Microvascular decompression of cranial nerves: lessons learned after 4400 operations. J Neurosurg. 1999;90(1):1–8.
4. Barker FG 2nd, Jannetta PJ, Bissonette DJ, Shields PT, Larkins MV, Jho HD. Microvascular decompression for hemifacial spasm. J Neurosurg. 1995;82(2):201–10.
5. Ying TT, Li ST, Zhong J, Li XY, Wang XH, Zhu J. The value of abnormal muscle response monitoring during microvascular decompression surgery for hemifacial spasm. Int J Surg. 2011;9(4):347–51.
6. Liu MX, Zhong J, Xia L, Dou NN, Li ST. A correlative analysis between inflammatory cytokines and trigeminal neuralgia or hemifacial spasm. Neurol Res. 2019;41(4):335–40.
7. Mercier P, Sindou M. Introduction to primary hemifacial spasm: a neurosurgical disease. Neurochirurgie. 2018;64(2):79–81.
8. Zhong J, Li ST, Zhu J, Guan HX. Is entire nerve root decompression necessary for hemifacial spasm? Int J Surg. 2011;9(3):254–7.
9. Zhong J, Li ST, Zhu J, Guan HX, Zhou QM, Jiao W, et al. A clinical analysis on microvascular decompression surgery in a series of 3000 cases. Clin Neurol Neurosurg. 2012;114(7):846–51.
10. Zhong J, Xia L, Dou NN, Ying TT, Zhu J, Liu MX, et al. Delayed relief of hemifacial spasm after microvascular decompression: can it be avoided? Acta Neurochir. 2015;157(1):93–8; discussion 8–9.
11. Li S, Hong W, Tang Y, Ying T, Zhang W, Li X, et al. Re-operation for persistent hemifacial spasm after microvascular decompression with the aid of intraoperative monitoring of abnormal muscle response. Acta Neurochir. 2010;152(12):2113–8.
12. Zhu J, Li ST, Zhong J, Guan HX, Ying TT, Yang M, et al. Role of arterioles in management of microvascular decompression in patients with hemifacial spasm. J Clin Neurosci. 2012;19(3):375–9.
13. Li Y, Zheng X, Hua X, Ying T, Zhong J, Zhang W, et al. Surgical treatment of hemifacial spasm with zone-4 offending vessel. Acta Neurochir. 2013;155(5):849–53.
14. Yang XS, Li ST, Zhong J, Zhu J, Du Q, Zhou QM, et al. Microvascular decompression on patients with

trigeminal neuralgia caused by ectatic vertebrobasilar artery complex: technique notes. Acta Neurochir. 2012;154(5):793–7; discussion 7.
15. Nonaka Y, Hayashi N, Matsumae M, Fukushima T. Wedge-technique for transposition of the vertebral artery in microvascular decompression for hemifacial spasm: technical nuances and surgical outcomes. Acta Neurochir. 2019;161(7):1435–42.
16. Khoo HM, Yoshimine T, Taki T. A "sling swing transposition" technique with pedicled dural flap for microvascular decompression in hemifacial spasm. Neurosurgery. 2012;71(1 Suppl Operative):25–30; discussion -1.
17. Skrap M, Tuniz F. Use of the arachnoid membrane of the cerebellopontine angle to transpose the superior cerebellar artery in microvascular decompression for trigeminal neuralgia: technical note. Neurosurgery. 2010;66(3 Suppl Operative):88–91.
18. Melvill RL, Baxter BL. A tentorial sling in microvascular decompression for trigeminal neuralgia. Technical note. J Neurosurg. 1996;84(1):127–8.
19. Zhong J, Zhu J, Sun H, Dou NN, Wang YN, Ying TT, et al. Microvascular decompression surgery: surgical principles and technical nuances based on 4000 cases. Neurol Res. 2014;36(10):882–93.
20. Li ST, Zhong J, Sekula RF. In: Li ST, Zhong J, Sekula RF, editors. Microvascular decompression surgery. Cham: Springer; 2016.
21. Steinberg JA, Sack J, Wilson B, Weingarten D, Carter B, Khalessi A, et al. Tentorial sling for microvascular decompression in patients with trigeminal neuralgia: a description of operative technique and clinical outcomes. J Neurosurg. 2018;130:1315.
22. Masuoka J, Matsushima T, Inoue K, Nakahara Y, Takase Y, Kawashima M. Outcome of microvascular decompression for trigeminal neuralgia treated with the stitched sling retraction technique. Neurosurg Rev. 2015;38(2):361–5; discussion 5.
23. Masuoka J, Matsushima T, Kawashima M, Nakahara Y, Funaki T, Mineta T. Stitched sling retraction technique for microvascular decompression: procedures and techniques based on an anatomical viewpoint. Neurosurg Rev. 2011;34(3):373–9; discussion 9–80.
24. Stone JL, Lichtor T, Crowell RM. Microvascular sling decompression for trigeminal neuralgia secondary to ectatic vertebrobasilar compression. Case report. J Neurosurg. 1993;79(6):943–5.
25. Zhong J. An ideal microvascular decompression technique should be simple and safe. Neurosurg Rev. 2012;35(1):137–40. author reply 40.
26. Zhang X, Kang X, Jiang Q, Zhao H, Tang Y, Zhu J, et al. Efficacy of biomedical glue sling technique versus traditional technique for microvascular decompression for Hemifacial spasm with refractory hypertension. World Neurosurg. 2018;110:e473–e8.
27. Liu J, Chen Z, Feng T, Jiang B, Yuan Y, Yu Y. Biomedical glue sling technique in microvascular decompression for trigeminal neuralgia caused by atherosclerotic Vertebrobasilar artery: a description of operative technique and clinical outcomes. World Neurosurg. 2019;128:e74–80.
28. Lee SH, Park JS, Ahn YH. Bioglue-coated Teflon sling technique in microvascular decompression for Hemifacial spasm involving the vertebral artery. J Korean Neurosurg Soc. 2016;59(5):505–11.
29. Jha RT, Kumar J, Pressman E, Agazzi S. Arterial sling decompression for Hemifacial spasm. World Neurosurg. 2019;132:134.
30. Zhong J, Zhu J, Li ST, Guan HX. Microvascular decompressions in patients with coexistent hemifacial spasm and trigeminal neuralgia. Neurosurgery. 2011;68(4):916–20. discussion 20
31. Jiao W, Zhong J, Sun H, Zhu J, Zhou QM, Yang XS, et al. Microvascular decompression for the patient with painful tic convulsif after bell palsy. J Craniofac Surg. 2013;24(3):e286–9.
32. Wang YN, Dou NN, Zhou QM, Jiao W, Zhu J, Zhong J, et al. Treatment of hemimasticatory spasm with microvascular decompression. J Craniofac Surg. 2013;24(5):1753–5.
33. Wang YN, Zhong J, Zhu J, Dou NN, Xia L, Visocchi M, et al. Microvascular decompression in patients with coexistent trigeminal neuralgia, hemifacial spasm and glossopharyngeal neuralgia. Acta Neurochir. 2014;156(6):1167–71.
34. Dou NN, Zhong J, Liu MX, Xia L, Sun H, Li B, et al. Teflon might be a factor accounting for a failed microvascular decompression in Hemifacial spasm: a technical note. Stereotact Funct Neurosurg. 2016;94(3):154–8.
35. Zhong J, Zhu J, Li ST, Li XY, Wang XH, Yang M, et al. An analysis of failed microvascular decompression in patients with hemifacial spasm: focused on the early reoperative findings. Acta Neurochir. 2010;152(12):2119–23.
36. Kondo A, Akiyama O, Suzuki M, Arai H. Prosthetic material degeneration over time as a possible factor in delayed recurrence of hemifacial spasm after successful microvascular decompression. Surg Neurol Int. 2018;9:187.
37. Xia L, Zhong J, Zhu J, Dou NN, Liu MX, Li ST. Delayed relief of hemifacial spasm after microvascular decompression. J Craniofac Surg. 2015;26(2):408–10.
38. Sindou M, Mercier P. Microvascular decompression for hemifacial spasm : surgical techniques and intraoperative monitoring. Neurochirurgie. 2018;64(2):133–43.
39. Zhong J, Li ST, Xu SQ, Wan L, Wang X. Management of petrosal veins during microvascular decompression for trigeminal neuralgia. Neurol Res. 2008;30(7):697–700.
40. Zhu J, Zhong J, Jiao W, Zhou QM, Guan HX, Dou NN, et al. Via-cerebellar-fissures approach for microvascular decompression of trigeminal nerve. J Craniofac Surg. 2014;25(4):1438–40.
41. Liu MX, Zhong J, Xia L, Dou NN, Sun H, Li B, et al. The significance of abnormal muscle response monitoring during microvascular decompression for Hemifacial spasm. Acta Neurochir Suppl. 2017;124:297–301.

7 Avoiding Failure in Microvascular Decompression for Hemifacial Spasm

Alwyn Gomez and Anthony M. Kaufmann

7.1 Introduction

Hemifacial spasm (HFS) is a rare condition characterized by unilateral facial muscle contractions. While the condition is painless and nonfatal, it can have a significant impact on quality of life and result in social stigmatization [1]. The etiology of the condition is now more clearly understood to be from neurovascular compression (NVC) of the ipsilateral facial nerve and fortunately can be treated safely, effectively, and durably through microvascular decompression (MVD) surgery [2]. In fact, several published series have reported long-term spasm relief in up to 90% of cases with low morbidity or mortality rates [3–6]. Despite this, much of the medical community considers serial botulinum toxin injections (SBIs) to be the treatment of choice [7]. As a result, there remains very low utilization rates of MVD for HFS resulting in few neurosurgeons being able to establish a high-volume practice [8]. With limited experience, failure and complication rates of MVD for HFS may be unnecessarily high. This can result in referral patterns that favor SBIs and further limit surgical experience.

The aim of this chapter is to provide practical advice that may aid in the avoidance of failure in MVD surgery for HFS. Technical aspects will be the primary focus; however, as with all surgeries, success begins with appropriate diagnosis, workup, and patient selection. Key to this is understanding that the goal of surgery is improved quality of life and not simply spasm relief. Patients with minimal impact from their HFS or those unable to tolerate surgery due to medical comorbidity are therefore poor candidates.

7.2 The Surgical Target

The key to a technically successful MVD for HFS is a thorough alleviation of the causative NVC. However, a clear understanding of the anatomy of the facial nerve, and in particular the root entry zone (REZ) is critical in the avoidance of technical failure.

It is now widely accepted that HFS is caused by the pulsatile vascular compression of the REZ of the facial nerve. Vascular contact upon the cisternal portion of the nerve is common and rarely causes HFS outside of the setting of marked deformation. As such, translocation of the vessel away from this facial REZ is paramount to a successful procedure. However, all too often the REZ is considered synonymous with the Obersteiner-

A. Gomez
Section of Neurosurgery, Department of Surgery, University of Manitoba, Winnipeg, MB, Canada

Department of Human Anatomy and Cell Science, University of Manitoba, Winnipeg, MB, Canada

A. M. Kaufmann (✉)
Section of Neurosurgery, Department of Surgery, University of Manitoba, Winnipeg, MB, Canada
e-mail: AKaufmann@hsc.mb.ca

S.-T. Li et al. (eds.), *Microvascular Decompression Surgery*,
https://doi.org/10.1007/978-981-96-0767-9_7

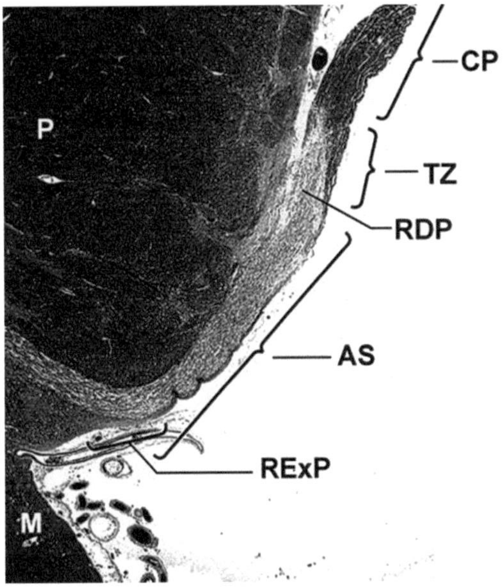

Fig. 7.1 Photomicrograph of a solochrome cyanin-stained longitudinal section of the pons (P) and medulla (M) showing the facial nerve. The central oligodendrocyte-derived myelin of the intraaxial facial nerve is seen to course through the pons and then exit at the pontomedullary sulcus at the root exit point (RExP), then remain strongly attached to the pontine surface as the attached segment (AS). At the root detachment point (RDP), a transition zone (TZ) or Obersteiner-Redlich zone (ORZ) is seen, with central myelin becoming replaced by the peripheral Schwann cell-derived myelin that continues in the distal cisternal portion (CP) of the facial nerve. (Figure and legend reproduced from Campos-Benitez and Kaufmann. J Neurosurg. 2008;109(9):416–420)

Redlich zone (ORZ). The ORZ is the transition zone (TZ) of central myelin of oligodendrocytes to peripheral myelin of Schwann cells. The REZ is more precisely defined as the entire length of the exposed central myelin of the facial nerve. It has previously been emphasized that the culprit NVC can occur at any point along the facial nerve REZ and not just at the ORZ [3, 9, 10].

The fibers of the facial nerve REZ emerge from the pontomedullary sulcus at the root exit point (RExP). Importantly, they then course superiorly, remaining exposed and adherent to the ventrolateral surface of the pons for approximately 8 mm. This is the attached segment (AS). At the root detachment point (RDP) these central fibers separate from the brainstem. Approximately 2 mm distal to the RDP, is located the transition zone (TZ or ORZ) where central myelin transitions to peripheral myelin. Beyond this is the cisternal portion of the facial nerve that traverses the subarachnoid space (Fig. 7.1) [9].

It is paramount to recognize that the minority of causative compression occurs at the ORZ or RDP, with one study reporting an incidence of just 23%. The successful procedures require the surgeon to direct their attention to more proximal aspects of the REZ. Of note, the most prevalent site of compression is along the AS, reported in 64% of cases and 10% of causative compression occurs at the RExP. Misguided efforts to "decompress" more distal aspects of the facial nerve are often to blame when MVD for HFS fails [9].

7.3 The Surgical Approach

Understanding the surgical target is only part of successful MVD for HFS. Appropriate translocation of the vessel without disruption of brain parenchyma or neurovascular injury along with avoidance of postoperative complications, such as infection and cerebrospinal fluid (CSF) leak, are all key aspects of success. Here is outlined the local institutional technique and approach that has been refined over numerous years and has been found to provide an optimal chance of a good patient outcome [1, 3].

A retrosigmoid approach has been found to provide appropriate exposure to successfully perform an MVD for HFS (Fig. 7.2). The patient is placed in the lateral decubitus position and maintained with lateral positioners. The knees are slightly bent with a cushion placed between them. Care is taken to ensure that the shoulders and lumbar region is perpendicular to the floor, with shoulders brought close to the edge of the operating table. Utilizing rigid fixation, the patient's head is drawn posteriorly and flexed while allowing two finger breaths between the chin and chest to avoid compromise of the airway or venous return. The vertex of the head is dropped 10–15 degrees and the ipsilateral shoulder taped inferiorly to gently open up the working area. Finally, the head is rotated in the contralateral direction so as to bring the mastoid

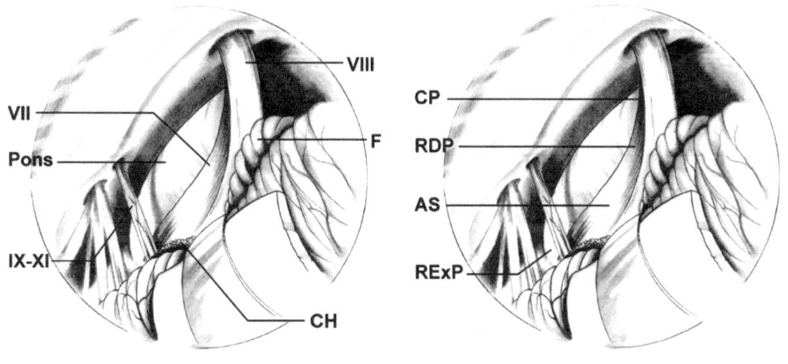

Fig. 7.2 Surgical exposure of the root entry zone (REZ) of the facial nerve. The labels VII, VIII, and IX–XI designate cranial nerves VII (facial nerve) and VIII (vestibulocochlear nerve) and the rootlets of cranial nerves IX–XI (glossopharyngeal, vagus, and accessory nerves), respectively. *CH* choroid plexus, *F* flocculus. (Figure and legend reproduced from Campos-Benitez and Kaufmann. J Neurosurg. 2008;109(9):416–420)

bone towards the horizontal plane. This also brings the ipsilateral petrosal surface of the posterior fossa to a near vertical orientation.

Maximal access is required of the junction of the posterior fossa floor and sigmoid sinus in the anterior-inferior aspect of the rectosigmoid space. The mastoid tip, which extends slightly below the floor of the posterior fossa, and the posterior edge of the mastoid process, which indicates the sigmoid sinus, are used as landmarks. Additionally, the transverse line, a straight line drawn between the lateral canthus, root of the zygoma, and inion, can be used to approximate the lateral transverse sinus. A linear cranial-caudal incision is marked 1 cm behind the mastoid process and spans from just above the transverse line to the level of the mastoid tip.

The incision is carried down through the skin and muscle layers to bone. Often the occipital artery is encountered and often coagulated and cut. Dissection is carried anteriorly in the subperiosteal plane to allow for retraction with a single self-retaining retractor. This includes clearing the digastric groove at the posterior aspect of the mastoid. During this dissection an emissary vein at the level of the mid-sigmoid sinus is typically encountered and can be controlled with bone wax.

Utilizing a high-speed burr and 3-5 mm angulated rongeurs, a low retrosigmoid craniectomy is performed. Typically, 3 × 2 cm in size, the anterior extent of the craniectomy must expose the posterior aspect of the sigmoid sinus while reaching inferior enough to view the floor of the posterior fossa end-on. Any mastoid air cells that are entered are sealed with a layer of wax to prevent CSF leak, without "stuffing" the air cells. The importance of an appropriately placed craniectomy cannot be overstated as this allows for access to the deep arachnoid cisterns and rootlets of the cranial nerves of the pons and medulla without any excessive brain retraction (Fig. 7.3).

A simple L-shaped dural opening is made and reflected anteriorly. To facilitate a watertight closure, it is important to place the dura on stretch using a couple of retaining sutures anchored to hemostats and maintain the dural flap moist by placing a saline-soaked Gelfoam under its reflected surface. Visualization of the posterior fossa floor can be improved though the placement of another retracting suture at the inferior dural edge.

Intradural work is carried out with the aid of the surgical microscope. To relax the cerebellum and facilitate further dissection, elevation of the cerebellum off the posterior fossa floor will give access to the lateral aspect of the cisterna magna, which can be opened to release CSF and relax the cerebellum. Minimal retraction is needed and can be achieved with a suction and bayonet overtop a ½-inch × 3-inch cottonoid and latex sheet "slider."

Further arachnoid dissection then continues from inferior to superior with the aim of separating the cerebellum from the rootlets of the lower

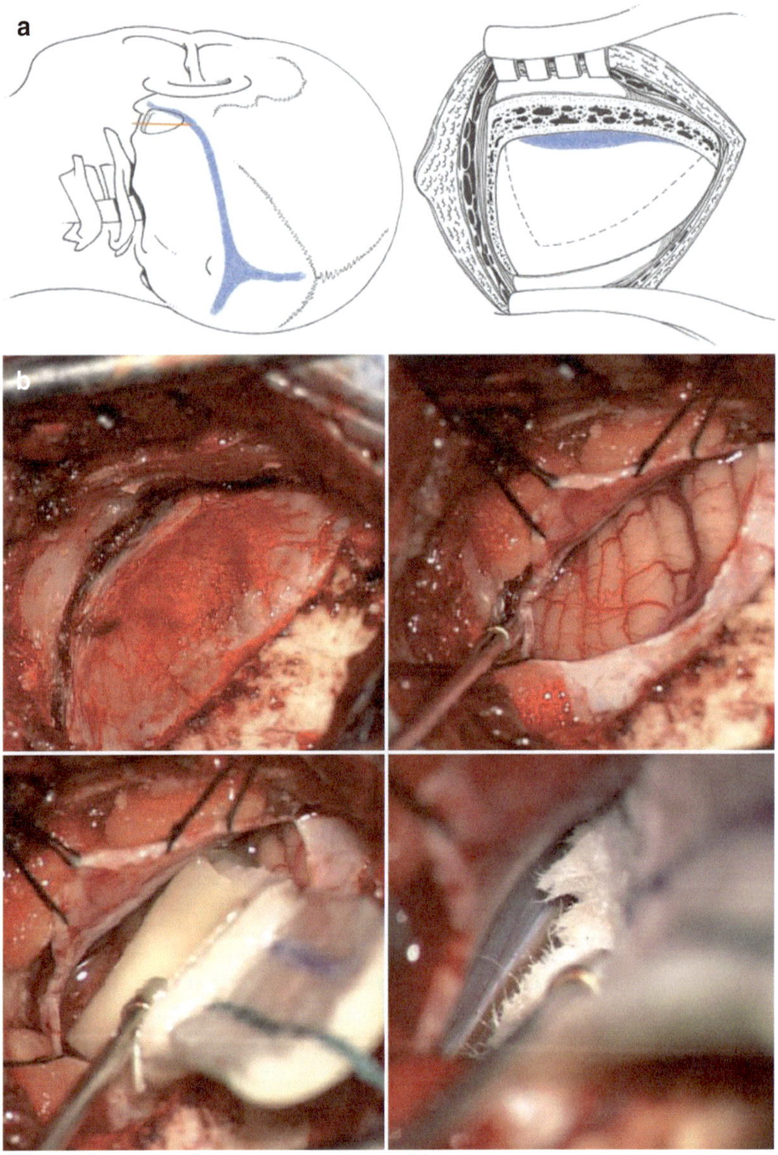

Fig. 7.3 (**a**) Left retromastoid craniectomy. A linear skin incision provides adequate exposure for a bony opening that extends to the sigmoid sinus laterally and the posterior fossa floor inferiorly. Soft tissue is held with a self-retaining retractor and bony opening completed. Importantly, the planned dural flap provides maximal anterior and inferior access. (**b**) Surgical microscope images of the approach through a left retromastoid craniectomy. Mastoid bone edges have been sealed with wax, and the sigmoid sinus edge is visible laterally (upper left). The dura has been opened in a curved fashion with an anterior flap reflected over moistened Gelfoam; a retraction stitch is placed inferiorly (upper right). The cerebellum is gently depressed with a folded "slider" fashioned with a sheet of latex beneath a 0.5 × 3–inch cottonoid (lower left). The slider has been unfolded and advanced beneath the cerebellum parallel to the posterior fossa floor (lower right). This corridor will provide access to the deep arachnoid cistern required for the procedure. Reproduced from Kaufmann AM, Sabit B. Microvascular decompression surgery for glossopharyngeal neuralgia. In: Li ST, Zhong J, Sekula RF Jr., eds. Microvascular Decompression Surgery. Springer Nature; 2016:103–122, with permission from Springer Nature Customer Service Centre GmbH (https://link-springer-com.uml.idm.oclc.org/chapter/10.1007/978-94-017-7366-9_9)

cranial nerves. A bridging vein may be encountered, entering dura in proximity to the ascending accessory nerve and should be handled with care, either by precise coagulation or sufficient mobilization through arachnoid dissection. On occasion, a rhomboid cyst may be encountered, sometimes misidentified as "thickened arachnoid" overlying these rootlets. Careful dissection of the tissue layers will achieve full mobilization of the cerebellum. Next, a subfloccular approach to the proximal vestibulocochlear and facial nerves is taken. This anterior-inferior approach is directed toward the facial nerve REZ. This is preferable to a more direct lateral approach that misdirects attention to the cisternal and meatal portions of the facial nerve and places unnecessary retraction stress upon the deliciated vestibulocochlear nerve (note its TZ is within the internal auditory canal).

Once access to the facial nerve REZ is obtained, attention is given to identifying and remedying the NVC. Since even light contact on centrally myelinated fibers by cerebellar arteries can result in HFS, it is paramount that all vascular contact is alleviated through vessel mobilization. The surgeon must also not be distracted by a close association of the anterior inferior cerebellar artery and the cisternal portion of the facial nerve. This common finding is rarely the cause of HFS (only 1–4% of the time) and is readily apparent when the cisternal facial nerve course is distorted by a compressing vessel [9].

Once all culprit vessels are identified, careful mobilization of the vessel away from the REZ should be performed. Transposition of the vessel is always favored over simple separation with an implant. This is best achieved through liberation of the vessel from its arachnoid tethers beginning away from the point of maximal compression. Special attention must be directed to identification and preservation of all the fine brainstem perforating vessels arising from the cerebellar arteries. These perforators arisng from the anterior-inferior cerebellar artery, coursing to pontine areas, may be quite short and limit culprit vessel mobilization. Conversely, when facial REZ compression is related to an elongated posterior-inferior cerebellar artery, the associated perforating vessels destined to the medulla are long. This will facilitate culprit mobilization, while care to avoid vessel kinking or stretching is always of paramont importance.

Shredded Teflon is the most used implant as only rarely does it cause any consequential reaction [11]. The implant should ideally be used to maintain the vessel in its new transposed position away from the nerve root without touching it and not simply interposing the implant between the nerve and vessel (Fig. 7.4). Whenever possible, Teflon placed upon the brainstem should "bridge" the facial REZ and avoid contact [12, 13]. In rare cases, slings of various forms can be attached to petrous dura and can aid in maintaining the vessels position away from the REZ (Fig. 7.5) [14].

A surgical adjunct in MVD for HFS is endoscopy to gain a fuller view of the facial REZ. Recently, entirely endoscopic MVD for HFS has been described [15]. A full description of this method is beyond the scope of this chapter; however, the interested reader is directed to various articles on the subject, found in the literature [16–18]. Endoscopy is, however, generally not necessary nor superior to the microsurgical view afforded through the described retrosigmoid approach.

Watertight closure is obtained to minimize complications related to CSF leak and infection. Dura is closed primary, which should be possible if the dura has remained moist throughout the case. Mastoid air cells are again checked for a wax seal. A large burr hole cover, hydroxyapatite, or acrylic can be used to reconstruct the craniectomy, and the soft tissues are meticulously closed in layers. Finally antibacterial ointment can be applied to the incision site [3].

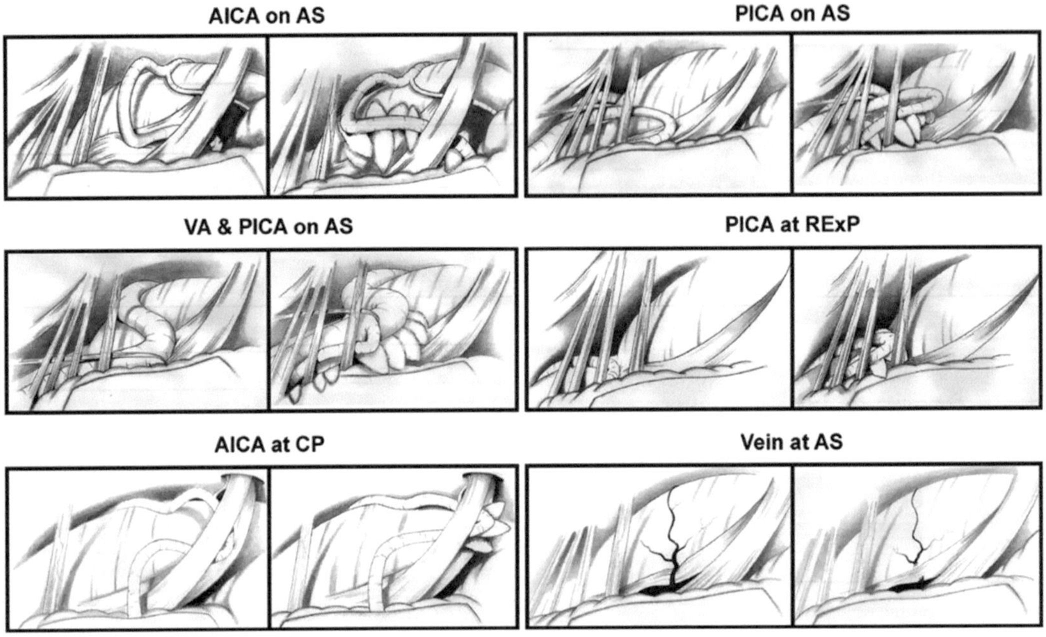

Fig. 7.4 Neurovascular compression in hemifacial spasm is usually related to the cerebellar arteries or ectatic vertebral artery impinging on the root entry zone (REZ) of the facial nerve. Multiple vessel contacts are not uncommon and should all be alleviated. The most prominent vessel contact is usually an arterial loop tightly apposed against the REZ. Important, vessel mobilization is initiated away from the point of maximal compression. This is facilitated best through wide arachnoid dissection. A series of shredded Teflon felt implants are sequentially placed to maintain the apex of the vessel loop in a new orientation, rather than to simply provide a cushion. *AICA* anterior inferior cerebellar artery, *CP* cisternal portion, *PICA* posterior inferior cerebellar artery, *VA* vertebral artery. (Reproduced from Campos-Benitez and Kaufmann. J Neurosurg. 2008;109(9):416–420)

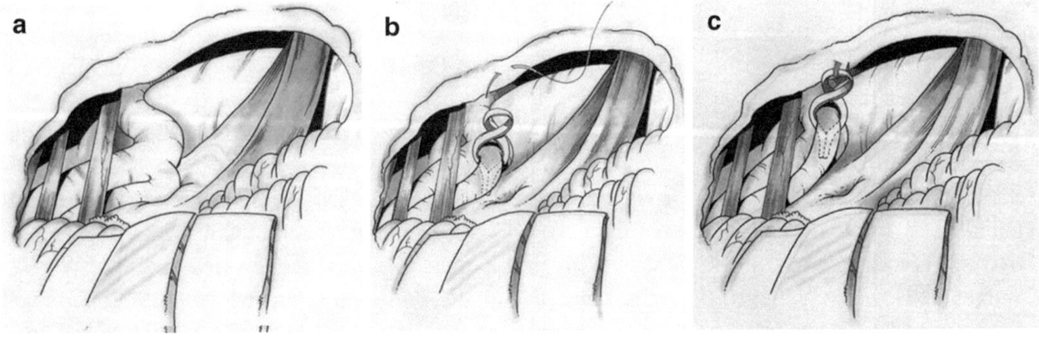

Fig. 7.5 (**a**) Significant facial nerve compression is caused by the posterior inferior cerebellar artery (PICA) originating from the ectatic vertebral artery, upon the attached segment (AS) of the root entry zone (REZ) of the facial nerve. (**b**) A fenestrated aneurysm clip is applied around the culprit PICA, and the suture is passed through the petrous dura. (**c**) Neurovascular coupling is alleviated with a clip sling secured to the dura. (Figure and legend reproduced from Attabib and Kaufmann. J Neurosurg. 2007;106(5):929–931)

7.4 Identifying Treatment Failure

Following MVD, spasms relief can take a variable course. Approximately a third of patients will have immediate spasm cessation. However, for the remaining two-thirds of patients, spasms may only resolve over the course of weeks, months, or rarely even beyond a year [19]. This delayed course may be attributable to reorganization of central neuronal hyperactivity that occurs following resolution of NVC. Conversely, immediate spasm resolution may be attributable to inadvertent traumatic manipulation of the nerve. As a result of this variability, early reoperation is rarely warranted, and procedural failure may not be readily apparent. Long-term follow-up is also crucial to determine success rates and treatment durability.

7.5 Conclusion

MVD is a safe, effective, and durable treatment for HFS and should be considered the gold-standard in the management of this debilitating condition [1]. High volume centers report achieving excellent procedural success rates. Paramount to this is an understanding of the surgical target and careful attention to the microsurgical approach that is focused on transposition of the vessel compressing the facial nerve REZ. In conjunction with adequate patient selection and complication avoidance, these principles can help avoid failure in MVD for HFS.

References

1. Kaufmann AM. Hemifacial spasm: a neurosurgical perspective. J Neurosurg. 2023;140:1–8.
2. Kaufmann AM, Price AV. A history of the Jannetta procedure. J Neurosurg. 2020;132:639–46.
3. Kaufmann AM, Wilkinson MF, Schmidek HH, Roberts DW. Microvascular decompression surgery for hemifacial spasm. Amsterdam: Elsevier; 2005. p. 1490.
4. Holste K, Sahyouni R, Teton Z, Chan AY, Englot DJ, Rolston JD. Spasm freedom following microvascular decompression for hemifacial spasm: systematic review and meta-analysis. World Neurosurg. 2020;139:e383–90.
5. Miller LE, Miller VM. Safety and effectiveness of microvascular decompression for treatment of hemifacial spasm: a systematic review. Br J Neurosurg. 2012;26:438–44.
6. Mizobuchi Y, Nagahiro S, Kondo A. Prospective, multicenter clinical study of microvascular decompression for hemifacial spasm. Neurosurgery. 2021;88:846–54.
7. Chaudhry N, Srivastava A, Joshi L. Hemifacial spasm: the past, present and future. J Neurol Sci. 2015;356:27–31.
8. Rosenstengel C, Matthes M, Baldauf J, Fleck S, Schroeder H. Hemifacial spasm: conservative and surgical treatment options. Dtsch Arztebl Int. 2012;109:667–73.
9. Campos-Benitez M, Kaufmann AM. Neurovascular compression findings in hemifacial spasm. J Neurosurg. 2008;109:416–20.
10. Bigder MG, Kaufmann AM. Failed microvascular decompression surgery for hemifacial spasm due to persistent neurovascular compression: an analysis of reoperations. J Neurosurg. 2016;124:90–5.
11. Bigder M, Matsuda K, Kaufmann A. Necrotizing Teflon granuloma after microvascular decompression and gamma knife. Can J Neurol Sci. 2017;44:757–8.
12. Liu JK, Shafiq A. Teflon bridge technique for endoscopic-assisted microvascular decompression of ectatic basilar artery and anterior inferior cerebellar artery for trigeminal neuralgia: operative video and technical nuances. Neurosurg Focus Video. 2020;3:V5.
13. Inoue T, Shitara S, Goto Y, Arham A, Prasetya M, Radcliffe L, Fukushima T. Bridge technique for hemifacial spasm with vertebral artery involvement. Acta Neurochir. 2021;163:3311–20.
14. Attabib N, Kaufmann AM. Use of fenestrated aneurysm clips in microvascular decompression surgery. Technical note and case series. J Neurosurg. 2007;106:929–31.
15. Zagzoog N, Attar A, Takroni R, Alotaibi MB, Reddy K. Endoscopic versus open microvascular decompression for trigeminal neuralgia: a systematic review and comparative meta-analysis. J Neurosurg. 2018;45:1–9.
16. Lang S-S, Chen HI, Lee JYK. Endoscopic microvascular decompression: a stepwise operative technique. ORL J Otorhinolaryngol Relat Spec. 2012;74:293–8.
17. Halpern CH, Lang S-S, Lee JYK. Fully endoscopic microvascular decompression: our early experience. Minim Invasive Surg. 2013;2013:1–5.
18. Flanders TM, Blue R, Roberts S. Fully endoscopic microvascular decompression for hemifacial spasm. J Neurosurg. 2018;131:813–9.
19. Lee JA, Kong DS, Lee S, Park SK, Park K. Chronological patterns of long-term outcomes after microvascular decompression for hemifacial spasm over 5 years. World Neurosurg. 2022;166:e313–8.

8 Teflon-Free MVD for Trigeminal Neuralgia: Advancing a Logical Technique

Devi P. Patra, Evelyn L. Turcotte, Kliment Donev, and Richard S. Zimmerman

8.1 Introduction

Often described as one of the most extremely agonizing conditions in human history, trigeminal neuralgia (TN) is a chronic pain syndrome characterized by sharp paroxysmal lancinating pain involving the face in the trigeminal nerve distribution. Despite the severity and gruesome nature of the disease, formal management guidelines lack a balanced view of medical and surgical options. Medical management is often considered as the primary treatment option, but the rate of significant side effects is not negligible [1, 2]. Surgical treatment in the form of microvascular decompression has been consistently shown to be effective in the majority of the patients, although recurrence of pain does occur. While following the general objective of "decompression" described by Jannetta using Teflon, refinement of surgical techniques have been developed to address both improved outcomes and address some of the limitations using Teflon. In this chapter we present the evolution of surgical procedures for TN, the rationale for further change, and illustrate our experience with the Teflon-Free MVD technique.

8.2 Historical Perspective and Early Operative Procedures

Although the initial description of TN dates back to four centuries ago, it took about another two centuries to establish the relationship of the pain to trigeminal nerve and another century to develop a surgical strategy to treat. Nevertheless, it is only in the last few decades the true form of microvascular decompression technique was described.

8.2.1 Gasserian Ganglionectomy

Most of the initial surgical procedures for TN focussed on the gasserian ganglion instead of the cisternal segment of the trigeminal nerve itself. In the Hartley-Krause appraoch described in 1892, the ganglion was accessed through an extradural, subtemporal approach, and the nerves

Supplementary Information The online version contains supplementary material available at https://doi.org/10.1007/978-981-96-0767-9_8.

D. P. Patra · R. S. Zimmerman (✉)
Department of Neurosurgery, Mayo Clinic, Phoenix, AZ, USA
e-mail: zimmerman.richard@mayo.edu

E. L. Turcotte
Mayo Clinic Alix School of Medicine, Mayo Clinic, Phoenix, AZ, USA

K. Donev
Department of Laboratory Medicine and Pathology, Mayo Clinic, Phoenix, AZ, USA

S.-T. Li et al. (eds.), *Microvascular Decompression Surgery*,
https://doi.org/10.1007/978-981-96-0767-9_8

were divided at their exit through the skull base foramina, and the ganglion was excised proximally up to the entrance of Meckle's cave [3]. This technique was further modified to include only the V2 and V3 branches to reduce the chance of corneal ulceration [4]. This selective sectioning of the nerve also called as Spiller-Frazier procedure proved to be effective and remained the preferred treatment for TN for about half a decade. Unfortunately, this procedure had a significantly higher risk of facial palsy. Nevertheless, this was pretty much accepted by the surgeons as well as the patients considering the morbidity associated with facial pain itself.

8.2.2 Trigeminal Nerve Sectioning

Walter Dandy, having performed several of dorsal gasserian rhizotomies, was unsatisfied with the results of the procedure due to high rate of facial palsy and facial anesthesia. He recognized the cause to be the undue traction of the geniculate ganglion from the greater superficial petrosal nerve during extradural exposure of the trigeminal nerve. Therefore, in the early 1920s, he developed a suboccipital retrosigmoid approach from the posterior fossa to exposure the cisternal segment of the trigeminal nerve. Not surprising enough, the procedure was relatively blood less with significantly lower risk of facial paralysis. Most importantly, with selective sectioning of the nerve he demonstrated preservation of the sensation to touch that particularly lessened the incidence of corneal anesthesia and also preservation of motor function of the trigeminal nerve.

8.2.3 Early Theory of Vascular Compression

In his early publication in 1929, Walter Dandy reported the results of his procedure in 88 patients where he mentioned regarding his observation of vascular loop compressing on the trigeminal nerve although he did not bring any inference from this observation [5]. However, in 1932, in his subsequent publication of 250 consecutive patients, he found a significant percentage of patients (in about 60%) having some sort of vascular compression including SCA loops or petrosal veins [4]. He also reported that he frequently observed the distortion of the nerve by the compression of this vascular loops and believed that this compression is the cause of the tic douloureux. However, his theory did not gain much traction with a majority of the surgeons around the world practicing the Frazier's approach. However, in early 1950s, Palle Taarnhoj from Denmark and then James Gardner from Clevaland Clinic, USA, used a combined extradural approach of Frazier and posterior fossa approach of Dandy to expose the dural sheath of the trigeminal nerve and brush the nerve with cotton pledget [6, 7]. Gardner was one of the earliest surgeon to believe demyelination of the nerve to be the cause of TN, which can occur due to "a prolonged period of the gentle compression" by vascular loops, tumors, aneurysms, etc.

8.3 Legacy of Peter Jennetta and Microvascular Decompression

Despite early recognition of vascular compression as the cause of the TN, this theory did not get popularized for decades until the development of microscopic surgery. Peter Jennetta was one of the early advocates of using microscope in neurosurgical procedures and through his experiments in the laboratory, he could expose the trigeminal nerve through retrosigmoid approach. Although, in the initial years he performed mainly nerve sectioning, he later became more convinced regarding the vascular compression theory and gradually moved towards isolated vascular decompression without nerve sectioning. In his first case with Robert Rand in 1966, the SCA loop was mobilized and was kept separated from the nerve using a small piece of Ivalon sponge. Subsequently, he chose Teflon that was easy to manipulate and produced minimal arachnoid scarring. Excellent visualization of the artery with the use of microscope and atraumatic mobilization with the use of arachnoid dissection was the key for his success.

Unfortunately, Jennetta's theory of vascular compression and microvascular decompression to alleviate the offending cause was looked at with skepticism by many of the prominent neurosurgeons at that time and therefore was not easily accepted by the neurosurgical community. After three decades of his initial MVD, Jennetta published his landmark paper in 1996 on a series of 1185 patients using his technique where he demonstrated success rate with complete pain relief in 82% of the patients and partial relief in 16% of the patients [8]. The long-term effect was also substantial, with about 68% of patients having excellent to good pain relief at 10 years of follow-up. Subsequently, this technique of microvascular decompression was extended to other similar pathologies including hemifacial spasm and glossopharyngeal neuralgia with excellent results. Over the years, microvascular decompression using Teflon became the standard open surgical treatment for trigeminal neuralgia.

8.4 Current Knowledge of Efficacy of Microvascular Decompression

Microvascular decompression has evolved as the most effective and durable intervention for drug-resistant TN [9]. Most notably, MVD provides immediate pain relief in most of the patients when compared to other intervention measures. The rate of acute pain relief immediately after the procedure has been reported to be ranging from 85% to 96.6% [10–12]. Similarly, the rate of acute pain relief in patients even with multiple sclerosis can be as high as 97% [13]. Carlo et al. performed a systematic review and meta-analysis on nine studies including 2102 patients and found immediate postoperative complete pain relief rate of 82.9% with surgical failure rate of 2.6% [14]. In another systematic review, Holste et al., analyzed 46 studies including 3897 patients undergoing MVD and found a overall 76% patients experiencing pain freedom over a follow-up of 1.7 ± 1.3 years [15]. The long-term effect of MVD is still promising as evidenced by multiple studies. Chen et al. reported a recurrence rate of 9.6%, while a slightly higher recurrence rate of 14.9% was noted by Mendelson et al. over a follow-up of 23 to 300 months [11, 16]. There are few available studies reporting long-term results after MVD showing about 64–74% complete pain relief at 10 years [8, 10]. Finally, in an umbrella review of meta-analyses and systematic reviews, Rapisarda and colleagues provide an overview comparing outcomes of surgical treatments for medically refractory trigeminal neuralgia. They consistently found MVD outcomes were superior and more durable than any of the percutaneous rhizotomies (glycerol, balloon compression, or radio frequency), stereotactic radiosurgery, or Gamma Knife treatment [9].

8.5 Recurrent Trigeminal Neuralgia and Teflon Granuloma

While the results of microvascular decompression are extremely satisfying for several years, overtime a significant number of patients develop recurrences. There are several factors that have been attributed to the recurrence of pain including longer duration of symptoms, multiple vessels, vertebrobasilar compressions, and atypical pain syndromes. Additionally, several other factors that are likely related to the surgery have also been frequently described including incomplete decompression, arachnoid scarring, and Teflon granuloma [17, 18]. After a remarkable discovery and success story from Jennetta's procedure, nearly all neurosurgeons adapted his Teflon interposition method. In the neurosurgical community, Teflon has long been thought to be an ideal inert material that produces minimal reaction, little tissue resorption, dislocation, and overall complication. However the true effects of Teflon are now being recognized as more patients are undergoing re-exploration after recurrence or initial failure.

This appears to be a repetition of the experiences elsewhere in the medical field. In

Orthopedics, Teflon was initially thought to be an ideal substance for hip replacement prostheses. However, the initial experiences had shown that tissue erosion and granuloma formation occurred and caused significant complications, with the discovery that the "inert" nature of Teflon did not hold true in this application [19]. In fact, Charnley had written a letter to the editor of the Journal of Bone and Joint Surgery stating, "I abandoned Teflon in November 1962. because of serious tissue reactions" [20].

The field of oral surgery also explored the utilization of a Teflon implant for a prosthetic replacement of the temporal-mandibular joint. Yet again, the outcome was dismal in that tissue erosion and destruction occurred with significant complications leading a complete abandonment of the technique [21].

At the gross structural level these surgical implants had mechanical forces which are quite different with dramatic weight and load bearing applications distinct from the use of Teflon pledgets in MVD. However the common finding at the histologic/microscopic (and subsequently gross anatomical level) was that Teflon elicited an inflammatory reaction leading to foreign body giant cell granuloma formation. This development is the same in response to the presence of solid Teflon particles, or Teflon fibers as seen in specimens of Teflon felt explanted in cases of recurrent TN (Fig. 8.1).

Teflon itself has been shown to produce scarring around vessels and nerves, and can produce distortion of the nerve. Teflon granuloma as a distinct entity is not frequently suspected in clinical practice. However, the foreign body reaction to Teflon can produce a tumor like mass with associated inflammation. Imaging with computed tomography (CT) and magnetic resonance imaging (MRI) shows a mass with heterogenous signal with irregular enhancement along the nerve. What exactly produces inflammatory reaction to Teflon in some patients is unclear. However, it has been postulated that contact with the tentorium and dura over time attracts blood supply to the mass inciting inflammation to the foreign body [17, 22]. Additional theories exist including scarring from contact of Teflon to brain stem as described by Premsagar et al [23]; On the other hand, Matsushima et al. thought that the contact with the nerve itself produces the fibrotic reaction [24]. Nevertheless, the common denominator is the development of chronic inflammation from Teflon producing a lesion that either compresses or irritates the nerve producing recurrent symptoms. This is evidenced by the histopathological findings of chronic inflammatory cells and giant cells surrounding the Teflon in the form of a granuloma formation. The reported rate of Teflon granuloma ranges from 1.1% to 7.3% in various studies although there are significant reporting bias therefore, the true incidence is unknown [17, 22–24]. However, Teflon granuloma has been observed in about 18–50% of the patients who were re-explored for recurrent pain after initial MVD [17, 22, 25]. In one study, Teflon granuloma was responsible in 71.4% of the patients for recurrence of pain [18]. Despite these observations, Teflon granuloma as a possible cause of recurrent TN is largely unrecognized. Many surgeons still practicing the Teflon interposition method swear on the inertness and benign nature of Teflon on tissues and continue to report good results. We now send all specimens of Teflon removed during repeat surgery for recurrent trigeminal neuralgia, and have found 100% contain reactive changes and granuloma formation. In more severe cases, turbid fluid (sterile purulence)

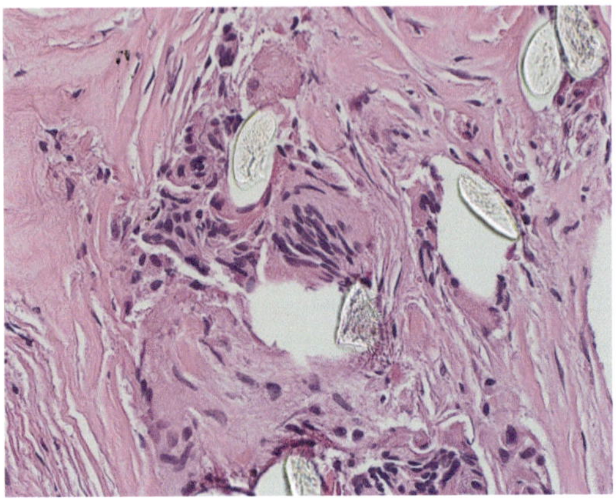

Fig. 8.1 Teflon granuloma removed from a patient after prior MVD demonstrating reactive changes and inflammatory cells including multinucleated giant cells (MGC) surrounding Teflon fibers

is seen during surgery (Video 8.1—granuloma with purulence). The technique necessary for Teflon removal requires a thoughtful surgical approach (Video 8.2—Teflon granuloma removal).

8.6 Need for Alternative Techniques

Although the role of microvascular decompression as an effective method of pain relief in TN is somewhat well established, there is rising controversy whether Teflon interposition is the most appropriate technique to achieve decompression. Arachnoid dissection and mobilization of the artery away from the nerve is the fundamental principle of microvascular decompression; however, there is a natural tendency of the artery to revert back to its original position, therefore additional technique is required to keep it separated from the nerve. The original method described by Jennetta is to interpose a Teflon pledget between the artery and the nerve, but considering the mechanical effects of the Teflon itself, and additional long-term complications, the alternative method is to transpose the artery to a different location and to secure it with a method that is durable, non-occlusive to the artery, and relatively atraumatic. Several alternative techniques have been described in the literature as summarized below,

8.7 Teflon-Free Decompression Techniques

8.7.1 Tentorial Sling

Melvill and Baxter reported their series of seven patients in 1995 where he described a tentorial sling technique to hold the SCA against the tentorium [26]. The sling is prepared with two parallel incisions along the tentorium and between the layers of tentorium, away from the superior petrosal sinus. That way a flap was created measuring about 15 mm in length and 3–4 mm in width. The medial end was kept attached to the tentorium and the lateral end was freed and passed below the SCA to bring the SCA loop superomedially and this way a sling was created. The sling was secured to the tentorium using a hemoclip. In this series they did not report any complications and six out of seven patients had complete pain relief although the follow-up duration was not reported. The tentorial sling technique has also been recently described by Steinberg et al. where they reported 45 patients using similar technique. At the last follow-up (2–36 months), 73% of patients remained pain free [27]. The complication rate was 6.6% although only one patient had neurologic complication with stroke in the SCA territory.

8.7.2 Sling/Suture Retraction

Masuoka et al., described a stitched sling retraction technique to mobilize the artery and transpose it to the tentorium [28, 29]. In this technique a 5–0 thread is placed on the central portion of the tentorium and is passed around the SCA and knotted to make a sling and transpose it superomedially, ensuring that the vessel is not kinked. It is important to avoid the medial boarder of the tentorium which often has vessels and nerves underneath. In case of compression from AICA, the stitch is placed on the petrous dura to transpose the artery inferolaterally. The important limitations of this technique are short perforators from SCA, vertebrobasilar compressions, etc. In a series of 50 patients, Masuoka et al. reported complete pain relief in 88% of patients at 1 year and 83% at 5 years [28]. In terms of neurological complications, 3 patients were reported to have transient cerebellar dysfunction from venous infarction. In another series of 12 patients using similar technique with a 2–0 silk suture, Meybodi et al. reported complete pain relief in all patients over a 24–38 months follow-up period with no incidence of complications [30]. A similar technique was described by Mitsos et al. which they described as "hanging technique" where they used autologous occipital fascia as the sling to "hang" the vessel to the tentorium using sutures [31]. In their report of four patients, all had complete pain relief over a follow-up period of 6–24 months with no complications. As acknowledged by the authors, this technique requires significant working room to manipulate instruments therefore needs a good brain relaxation or cerebellar retraction. Several other allograft materials including cord shaped Teflon felt, tape shaped Gore-Tex and expanded Polytetrafluoroethylene (ePTFE) have also been used as a sling for the vessel transposition. Kato et al. described 13 patients undergoing microvascular decompression using ion beam implanted ePTFE, which is produced by focussing a radiating ion beam at the surface of ePTFE to improve bondability to the tentorial surface when used with fibrin glue [32].

8.7.3 Fenestrated Clip

Instead of sutures and slings, fenestrated aneurysm clips have also been used to hold the SCA and other vessel to the tentorium. In this case a small rent in the tentorium is made to allow a lip of tissue to hold between the clip blades where the vessel is taken within the clip fenestration. We have published our experience on use of fenestrated clips in few cases with good results [33–35]. Similarly, Kauffman et al. have reported their experience on 2 cases of trigeminal neuralgia and 6 patients of hemifacial spasm with good clinical results without complications [36]. Use of fenestrated clips obviates the need of suture placement in a narrow filed; however, it is important to recognize the aneurysm clip itself can twist and compress on the nerve if sufficient care is not taken to properly orient the clip during placement.

8.7.4 Tissue Sealant

Tissue sealants like TachoSil (CSL Behring K.K) are surgical patches with a white collagen sponge coated with fibrinogen and thrombin on one side that are used for hemostasis and to seal the dural surface to prevent CSF leak. A "Double stick tape" technique was described by Ichikawa et al. where two pieces of collagen fleece were adhered using fibrin glue on the nonadhesive side to form a double sticky tape that was used to transpose vertebral artery to petrous bone in a patient with hemifacial spasm [37]. A modified technique was described by Otani et al. where a sponge of TachoSil sheet was trimmed and soaked with fibrin glue using fingers to make a bead similar to birdlime [38]. The bead is then placed on the tentorium at the attachment site and the vessel is adhered to the TachoSil bead using microfine forceps for 3 minutes. In 19 patients with hemifacial spasm and 8 patients with TN, stable adhesion with remission of symptoms was achieved in all patients.

8.8 Author's Preferred Technique—Teflon-Free MVD

Considering the persistent mass effect from Teflon interposition method and its long-term complications, the senior author (RZ) is a strong advocate for Teflon-free transposition technique. Although using sling, sutures, surgical clips are promising techniques, we believe that these techniques require significant maneuvering of surgical instruments in a deep and narrow surgical corridor. This requires a generous brain relaxation and therefore challenging in patients with relatively narrow cerebellopontine angle. Additionally cerebellar retraction may result in postoperative edema and resultant neurological deficit. In this regard, we prefer surgical glue to transpose the vessels to the tentorium. Fibrin glue has been shown as a strong and reliable tissue sealant and been used for dural repair and hemostasis. Instead of commercially available fibrin sealants, we prefer the use of thrombin and cryoprecipitate, which when used in combination produces a natural hemostatic coagulum that is reliable, strong, and durable. Additionally, this is readily available in hospital settings and more economical than commercial glues. Finally, as a biological product, the "fibrin glue" is slowly dissolved and broken down, yet is replaced by the patient's own newly formed arachnoid scar and adhesions. Thus, the patient's own healing tissue provides the long-term regenerative solution to maintain vascular transposition.

In our standard technique, position the patient in lateral park bench position resting on a beanbag and gel pad with an axillary roll supporting the chest wall. The head is gently flexed, slightly rotated to the side of surgery, and tilted away from the side of surgery. The OR table is placed in mild reverse Trendelenburg during surgery to help with brain relaxation. Using a straight incision two fingerbreadth behind the ear, a standard retrosigmoid suboccipital craniectomy is made exposing the transverse and sigmoid sinuses at the superior and lateral borders of craniectomy. The dura is opened in a lazy-T-shaped incision reflecting the two leaflets of the dura based on transverse and sigmoid sinuses to expose the petrotentorial junction. Reverse Trendelenburg position, use of hypertonic saline, mannitol, and CSF release allow significant brain relaxation obviating the need of any fixed cerebellar retraction. Initial division of arachnoid bands along the tentorial surface of the cerebellum and along the 7–8 CN complex allows medial mobilization of the cerebellum to expose the trigeminal nerve along its entirety with good visualization of the root entry zone. We coagulate and divide a branch, or the entire superior petrosal vein as needed to improve visualization. A careful and generous arachnoid dissection is performed to isolate and separate the vascular conflict from the trigeminal nerve. We usually continue the dissection all along the visualized segment of the artery distally up to and beyond the bifurcation to allow complete mobilization. Careful observation of the perforators to the brainstem is required during mobilization. After satisfactory mobilization of the artery, a thorough inspection around the root entry zone and along the ventral aspect of the nerve is made to rule out any additional vascular contact. Subsequently, the vascular loop is transposed to the tentorial surface and held against using an instrument (either suction or fine dissector). Then cryoprecipitate and thrombin are applied drop by drop in alternate fashion over the artery and along the contacting surface of the tentorium to form a stable coagulum. After allowing some time to stabilize the coagulum, rapid jet of irrigation is applied over the artery to confirm stability and strong adherence to the tentorial surface. Once hemostasis is confirmed, duroplasty using grafts and a cranioplasty is performed in standard fashion. Recently the senior author (RZ) has published his 17-year experience on Teflon-free microvascular transposition on 102 patients with 1-year, 5-year, and 10-year pain-free estimates of 94.1%, 94.1%, and 83.0% [39]. These findings further support the use of Teflon-free technique using fibrin glue to permanently maintain the transposition away from the vessel with a significantly higher rate of long-term pain relief. This reproducible and standardized procedure for a Teflon-free MVD is demonstrated in 6 cases in this compilation (Video 8.3—Teflon-free MVD compliation). The robust nature of fibrin glue as an intraoperative adhesive is tested in all cases (Video 8.4—Irrigation after application of fibrin glue). Finally, the use of fibrin glue to secure vessel transposition is also useful as an adjunct for surgical exposure. Video 8.5 demonstrates how this technique provides an additional option to gain access to the trigeminal nerve as well as transposing a long vessel loop.

8.9 Conclusion

The contribution of Dr. Jannetta to those who suffer from trigeminal neuralgia is immeasurable. Not only has he championed the procedure that provides relief for so many patients, he has educated countless neurosurgeons and other physicians about this unusual condition. His initial technique has been proven to work very well; however, there are clearly failures, recurrences, and complications. It is also more likely than not that we have underestimated the recurrence rates for MVD. As we strive to improve the care for patients and our surgical outcomes, we must consider all opportunities to incrementally do better. While Teflon has been the initial substrate chosen by Dr. Jannetta for MVD, there is an undeniable amount of medical literature that substantiates the potential for Teflon related problems. The desire to innovate and achieve even relatively small gains are our mandate whenever possible. A case in point is the dramatic efforts put forth to reduce or eliminate surgical site infections, even though the magnitude of improvement may be small. Looking from the opposite perspective, our failures or recurrences have significant morbidity for those affected. If we are to maximize the potential good we offer patients, we should try to eliminate any potential for recurrences of trigeminal neuralgia. The literature clearly identifies the association between implanted Teflon and the potential for granuloma formation and recurrence of pain. In summary, the logical step in the evolution of MVD would be to consider methods that avoid the use of Teflon, such as the Teflon-free MVD technique or others as described above.

References

1. Gronseth G, Cruccu G, Alksne J, et al. Practice parameter: the diagnostic evaluation and treatment of trigeminal neuralgia (an evidence-based review): report of the quality standards Subcommittee of the American Academy of neurology and the European Federation of Neurological Societies. Neurology. 2008;71(15):1183–90. https://doi.org/10.1212/01.wnl.0000326598.83183.04.
2. Maarbjerg S, Di Stefano G, Bendtsen L, Cruccu G. Trigeminal neuralgia—diagnosis and treatment. Cephalalgia. 2017;37(7):648–57. https://doi.org/10.1177/0333102416687280.
3. Patel SK, Liu JK. Overview and history of trigeminal neuralgia. Neurosurg Clin N Am. 2016;27(3):265–76. https://doi.org/10.1016/j.nec.2016.02.002.
4. Shelton ML. Working in a very small place: the making of a neurosurgeon. Vintage; 1990.
5. Dandy WE. An operation for the cure of tic douloureux: partial section of the sensory root at the pons. Arch Surg. 1929;18(2):687–734.
6. Taarnhøj P. Decompression of the trigeminal root. J Neurosurg. 1954;11(3):299–305.
7. Gardner WJ, Pinto JP. The tarrnhoj operation; relief of trigeminal neuralgia without numbness. Cleve Clin Q. 1953;20(2):364–7.
8. Barker FG, Jannetta PJ, Bissonette DJ, Larkins MV, Jho HD. The long-term outcome of microvascular decompression for trigeminal neuralgia. N Engl J Med. 1996;334(17):1077–84.
9. Rapisarda A, Battistelli M, Izzo A, et al. Outcome comparison of drug-resistant trigeminal neuralgia surgical treatments—an umbrella review of meta-analyses and systematic reviews. Brain Sci. 2023;13(4):530.
10. Diana C, Kumar RD, Bodh R, Kumari S. Does the surgical intervention for trigeminal neuralgia refractory to pharmacotherapy improve quality-of-life?–a systematic review. J Oral Maxillofac Surg. 2021;79(11):2227–39.
11. Mendelson ZS, Velagala JR, Kohli G, Heir GM, Mammis A, Liu JK. Pain-free outcomes and durability of surgical intervention for trigeminal neuralgia: a comparison of gamma knife and microvascular decompression. World Neurosurg. 2018;112:e732–46.
12. Sharma R, Phalak M, Katiyar V, Borkar S, Kale SS, Mahapatra AK. Microvascular decompression versus stereotactic radiosurgery as primary treatment modality for trigeminal neuralgia: a systematic review and meta-analysis of prospective comparative trials. Neurol India. 2018;66(3):688.
13. Nascimento RFV, Pipek LZ, de Aguiar PHP. Is percutaneous balloon compression better than microvascular decompression to treat trigeminal neuralgia? A systematic review and meta-analysis. J Clin Neurosci. 2023;109:11–20.
14. Di Carlo DT, Benedetto N, Perrini P. Clinical outcome after microvascular decompression for trigeminal neuralgia: a systematic review and meta-analysis. Neurosurg Rev. 2022;46(1):8.
15. Holste K, Chan AY, Rolston JD, Englot DJ. Pain outcomes following microvascular decompression for drug-resistant trigeminal neuralgia: a systematic review and meta-analysis. Neurosurgery. 2020;86(2):182–90. https://doi.org/10.1093/neuros/nyz075.
16. Chen F, Niu Y, Meng F, et al. Recurrence rates after microvascular decompression in patients with primary trigeminal neuralgia and its influencing factors: a systematic review and meta-analysis based on 8,172 surgery patients. Front Neurol. 2021;12:738032. https://doi.org/10.3389/fneur.2021.738032.
17. Capelle H-H, Brandis A, Tschan CA, Krauss JK. Treatment of recurrent trigeminal neuralgia due to Teflon granuloma. J Headache Pain. 2010;11(4):339–44.
18. Sun T, Wang W, Huang Q, et al. Teflon granuloma: a common cause of recurrent trigeminal neuralgia. World Neurosurg. 2022;158:e612–7.
19. Gheorghiu D, Peter V, Lynch M. Living history in current orthopaedic hip surgery: intrapelvic teflon granuloma after total hip replacement. Acta Orthop Belg. 2010;76(1):129–31.
20. Charnley J. Using Teflon in arthroplasty of the hip-joint. J Bone Joint Surg Am. 1966;48(4):819.
21. Chuong R, Piper MA, Boland TJ. Recurrent giant cell reaction to residual proplast in the temporomandibular joint. Oral Surg Oral Med Oral Pathol. 1993;76(1):16–9. https://doi.org/10.1016/0030-4220(93)90286-d.
22. Chen J-F, Lee S-T, Lui T-N, Yeh Y-S, Chen T-Y, Tzaan W-C. Teflon granuloma after microvascular decompression for trigeminal neuralgia. Surg Neurol. 2000;53(3):281–7.

23. Premsagar IC, Moss T, Coakham HB. Teflon-induced granuloma following treatment of trigeminal neuralgia by microvascular decompression: report of two cases. J Neurosurg. 1997;87(3):454–7.
24. Matsushima T, Yamaguchi T, Inoue T, Matsukado K, Fukui M. Recurrent trigeminal neuralgia after microvascular decompression using an interposing technique. Teflon felt adhesion and the sling retraction technique. Acta Neurochir. 2000;142:557–61.
25. Liu J, Wu G, Xiang H, et al. Long-term retrospective analysis of microvascular decompression in patients with recurrent trigeminal neuralgia. Front Neurol. 2020;11:584224.
26. Melvill RL, Baxter BL. A tentorial sling in microvascular decompression for trigeminal neuralgia. J Neurosurg. 1996;84(1):127–8.
27. Steinberg JA, Sack J, Wilson B, et al. Tentorial sling for microvascular decompression in patients with trigeminal neuralgia: a description of operative technique and clinical outcomes. J Neurosurg. 2018;130(4):1315–20. https://doi.org/10.3171/2017.10.JNS17971.
28. Masuoka J, Matsushima T, Inoue K, Nakahara Y, Takase Y, Kawashima M. Outcome of microvascular decompression for trigeminal neuralgia treated with the stitched sling retraction technique. Neurosurg Rev. 2015;38(2):361–5. discussion 365. https://doi.org/10.1007/s10143-015-0607-5.
29. Masuoka J, Matsushima T, Kawashima M, Nakahara Y, Funaki T, Mineta T. Stitched sling retraction technique for microvascular decompression: procedures and techniques based on an anatomical viewpoint. Neurosurg Rev. 2011;34(3):373–9; discussion 379–80. https://doi.org/10.1007/s10143-011-0310-0.
30. Meybodi AT, Habibi Z, Miri M, Tabatabaie SA. Microvascular decompression for trigeminal neuralgia using the 'Stitched sling Retraction' technique in recurrent cases after previous microvascular decompression. Acta Neurochir. 2014;156(6):1181–7; discussion 1187. https://doi.org/10.1007/s00701-014-2092-y.
31. Mitsos AP, Georgakoulias N, Lafazanos SA, Konstantinou EA. The "hanging technique" of vascular transposition in microvascular decompression for trigeminal neuralgia: technical report of four cases. Neurosurg Rev. 2008;31(3):327–30. https://doi.org/10.1007/s10143-008-0144-6.
32. Kato K, Ujiie H, Nakano H, et al. Application of ion-beam implanted expanded polytetrafluoroethylene to microvascular decompression and the surgical outcome. Neurol Med Chir (Tokyo). 2017;57(11):601–6. https://doi.org/10.2176/nmc.oa.2017-0007.
33. Abi-Aad KR, Turcotte E, Patra DP, et al. Vascular transposition of the superior cerebellar artery using a fenestrated clip and fibrin glue in trigeminal neuralgia: 2-dimensional operative video. Oper Neurosurg (Hagerstown). 2020;19(1):E50–e51. https://doi.org/10.1093/ons/opz291.
34. Patra DP, Rahme RJ, Zimmerman R, Bendok BR. In reply: vascular transposition of the superior cerebellar artery using a fenestrated clip and fibrin glue in trigeminal neuralgia: 2-dimensional operative video. Oper Neurosurg (Hagerstown). 2020;19(1):E98. https://doi.org/10.1093/ons/opaa069.
35. Patra DP, Turcotte EL, Krishna C, Zimmerman RS, Batjer HH, Bendok BR. Microvascular decompression technique for trigeminal neuralgia using a vascular clip. World Neurosurg. 2021;154:1. https://doi.org/10.1016/j.wneu.2021.06.124.
36. Attabib N, Kaufmann AM. Use of fenestrated aneurysm clips in microvascular decompression surgery: technical note and case series. J Neurosurg. 2007;106(5):929–31.
37. Ichikawa T, Agari T, Kurozumi K, Maruo T, Satoh T, Date I. "Double-stick tape" technique for transposition of an offending vessel in microvascular decompression: technical case report. Oper Neurosurg. 2011;68:onsE377–82.
38. Otani N, Toyooka T, Fujii K, et al. "Birdlime" technique using TachoSil tissue sealing sheet soaked with fibrin glue for sutureless vessel transposition in microvascular decompression: operative technique and nuances. J Neurosurg. 2017;128(5):1522–9.
39. Pines AR, Butterfield RJ, Turcotte EL, et al. Microvascular transposition without teflon: a single institution's 17-year experience treating trigeminal neuralgia. Oper Neurosurg. 2021;20(4):397–405.

9 Pure Endoscopic Microvascular Decompression Using the Transposition Technique for Trigeminal Neuralgia and Hemifacial Spasm

Fuminari Komatsu and Yoko Kato

9.1 Introduction

Trigeminal neuralgia (TN) is a condition characterized by intense, unilateral, paroxysmal pain in the face commonly due to compression of the trigeminal nerve (CN V), while hemifacial spasm (HFS) is a common neurological disorder with involuntary, paroxysmal tetany or clonic movement of unilateral facial muscles due to compression of the facial nerve (CN VII).

Microvascular decompression (MVD) has become the accepted surgical technique for the treatment of TN and HFS because of the positive surgical outcomes and prevention of long-term recurrence [1, 2]. Although MVD is traditionally performed under microscopic visualization, microscopes have certain theoretical limitations, in that the operator can observe only the objects that are directly in front of the microscope, and observation of structures behind obstacles is restricted. In contrast, use of endoscopes in MVD surgery can apparently improve visibility of neurovascular conflict (NVC), since endoscopy provides panoramic views even in deep surgical fields, with minimal invasiveness [3]. Some authors have reported excellent surgical outcomes following endoscopic MVD, and the procedure is now becoming the standard procedure in MVD surgery [4–6].

In addition to securing observation of NVC, another important element for successful MVD is the method of decompression. Decompressive procedures are mainly classified as two types, interposition and transposition. For interposition, a prosthesis is placed between the cranial nerve and the offending artery. In contrast, in transposition, the offending artery is moved away from the cranial nerve and fixed to surrounding structures, such as the tentorium cerebelli or petrosal dura mater, with a prosthesis and fibrin glue. Although interposition is technically easier than transposition, its recurrence rate is higher than that of transposition. On the other hand, transposition is technically more difficult and complicated than interposition, although it provides superior outcomes in terms of reducing recurrence [7].

Here, we describe purely endoscopic MVD with transposition for TN and HFS, especially focusing on the technical nuances, and discuss the advantages of endoscopic MVD described in the literature.

9.2 Methods

9.2.1 Preoperative 3D Fusion Image

Three-dimensional (3D) fusion images for preoperative surgical simulation of MVD are digital

F. Komatsu (✉) · Y. Kato
Department of Neurosurgery, Fujita Health University Bantane Hospital, Nagoya, Japan

S.-T. Li et al. (eds.), *Microvascular Decompression Surgery*,
https://doi.org/10.1007/978-981-96-0767-9_9

models reconstructed from computed tomography (CT) and magnetic resonance (MR) images. In this technique, CT images for data collection are obtained using a 320-row multidetector CT scanner (Aquilon One; Toshiba, Tokyo, Japan) with a slice thickness of 0.5 mm. CT angiography with immediate and delayed scanning sessions after injection of iodized contrast media is used for acquiring information on the arteries and veins. MR images are obtained using a 1.5-T system (Orian; Canon, Tochigi, Japan), and MR cisternography is also performed. All the digital imaging and communication in medicine (DICOM)-formatted data are processed using image analysis software (Ziostation2; ZIOSOFT, Tokyo, Japan) to create 3D fusion images. Data on the brainstem and cranial nerves are extracted from MR cisternography, and data on the arteries, veins and skull are extracted from CT angiography. All the extracted models are automatically fused using image analysis software, and the targeted structures are determined by the extent of interest and by adjusting the window level. Finally, creation of each structural 3D model of the brainstem, cranial nerves, vessels (arteries and veins), and skull is completed (Figs. 9.1b and 9.2b).

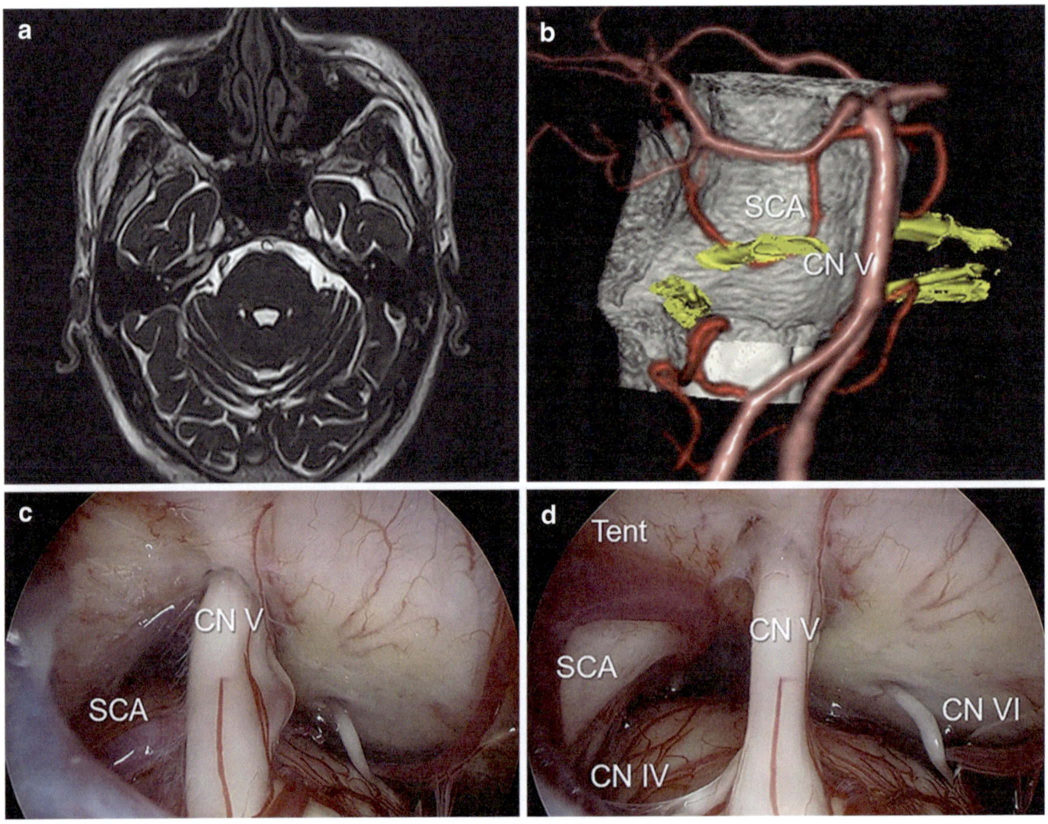

Fig. 9.1 Endoscopic microvascular decompression (MVD) for trigeminal neuralgia (TN) in an illustrative case. (**a**) MR cisternography revealed that the CN V was compressed by the SCA and the CN V was deformed by the compression. (**b**) A 3D fusion image indicated the deep caudal loop of the SCA and neurovascular conflict. (**c**) Endoscopic view before decompression demonstrated that the CN V was severely compressed by the SCA. (**d**) Endoscopic view after transposition showed secure fixation of the SCA at the tentorium cerebelli with fibrin glue, with straightening of the CN after decompression. *Arrow* neurovascular conflict, *CN IV* trochlear nerve, *CN V* trigeminal nerve, *CN VI* abducens nerve, *SCA* superior cerebellar artery

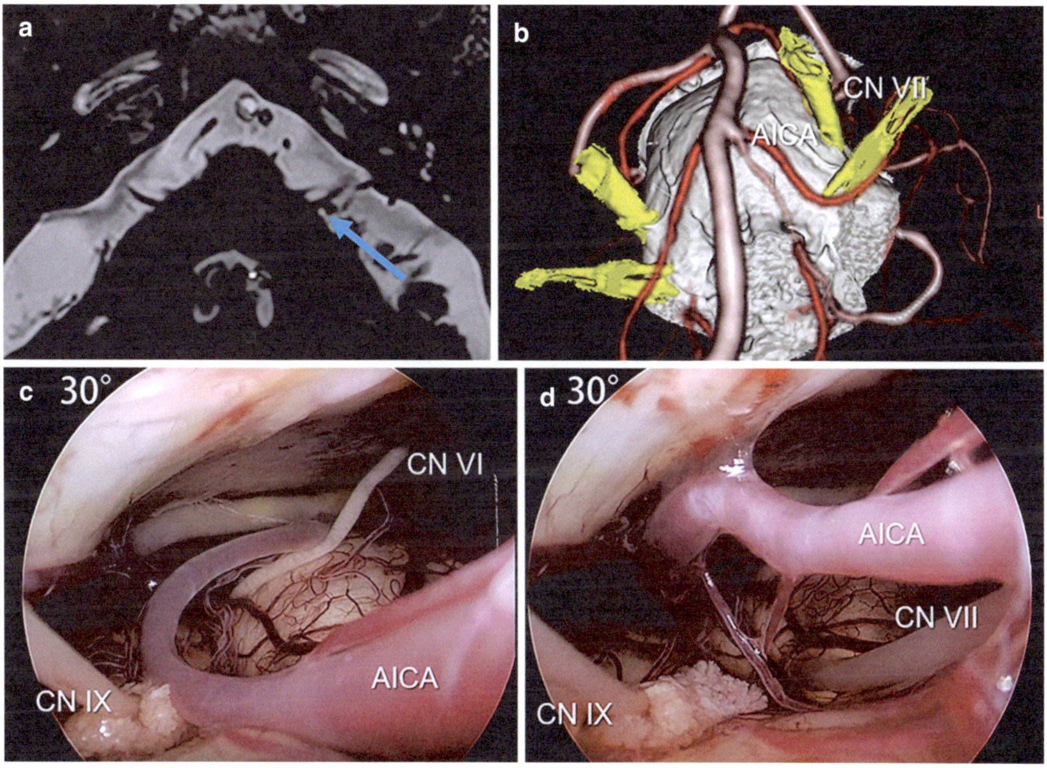

Fig. 9.2 Endoscopic microvascular decompression (MVD) for hemifacial spasm (HFS) in an illustrative case. (**a**) MR cisternography showed the AICA running toward the CN VII. (**b**) A 3D fusion image revealed the AICA compressing the root exit zone of the CN VII. (**c**) A 30-degree angled endoscopic view before decompression clearly demonstrated the AICA running along the root exit zone of the CN VII. (**d**) A 30-degree angled endoscopic view after transposition demonstrated secure decompression of the CN VII and the structures around the ponto-medullary junction. The AICA was fixed to the petrosal dura mater using fibrin glue, with preservation of the perforators. *AICA* anterior inferior cerebellar artery, *Arrow* neurovascular conflict, *CN VI* abducens nerve, *CN VII* facial nerve, *CN IX* glossopharyngeal nerve

9.2.2 Surgical Setting of Endoscopic MVD

The patient is placed in the park-bench position under general anesthesia. After making a 30–40 mm straight skin incision, a small 15 mm craniotomy is created at the transverse-sigmoid junction. The same craniotomy is used for both TN and HFS. Then, 4 mm, 0- and 30-degree endoscopes are fixed using a pneumatic endoscope holder for performance of MVD using a bimanual technique. Single-shaft instruments, including dissectors, alligator forceps and scissors, and slim-type bipolar forceps are used in the procedure. A brain retractor is not used. Brainstem auditory evoked potential (BAEP) is continuously monitored during the procedure.

9.2.3 Decompression under Endoscopy

Basically, transposition is performed as the decompression procedure, and the offending arteries are directly fixed at the tentorium cerebelli or petrosal dura without the use of Teflon felt strings [8]. The birdlime method, in which a gelatin sponge is braced between the offending artery and dura mater, is performed if the distance between the offending artery and dura is very wide, such that their direct fixation is not possible [9].

9.2.4 Case Series

We performed 195 endoscopic MVD procedures, including 156 for TN, 37 for HFS, and two for glossopharyngeal neuralgia, at our institute from January 2021 to December 2022.

9.3 Results

9.3.1 Endoscopic MVD for TN

The 0-degree endoscope is inserted into the intradural space through the retrosigmoid keyhole. After gradual drainage of the cerebrospinal fluid (CSF), the endoscope is inserted up to the cerebellopontine angle. Then, the superior petrosal vein (SPV) and acousticofacial nerve bundle (CN VII/VIII) are identified, and the arachnoid membrane between the SPV and CN VII/VIII is sharply opened using single-shaft micro-scissors, with preservation of the SPV. Next, the endoscope is advanced, and the trigeminal nerve (CN V) is well visualized in a panoramic view under endoscopy from the root entry zone (REZ) to the porus trigeminus, and NVCs by offending arteries are investigated. The superior cerebellar artery (SCA) is the most common offending artery, which usually forms a caudal loop that compresses the REZ of CN V from the medial aspect. The arachnoid trabecula between the SCA and CN V is completely dissected to prepare for decompression by transposition. The SCA is separated from the CN V by a dissector or micro-suction, taking great care to preserve the perforators arising from the SCA. Once the SCA is safely mobilized, it is fixed to the tentorium cerebelli using only fibrin glue, which is applied by special droppers that allow the glue to be applied drop by drop. Next, secure fixation of the offending artery to the tentorium cerebelli, and decompression of the CN V is confirmed. Appropriate decompression by transposition leads to relief of the deformity of the CN V by the artery and straightening of the nerve from the REZ to Meckel's cave.

9.3.2 Endoscopic MVD for HFS

The 0-degree endoscope is advanced into the intradural space of the cerebellopontine angle through the retrosigmoid keyhole. The CN VII/VIII and lower cranial nerves, including the glossopharyngeal (CN IX), vagus, and accessory nerves, are identified, and the arachnoid membrane between the CN VII/VIII and CN IX and the arachnoid membrane around the jugular foramen are sharply incised and opened. Next, the 0-degree endoscope is replaced by the 30-degree endoscope, which is then introduced into the space between CN VII/VIII and CN IX. The angled endoscopic view enables clear visualization of the offending artery running along the root exit zone of the CN VII. The offending artery in most HFS cases is the anterior inferior cerebellar artery (AICA). After identification of the AICA as the offending artery, it is separated from the root exit zone of CN VII, and perforators from the AICA are carefully observed. Once safe mobilization of the AICA is confirmed, it is lifted and fixed to the petrosal dura mater with only fibrin glue applied using a dropper. Next, secure fixation of the offending artery to the petrosal dura mater and decompression of the CN VII are confirmed. Finally, after proper decompression, the pontomedullary junction and the supraolivary fossette are exposed under the angled endoscopic view.

9.3.3 Surgical Results

In TN cases, a good outcome (no pain or occasional pain without medication) was achieved in 91.0% (142/156) of cases. The spasm-free rate in HFS case was 94.2% (33/35 cases). The overall complication rate was hearing loss in 2.5% (5/195 cases), diplopia due to trochlear nerve palsy in 0.5% (1/195 cases), and CSF rhinorrhea requiring reconstruction surgery in 1.5% (3/195) of cases.

9.4 Discussion

During endoscopic MVD, since the endoscope facilitates visualization of the NVCs, appropriate decompression is feasible with minimal invasiveness purely under endoscopic MVD. Some authors have described the advantages of endoscopic MVD compared to microscopic MVD. Zagzoog N et al. conducted a systematic review and comparative meta-analysis between endoscopic and microscopic MVD in 6749 TN cases from 23 previously reported articles, and concluded a low recurrence rate in endoscopic MVD cases [1]. In addition, Zhao Z et al. [2] conducted a meta-analysis and systematic review of 1122 HFS cases reported in 12 previous articles, and described that endoscopic MVD is better than microscopic MVD in terms of treatment effect, overall complications, and recurrence rate. However, although these systematic reviews have indicated the superiority of endoscopic MVD over microscopic MVD, a significant difference between endoscopic and microscopic MVD has not been proven in retrospective single center studies. Xiang et al. conducted a prospective study of 213 TN cases at a single institute, and concluded no significant superiority between endoscopic and microscopic MVD [10]. Zhu et al. conducted a retrospective cohort study of 116 HFS cases at a single institute, and concluded no significant superiority between endoscopic and microscopic MVD [11].

From another point of view, Lee et al. conducted a single center retrospective study of 167 TN cases, and concluded that endoscopic and microscopic MVD provide patients with equivalent pain outcomes and complication rates. On the other hand, the rate of headaches 1 month postoperatively was significantly lower in the endoscopic MVD group, suggesting the minimal invasiveness of endoscopic MVD [12]. However, the endoscopic MVD procedure is still under development, and further study is needed to conclude its superiority compared to conventional microscopic MVD.

With respect to the decompression method, studies focusing on decompression under endoscopy have not been performed so far. Most previous endoscopic MVD series seem to have achieved decompression by the interposition technique [4–6]. Our results in this study suggest that direct fibrin glue fixation is a simple and easy technique and can be successfully performed even in a narrow corridor under endoscopy. The results are effective and safe enough in the short-term. However, the long-term outcomes of endoscopic MVD have not yet been validated, and follow-up studies need to be performed in the future. Evaluation of the optimal decompression method under endoscopy is also an issue for the future.

9.5 Conclusion

Fully endoscopic MVD for TN and HFS by transposition of the offending artery away from the nerve is safe and effective, with minimal invasiveness. Further improvement of the endoscopic MVD procedure can be expected with advances in relation to endoscopes, instruments, and surgical techniques.

Declarations Funding

No funding was received for conducting this study.

Ethics Approval

The institutional ethics committee approved this study (No. HM18–447), and the study was conducted in accordance with the guidelines of the 1964 Declaration of Helsinki.

Consent to Participate

Informed consent was obtained from all individual participants included in this study.

Conflicts of Interest The authors have no relevant financial or nonfinancial interests to disclose.

References

1. Zagzoog N, Attar A, Takroni R, Alotaibi MB, Reddy K. Endoscopic versus open microvascular decompression for trigeminal neuralgia: a systematic review and comparative meta-analysis. J Neurosurg. 2018;131:1532. https://doi.org/10.3171/2018.6.Jns172690.
2. Zhao Z, Chai S, Xiao D, Zhou Y, Gan J, Jiang X, et al. Microscopic versus endoscopic microvascular decompression for the treatment of hemifacial spasm in China: a meta-analysis and systematic review. J Clin

Neurosci. 2021;91:23–31. https://doi.org/10.1016/j.jocn.2021.06.034.

3. Komatsu F, Imai M, Hirayama A, Hotta K, Hayashi N, Oda S, et al. Endoscopic microvascular decompression with transposition for trigeminal neuralgia and Hemifacial spasm: technical note. J Neurol Surg A Cent Eur Neurosurg. 2017;78(3):291–5. https://doi.org/10.1055/s-0036-1592077.
4. Bohman LE, Pierce J, Stephen JH, Sandhu S, Lee JY. Fully endoscopic microvascular decompression for trigeminal neuralgia: technique review and early outcomes. Neurosurg Focus. 2014;37(4):E18. https://doi.org/10.3171/2014.7.Focus14318.
5. Kabil MS, Eby JB, Shahinian HK. Endoscopic vascular decompression versus microvascular decompression of the trigeminal nerve. Minim Invasive Neurosurg. 2005;48(4):207–12. https://doi.org/10.1055/s-2005-870928.
6. Kher Y, Yadav N, Yadav YR, Parihar V, Ratre S, Bajaj J. Endoscopic Vascular Decompression in Trigeminal Neuralgia. Turk Neurosurg. 2017;27(6):998–1006. https://doi.org/10.5137/1019-5149.Jtn.17046-16.1.
7. Sindou M, Leston JM, Decullier E, Chapuis F. Microvascular decompression for trigeminal neuralgia: the importance of a noncompressive technique--Kaplan-Meier analysis in a consecutive series of 330 patients. Neurosurgery. 2008;63(4 Suppl 2):341–50; discussion 50–1. https://doi.org/10.1227/01.neu.0000327022.79171.d6.
8. Komatsu F, Kato Y, Hirose Y. How I do it: two-step transposition technique during endoscopic microvascular decompression for trigeminal neuralgia. Acta Neurochir. 2022;164(3):823–6. https://doi.org/10.1007/s00701-021-05080-y.
9. Otani N, Toyooka T, Fujii K, Kumagai K, Takeuchi S, Tomiyama A, et al. "birdlime" technique using TachoSil tissue sealing sheet soaked with fibrin glue for sutureless vessel transposition in microvascular decompression: operative technique and nuances. J Neurosurg. 2018;128(5):1522–9. https://doi.org/10.3171/2017.1.jns161243.
10. Xiang H, Wu G, Ouyang J, Liu R. Prospective study of Neuroendoscopy versus microscopy: 213 cases of microvascular decompression for trigeminal neuralgia performed by one neurosurgeon. World Neurosurg. 2018;111:e335–e9. https://doi.org/10.1016/j.wneu.2017.12.051.
11. Zhu J, Sun J, Li R, Yu Y, Zhang L. Fully endoscopic versus microscopic vascular decompression for hemifacial spasm: a retrospective cohort study. Acta Neurochir. 2021;163(9):2417–23. https://doi.org/10.1007/s00701-021-04824-0.
12. Lee JYK, Pierce JT, Sandhu SK, Petrov D, Yang AI. Endoscopic versus microscopic microvascular decompression for trigeminal neuralgia: equivalent pain outcomes with possibly decreased postoperative headache after endoscopic surgery. J Neurosurg. 2017;126(5):1676–84. https://doi.org/10.3171/2016.5.Jns1621.

10 Posterior Fossa Re-Exploration for Recurrent Trigeminal Neuralgia

Joachim K. Krauss and Filipe Wolff Fernandes

10.1 Introduction

Microvascular decompression (MVD) is the only non-ablative procedure that can provide a potentially causative cure for trigeminal neuralgia, as reflected by its high success rate and its minimal operative morbidity. Nevertheless, despite initial pain relief, patients might experience recurrence of pain, with an estimated mean annual risk between 1% and 4% [1, 2]. There is controversy on what is the best treatment strategy for the treatment of recurrent trigeminal neuralgia. Treatment strategies include percutaneous trigeminal ganglion ablation (by thermocoagulation, balloon compression, or glycerol injection), stereotactic radiosurgery, or peripheral nerve field stimulation [3–6]. But also MVD for those patients who underwent a previous destructive procedure, or "repeat MVD"/posterior fossa re-exploration for patients who had a previous MVD is a viable therapeutical option in this scenario [7–9].

The attention was already directed to this topic by Jannetta and Bissonette in [10], when they documented the intraoperative results in a series of 51 patients, who underwent posterior fossa re-exploration for trigeminal neuralgia after previous MVD, concluding that re-exploration is an overall safe and effective strategy [10]. Since then, several studies reported on intraoperative findings and discussed various potential operative strategies to achieve effective and durable relief of pain [8–16].

Posterior fossa re-exploration has the advantage of addressing directly the causative factors for recurrence in trigeminal neuralgia after previously successful MVD in most instances. In this chapter, we present an overview of the definition, epidemiology, and pathophysiology of the recurrence of trigeminal neuralgia after a previous successful MVD. Furthermore, we describe our surgical technique and provide an overview on other surgical options, and on clinical outcome.

10.2 Definition of Recurrence of Trigeminal Neuralgia

Recurrence of trigeminal neuralgia is defined as the reoccurrence of neuralgic pain after a previous successful surgical procedure, which provided a period of absence or improvement of pain. This should be distinguished from "persisting pain" or "intractable pain" since these scenarios imply different mechanisms [17].

Recurrent pain may present either as a "classical trigeminal neuralgia" or it may be accompanied by atypical features, such as a continuous background type of pain. Also, recurrent trigeminal neuralgia may affect new branches of the

J. K. Krauss (✉) · F. Wolff Fernandes
Department of Neurosurgery, Hannover Medical School, Hannover, Germany
e-mail: krauss.joachim@mh-hannover.de

S.-T. Li et al. (eds.), *Microvascular Decompression Surgery*,
https://doi.org/10.1007/978-981-96-0767-9_10

Table 10.1 Barrow Neurological Institute Pain Score for trigeminal neuralgia. Barrow Neurological Institute (BNI) pain intensity score (adapted from [20]) to assess the level of pain in patients with trigeminal neuralgia

Pain score	Definition
I	No pain, not taking medication
II	Occasional pain, not requiring medications
IIIa	No pain, with medication
IIIb	Acceptable pain relief with medication
IV	Minimal pain relief, not adequately controlled by medication
V	No relief

trigeminal nerve where the pain did not occur prior to the first surgical procedure. However, the appearance of atypical features associated with pain should always lead one to reconsider the clinical diagnosis.

The definition of recurrence is variable in the literature. Burchiel et al. categorized recurrence of pain as minor (neuralgic pain as transient, infrequent, mild, or controlled by medication alone) or major recurrence (typical neuralgic pain, not adequately controlled by medication) [18]. Barker et al., on the other hand, defined recurrence as a transition from excellent outcome (absence of pain, reduction of pain of at least 98% compared to the preoperative level as assessed by the patient) to either good outcome (75% reduction in pain, intermittent treatment with low doses of medication), or poor outcome (25% reduction in pain, or long-term medication resumed) [1]. Sun et al. classified recurrence as the development of recurrent pain at least 1 month following MVD [19]. Recent studies applied the Barrow Neurological Institute (BNI) pain intensity score [20] (Table 10.1) to measure the outcome. Recurrence was defined as the return of neuralgic pain (BNI III-V) after a specific period of pain relief [12, 14–16, 21–24].

10.3 Frequency of Recurrence of Trigeminal Neuralgia

Recurrences occur more frequently after percutaneous procedures than after MVD [25–28]. In the following, we will concentrate on recurrences after MVD.

The rate of recurrence of trigeminal neuralgia after successful MVD varies, according to a recent systematic review, between 5% and 53% [29]. The recurrence rate after MVD is both related to the surgical methods and to the experience of the surgeon. Also, it depends much on the length of follow-up, since most recurrences occur within 2 years. In the systematic review by Jiao et al. a mean pain-free interval after MVD of 27.75 months has been reported, ranging between 2.4 and 60 months [29].

In a cohort of 63 patients with recurrent TN after MVD, Inoue et al., reported a mean and a median pain-free interval of 20 and 9 months, respectively [9]. Such a difference was corroborated also by the Kaplan-Meier curves in the large patient series of Pittsburgh and Lyon [1, 30]. The different recurrence rates and their respective follow-up are presented in Table 10.2.

In a cohort of 1185 patients, Barker et al. reported a 2% annual risk of recurrence 5 years after MVD, and less than 1% in 10 years [1]. Bederson and Wilson described recurrence in 31 out of 252 patients (12%) after successful MVD with an average follow-up of 5.1 years [33]. Similarly, in a cohort of 291 patients with successful MVD, 14% had a recurrence after a mean follow-up period of 5 years (1–12 years range) [36]. Liao et al. reported 5 cases of recurrence out of 80 MVD procedures within 12 months of follow-up [39]. More recently, in 102 patients undergoing MVD, 21 presented with recurrence at an average follow-up of 44.6 months [45], while Andersen et al. reported a rate of 5 cases of major recurrence (BNI IV-V) and 9 cases of minor recurrence (BNI II-III) in 87 patients that had complete pain relief without medication after MVD [46].

Different factors were reported to be associated with the rate of recurrence. In a large cohort of 281 patients, Kondo showed that a variation in technique could diminish the rate of recurrence [40]. By performing a resection of the arachnoid membrane around the nerve to straighten its axis, the recurrence rate fell from 10.2% to 6.5%. Sindou et al. highlighted the importance of a non-compressive technique, showing that 214 out of 260 patients remained pain-free 15 years after inserting an implant without touching the root, compared to 47 out of 70 patients who received

Table 10.2 Rate of recurrence and respective follow-up in the literature. Summary of the literature regarding the rate of recurrence and respective follow-up (adapted from [9]). *MVD* microvascular decompression

Author & year	MVD No. of patients	Recurrence rate	Mean follow-up (range)
Van Loveren et al. [31]	50	12%	3 years (3–6 years)
Zorman and Wilson [32]	125	16%	2.4 years (6 months–13 years)
Burchiel et al. [18]	36	47%	8.5 years (7.5–11.5 years)
Bederson and Wilson [33]	246	12%	5.1 years (6 months–16 years)
Klun [34]	178	6%	5.2 years (6 months–12 years)
Sun et al. [19]	61	16%	2 years (1.1–10.5 years)
Cutbush and Atkinson [35]	109	20.4%	57 months
Sindou et al. [36]	291	14%	5 years (1–12 years)
Mendoza and Illingworth [37]	133	16%	5.3 years (6 months–15 years)
Barker et al. [1]	1185	23.8%	6.2 years (1–10 years)
Rath et al. [38]	135	16.7%	1.4 years (3 months–5 years)
Liao et al. [39]	80	6.25%	1 year (9 months–4 years)
Kondo [40]	281	8.2%	10.1 years (5–20 years)
Lee et al. [41]	146	8.6%	5.7 years (2–6 years)
Chen and Lee [25]	114	15.7%	2 years
Zhong et al. [42]	1274	1.2%	3 years
Haridas et al. [43]	83 78 73	14.4% 15.4% 17.7%	36 months 48 months 60 months
Jafree and Zakrzewska [44]	169	16.6%	5 years
Greve et al. [45]	102	20.6%	44.6 months (26.7–72.3 months)
Andersen et al. [46]	115	10.4%	24 months follow-up

an implant that was left in contact with the trigeminal nerve root [47]. In a series of 50 patients with TN that underwent the stitched sling retraction technique, in which a stitch made in the dura or tentorium kept the offending vessel away from the nerve, only 2 patients (4%) had a recurrence 1 and 3.8 years after, respectively [48].

More recently, in a 2-center retrospective cohort study of MVD in TN patients using Teflon or Ivalon, Pressman et al. found that the implant type had no impact on the final outcome score or risk of recurrence [24].

Studies present contradictory results regarding clinical aspects. This concerns factors such as age, sex, side of pain, duration of symptoms, distribution of pain, or other previous surgical procedures [2, 45, 47]. When focusing on operative findings, venous conflict and a less severe degree of compression by a culprit vessel at the primary MVD surgery had a higher rate of recurrence [1, 30]. Sun et al. noted that only the presence of venous compression or combined venous and arterial compression was correlated with a higher rate of recurrence when compared to arterial compression only (80% vs. 11% rate of recurrence) [19]. Additionally, the rate of recurrence is higher in patients with trigeminal neuralgia and multiple sclerosis undergoing MVD, when compared to classical trigeminal neuralgia [49, 50]. Overall, the variable number of patients, different types of assessment, and statistical calculations make it difficult to define potential risk factors for recurrence.

10.4 Local Findings Associated with Recurrence of Trigeminal Neuralgia

The causative factors responsible for the recurrence of TN after a previous MVD depend on both previous surgical technique and the material used for interposition. The descriptions of the intraoperative findings upon re-do surgery are highly variable, depending much on the eye of the beholder performing posterior fossa re-exploration. Sindou et al. highlighted this fact when commenting on the rarity of negative explorations in a large series of MVD for trigeminal neuralgia [51].

Causes thought to be responsible for recurrence include new vascular contact, scarring/adhesions, and Teflon granuloma [13, 52–56]. According to the review by Jiao et al., in a total of 193 patients that underwent posterior fossa re-exploration, the following distribution was noted: granulomatous lesions or arachnoid adhesions (31%), vascular conflict (36%), slippage of Teflon felt (9%), and no identifiable cause (29%) [29]. A summary of intraoperative findings as reported in the literature is presented in Table 10.3. We have analyzed the variety of findings in a series of 26 patients as outlined in Table 10.4.

10.4.1 Vascular Conflict

Several studies on redo posterior fossa exploration reported the findings of a vascular conflict, occasionally attributed to a missed culprit vessel.

Table 10.3 Intraoperative findings during posterior fossa re-exploration in the literature. Summary of the intraoperative findings during posterior fossa re-exploration described in the literature (adapted from [9]). *MVD* microvascular decompression, *NR* not reported

Author and Year	Number of redo cases	Interval from previous MVD	Causative findings			
			Artery	Vein	Implant	Adhesion
Bederson and Wilson [33]	20	NR	NR	NR	NR	1 (5%)
Cho [17]	31	1 week–4 years	7 (22%)	4 (13%)	4 (13%)	16 (52%)
Barker et al. [1]	132	30 days–2 years	79 (60%)	95 (72%)	NS	NS
Rath et al. [38]	16	17 months (4–62 months)	9 (56%)	0 (0%)	0 (0%)	7 (44%)
Liao et al. [39]	5	1 day–32 months	2 (40%)	1%)	2 (40%)	0 (0%)
Kureshi and Wilkins [57]	23	11 days–12 years	1 (4%)	0 (0%)	5 (22%)	16 (70%)
Chen et al. [58]	10	1–42 months	3 (30%)	1 (10%)	5 (50%)	1 (10%)
Matsushima et al. [59]	6	19 months (2–48 months)	0 (0%)	0 (0%)	6 (100%)	0 (0%)
Amador et al. [60]	29	70 months (4 days–29 years)	13 (45%)	4 (14%)	7 (24%)	NR
Zhong et al. [42]	46	2–5 days	46 (73%)	17 (27%)	NR	NR
Bakker et al. [7]	33	30 days–2 years	7 (21%)	6 (18%)	16 (48%)	4 (12%)
Gu et al. [61]	12	57 months (10–144 months)	6 (50%)	1 (8%)	4 (33%)	1 (8.3%)
Yang et al. [62]	15	NR	4 (27%)	0 (0%)	1 (7%)	11 (73%)
Feng et al. [63]	15	NR	9 (29%)	2 (6.5%)	14 (32%)	6 (19%)
Hussain et al. [13]	32	NR	6 (19%)	3 (9.4%)	6 (19%)	11 (34%)
Cheng et al. [53]	41	55 months (18–144 months)	15 (37%)	6 (15%)	8 (20%)	12 (29%)
Huang et al. [64]	8	6 days–3 months	7 (88%)	1 (13%)	0 (0%)	0 (0%)
Inoue et al. [9]	63	62 months (2–240 months)	13 (21%)	11 (17%)	25 (40%)	14 (22%)
Wang et al. [55]	137	NR	46 (34%)	18 (13%)	37 (27%)	137 (100%)

Table 10.4 Intraoperative findings and respective measures of 26 patients with recurrent trigeminal neuralgia undergoing posterior fossa re-exploration after previous microvascular decompression

Intraoperative findings and measures	No. of patients (total 26)
Intraoperative findings	
Dislocation of Teflon	0 (0%)
Arachnoid scar tissue	22 (84.6%)
Arterial compression	1 (3.8%)
Venous contact	8 (30.8%)
Teflon granuloma	14 (53.8%)
Cavum Meckeli electrode	1 (3.8%)
Piston effect	15 (57.7%)
Intraoperative measures	
Total removal of Teflon	9 (34.6%)
Partial removal of Teflon	16 (61.5%)
Removal of adhesions	22 (84.6%)
Removal of electrode	1 (3.8%)
Coagulation of vein	5 (19.2%)
New Teflon inserted	10 (38.5%)

In the review by Jiao et al. on redo MVD, in a total of 193 patients with recurrent TN, 12 had a primary vascular compression (4.4%) and 72 had an arterial conflict with the trigeminal nerve (26.7%) [29]. That means that in some cases, recurrence may result from a missed vessel during the first MVD, an insufficiently interposed implant between artery and nerve, and slippage of the implant. Missed culprit vessels must be avoided by inspection of the whole course of the trigeminal nerve from the root entry zone to its entrance into the cavum Meckeli and adequate interposition of Teflon between nerve and artery [9, 30, 65, 66].

Venous compression has a higher degree of recurrence compared to arterial compression. When pain recurs in this scenario, it is likely to occur within 1 year after MVD, as shown in 24 of 31 patients from the series in Pittsburgh [67]. Remarkably, in a systematic review, Soni et al. reported 39 out of 169 operated patients, that had a recurrence after 4 years, regardless of whether veins were coagulated and transected, or simply mobilized [68]. Additionally, Lee et al. reported the appearance of a new vein in 20 out of 31 patients, and new veins under the Teflon felt were observed in 6 patients. In the 31 reoperated patients, 19 had an offending vein in the proximal part of the nerve root (59.4%), 10 at both proximal and distal parts (31.3%), 3 next to the cavum Meckeli (9.4%), and 4 patients exhibited intraneural veins (12.5%) [67].

10.4.2 Teflon Granuloma, Arachnoid Adhesions, and Nerve Distortion

Teflon is the most frequently used material when performing MVD. Initially, Peter J. Jannetta introduced Teflon in 1985 after noting several patients with recurrent TN with stiffened Ivalon implants during repeat surgery, which caused transmission of pulsations to the trigeminal nerve, which he named as the "second missile phenomenon" [57]. Teflon was thought to be an inert material with a low rate of tissue reaction. Despite this, however, granulomatous reactions of implanted Teflon have been reported to occur between 1.1% and 7.3% in patients undergoing MVD [17, 52, 58–60, 69, 70]. Teflon is usually moistened in saline solution and shaped in different tailored forms, avoiding thus the potential adhesion to adjacent structures. Some surgeons use fibrin glue to fixate the Teflon.

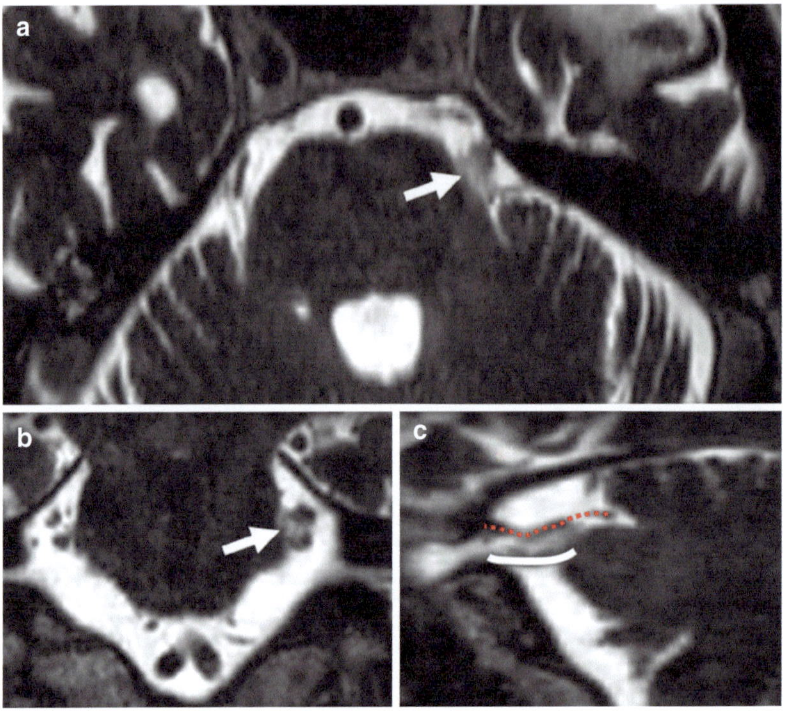

Fig. 10.1 T2-weighted MRI in a 54-year-old patient with recurrent trigeminal neuralgia on the left side after previous successful microvascular decompression 1 year before. (**a**) The axial scan shows the Teflon granuloma (white arrow) distorting the trigeminal nerve from medial and superior. (**b**) coronal and (**c**) sagittal images depict the Teflon granuloma adherent to the trigeminal nerve (white line) and the superior cerebellar artery (red dotted line)

In magnetic resonance imaging (MRI), Teflon granuloma presents as an iso- or hypointense mass in T1-sequences, hyperintense in T2-sequences, and it can show contrast enhancement with gadolinium (Fig. 10.1). Intraoperatively, Teflon granuloma appears as a dense yellow-brown mass with nonelastic consistency, accompanied by arachnoid scar tissue, and adherent to both the offending vessel and the trigeminal nerve, and it may also distort the trigeminal nerve by compressive mass effect (Fig. 10.2).

In the authors' series, the removed Teflon felt was analyzed histologically in 13 patients undergoing posterior fossa re-exploration for recurrent trigeminal neuralgia. Each specimen presented with scar tissue and an amorphous matrix with enlarged collagen fibers intertwined between the Teflon fibers, which appeared birefringent in polarized light (Fig. 10.3). Histologically, the specimens were characterized by multinuclear giant cells (10/13), lymphocytes (10/13), sidero-

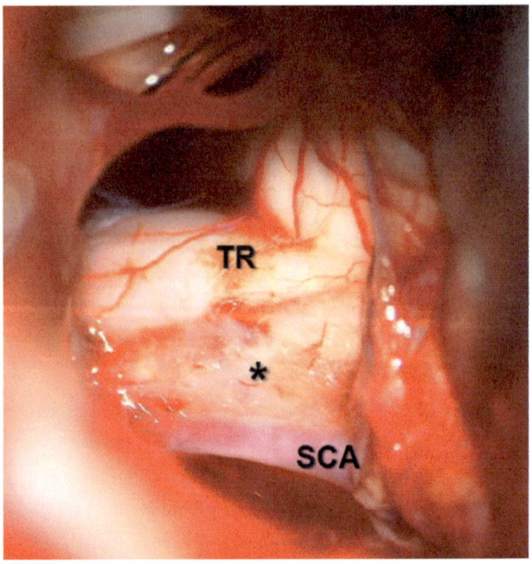

Fig. 10.2 Intraoperative example of a patient with right-sided recurrent trigeminal neuralgia after successful microvascular decompression. Note the yellow-brown color of the Teflon granuloma (asterisk), and its strong adherence to the trigeminal nerve root (TR) and superior cerebellar artery (SCA). Patient is in prone position

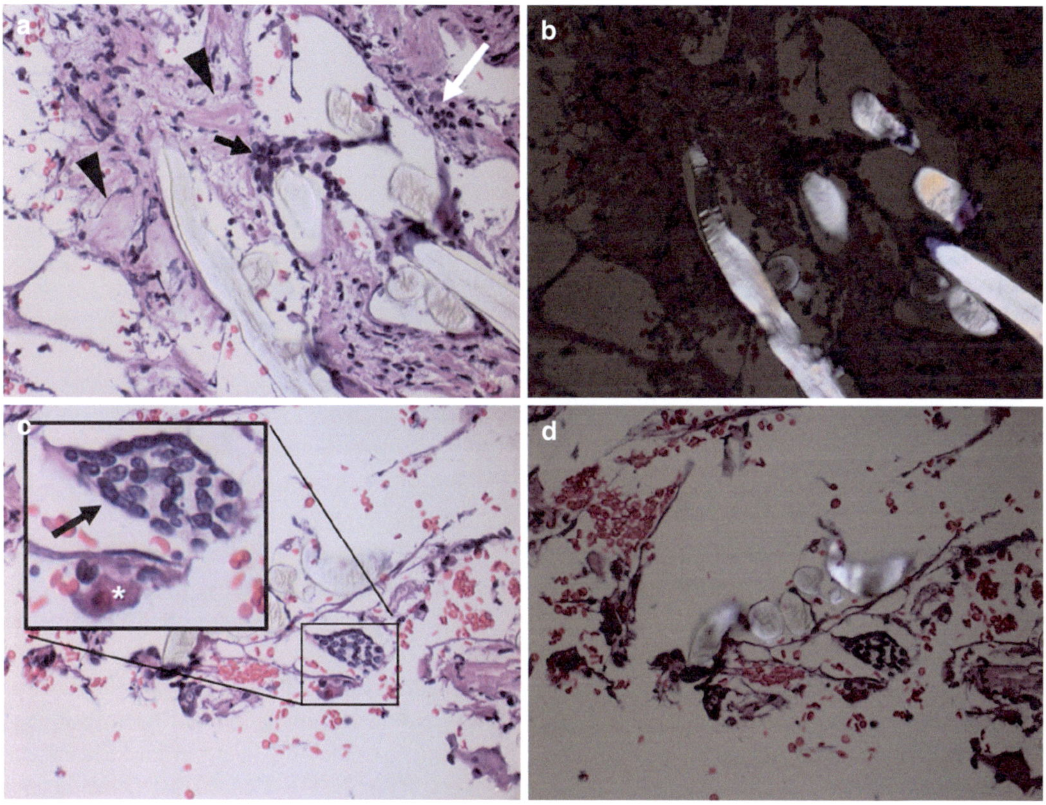

Fig. 10.3 Photomicrographs of the removed Teflon felt in an 80-year old patient with recurrent trigeminal neuralgia after successful microvascular decompression 1 year before. (**a**, **c** H&E, 400×) dense infiltrates of lymphocytes (white arrow), multinuclear giant cells (black arrow), and occasional siderophages (white asterisk) surrounding the Teflon fibers, intertwined between congestive scar tissue (black arrowhead). (**b**, **d** H&E and polarized light 400×) birefringent Teflon fibers displayed in multiple directions. H&E: Hematoxylin and eosin

phages (5/13), microcalcifications (5/13), and macrophages (3/13). The presence of macrophages and siderophages was correlated with a longer duration of recurrence [70]. Siderophages were also associated with older bleeding in the tissue before the operation. It has been postulated, that this reaction is triggered due to contact with the tentorium or dura [58], contact with the trigeminal nerve itself [59], or the brainstem [69]. The presence of siderophages indicates blood supply from smaller vessels, most probably the ones located within the dura and tentorium. Capelle et al., however, suggested that this reaction may also be triggered by a small bleeding into the Teflon felt during MVD, leading to a foreign body reaction [52]. Additionally, fibrin glue may add up to the risk of developing a Teflon granuloma [52, 70].

Different pathophysiological mechanisms concerning recurrent trigeminal neuralgia in the presence of Teflon granuloma have been proposed. One includes its mass effect, especially when too much Teflon is added. Scarring and distortion of the trigeminal nerve are more common. Another mechanism receiving less attention, described in detail in the authors' series, is what we call the "piston effect," in which the granulomatous Teflon felt is adherent to both artery and trigeminal nerve, enabling the transmission of arterial pulsations, leading to recurrent pain (Fig. 10.4). Two key elements leading to this phenomenon have been identified: hardening of the Teflon felt, and a tight adhesion between nerve, Teflon, and artery [8].

Arachnoid membranes are a coexistent intraoperative finding in MVD. Indeed, surrounding

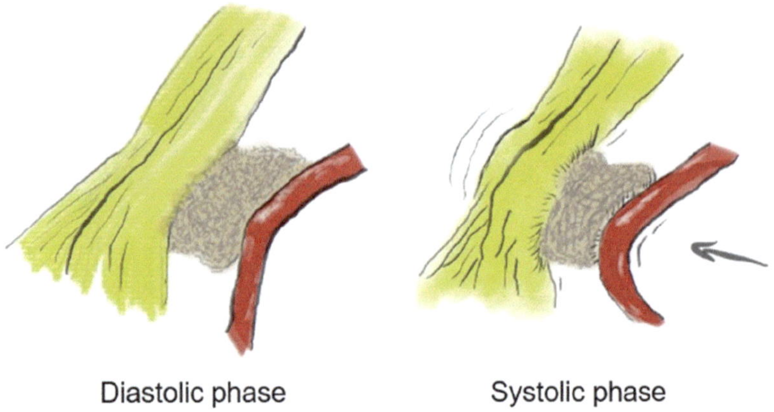

Fig. 10.4 Graphical demonstration of the "piston effect," which is defined as the transmission of pulsations to the trigeminal nerve via the interposed and hardened Teflon from systole to diastole from an arterial vessel (reprinted from [8] with permission)

arachnoid membranes tend to thicken and adhere, altering the anatomy of the structures in situ [14]. Similarly, arachnoid membranes or adhesions are a frequently reported finding in recurrent TN after previously successful MVD [53, 55], and their presence is correlated with a favorable outcome after posterior fossa re-exploration [8].

10.5 Treatment Considerations

For decision-making, a detailed clinical history and physical examination are mandatory. MRI should be performed in all these patients in the same manner as a primary evaluation of trigeminal neuralgia [71]. Imaging aids for the detection of possible causes for recurrent TN and surgical planning. However, the absence of any visible imagiological causative finding, such as new neurovascular conflict, or Teflon granuloma, should not withhold the decision to perform posterior fossa re-exploration.

The first step in recurrence is to start or increase the effective medication for TN, as recommended [72]. If these prove to be insufficient, whether by inadequate control of pain or undesirable side effects, the patient should be considered for a second surgery. There is no standard surgical treatment for recurrent TN after a previously successful MVD. As stated above, surgical options besides posterior fossa re-exploration, include percutaneous techniques (thermocoagulation, balloon compression, glycerol injection), stereotactic radiosurgery, and peripheral nerve stimulation [6, 29].

Besides the treatment of a neurovascular conflict, not all centers address recurrence in the same way. "Negative explorations" or "negative findings" are currently sometimes also treated via "mechanical injuries" aiming to alter the function of the nerve, including internal neurolysis (e.g. combing, or pinching) and partial sensory rhizotomy ([7, 13, 33]; Lee 2014). Other centers recognize adhesions and arachnoid membranes as the main cause for recurrence and thus aim for adhesiolysis without violating the trigeminal nerve [14, 53, 54].

10.6 Posterior Fossa Re-exploration: Hannover Surgical Technique and Intraoperative Findings

In the authors' department, patients with recurrent and therapy-refractory trigeminal neuralgia are always offered a posterior fossa re-exploration, including patients with multiple sclerosis [8, 50, 52, 73]. The preparation and positioning of the patient is the same as with a first MVD in our department, as described elsewhere [50, 52, 74–77]. Under general anaesthesia, the patient is placed in the prone position with the head in a three-pin holder, slightly flexed, and rotated 45° to the contralateral side. After positioning, the skin incision is directed through the existing scar of the first MVD, the site of the previous craniotomy is exposed, and the cranioplasty material is removed. If necessary, additional bone is drilled for the identification of the edges of both sigmoid and transverse sinus.

The durotomy is prepared in an L-shaped form. Adhesions between the cerebellum and dura are carefully dissected. A self-retaining retractor blade is placed gently over the lateral cerebellar hemisphere to open the way to the pontomedullary cistern. Already along this pathway, scar tissue and thickened and adhesive arachnoid membranes can be found. Care is taken when retracting the cerebellum medially, because the arachnoid membranes may increase the risk of stretching the facial-vestibulocochlear nerve complex. Any adhesions are meticulously dissected using microscissors, to fully expose the whole length of the trigeminal nerve. Additionally, to further decrease the risk of stretching, the arachnoid membranes next to the facial-vestibulocochlear complex are dissected. Similar to first MVD, a wide adhesiolysis and adequate drainage of CSF achieve a good exposure of the trigeminal nerve. No mannitol or lumbar drainage is necessary.

During the first MVD in the authors' institution, the superior petrosal vein is usually coagulated and cut in a way that its contributing veins are preserved and form a "natural" anastomotic connection. This facilitates the full exposure of the trigeminal nerve when performing posterior fossa re-exploration. In the case, this has not been done and if collateralization is secured, the same procedure can be done during posterior fossa re-exploration. In the authors' series, this practice has not resulted in any case of venous infarction or cerebellar swelling (unpublished data).

The trigeminal nerve is fully inspected from its root entry zone to its entrance to Meckel's cave. All adherent arachnoid membranes between the trigeminal nerve and the Teflon felt are carefully dissected. Then, small amounts are gently cut from the center of the Teflon felt to achieve a good distance between the adherent Teflon to the artery and the trigeminal nerve, assuring an adequate decompression and preserving the integrity of the trigeminal nerve (Fig. 10.5). It is to note that the total removal of Teflon is not always necessary to achieve a good outcome [8]. Also after removing partially or completely the previously placed Teflon, the site is inspected for new neurovascular conflicts, along the trigeminal nerve up to its entrance to the cavum Meckeli.

In the case of the "piston effect," a satisfactory result is achieved, when arterial pulsations are not transmitted towards the nerve. If, after the Teflon removal there is not sufficient decompressed space, new Teflon may be placed between the artery and the nerve. Alternatively, a "sling strategy" can be pursued, by suturing Teflon which is adherent to the artery to the tentorium or dura, keeping it away from the trigeminal nerve ("tefling"). Internal neurolysis, or "pinching and combing" the trigeminal nerve is strictly avoided.

After ensuring adequate local hemostasis, the dura is closed with single stitches. For a watertight closure, a piece of periost or Tachosil is affixed externally to the dura. Open mastoid cells are always waxed ("wax your way in, wax your way out"). The same cranioplasty is used, and new titanium screws are placed. Finally, the muscular and subcutaneous layers are closed with interrupted sutures and the cutaneous layer with a continuous suture.

10.6.1 Intraoperative Findings

In the authors' series several findings were noted. A combination of findings was noted in 18 out of the 26 operated patients (69.2%). Dislocation or slippage of Teflon could not be identified in any case. One patient had compression of the trigeminal nerve due to an electrode in the cavum Meckeli (3.8%). One patient with arterial compression had previous surgery in another hospital 70 months earlier (3.8%). The "piston effect" was identified in at least 15 patients (57.7%). The intraoperative findings and tailored surgical measures are displayed in Table 10.4.

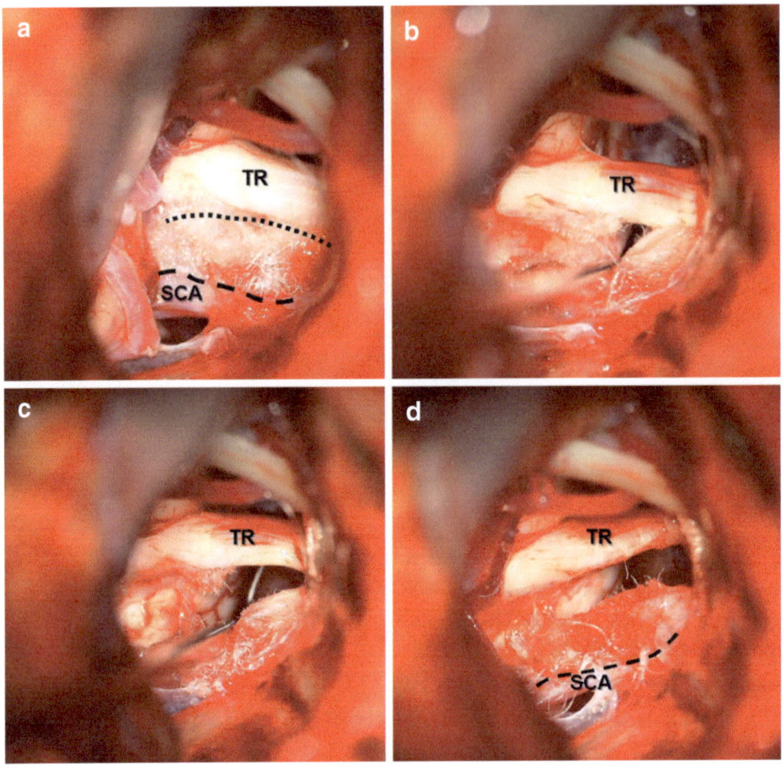

Fig. 10.5 Overview of the posterior fossa re-exploration in prone position in patients with left-sided recurrent trigeminal neuralgia. (**a**) The yellow-brown-colored and hardened Teflon remains adherent to the trigeminal nerve root (TR) and transmits pulsations from the superior cerebellar artery (SCA). The dissection plane for removal of Teflon felt is shown in the black dotted line. (**b**) and (**c**) demonstrate the meticulous dissection and removal of the Teflon felt, in order to achieve a complete decompression. (**d**) the rest of Teflon is adherent to the SCA and has no contact with the TR, thus achieving a resolution of the "piston effect"

10.7 Posterior Fossa Re-exploration: Outcome Hannover Series

In the authors' series, 26 patients with recurrent trigeminal neuralgia underwent posterior fossa re-exploration. Postoperative side effects included new sensory deficit in 5 patients (19.2%), from which 2 were transient, one patient with transient diplopia secondary to trochlear palsy (3.8%), and one with delayed facial palsy (3.8%). No severe side effects occurred.

Early postoperative pain relief was achieved in all instances. The individual BNI scores for the 3-, 6-, 12-, and 24-month and long-term follow-up are shown in Fig. 10.6. At long-term follow-up (mean 79.5 months, range 29–184 months), 38.5% had complete pain relief (BNI I), 42.3% had pain relief but continued taking medication (BNI IIIa), 12% had a BNI score of IV, and 8% had a BNI score V. The exact cause of re-recurrence could not be determined, since none of the patients underwent secondary posterior fossa re-exploration [8].

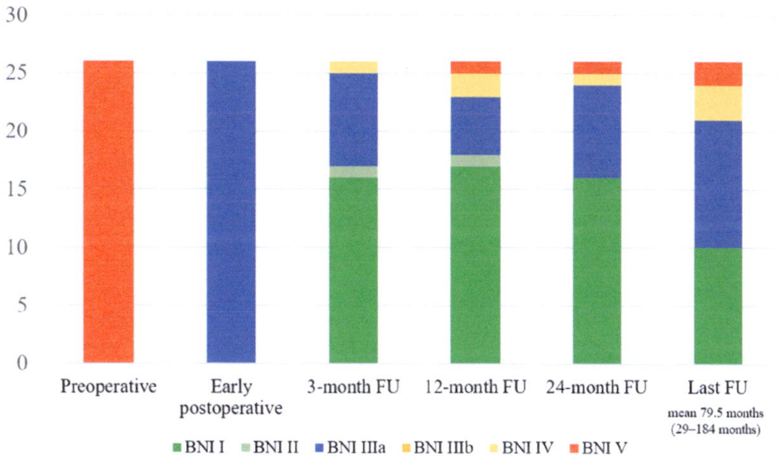

Fig. 10.6 Severity of pain according to the Barrow Neurological Institute (BNI) pain intensity score in a series of 26 patients before and after posterior fossa re-exploration after previous successful microvascular decompression (adapted from [8]). *FU* follow-up

10.8 Posterior Fossa Re-exploration: Outcome in the Literature

Published outcome after posterior fossa re-exploration has been quite variable, depending on the different frequency of intraoperative findings and surgical techniques, as well as pain assessment methods. Operative techniques include partial or total removal of the implant, placement of new implant material, sling technique, coagulation of veins, adhesiolysis, and in the presumed absence of a causative finding by the surgeon, partial sensory rhizotomy or nerve combing. According to a systematic review of patients undergoing posterior fossa re-exploration, the majority of patients reported relief of pain at a similar frequency like after the MVD. Long-term follow-up studies, however, have rarely been performed [29].

Posterior fossa re-exploration, in general, has been described to be relatively safe. The mean rate of facial numbness was reported as 24%, ranging from 0% to 52% in the literature [7, 9, 17, 29, 33, 60]. Other much more infrequent complications include bothersome dysesthesia, hearing loss, abducens nerve palsy, facial palsy, ataxia, CSF leak, aseptic meningitis, and wound infection [9, 29].

In the largest study with patients with TN undergoing MVD, Barker et al. reported an excellent outcome in 42%, and a good outcome in 5% of patients. In this series of 132 reoperated patients, veins or small arteries were the compressing vessels most frequently found, but this included cases performed within 30 days after the initial surgery [1]. Kureshi and Wilkins, having found no new causative factor for recurrence in 16 out of 23 reoperated patients performed a partial sensory rhizotomy, and reported complete pain relief in 15 patients, and partial relief in 6 patients at a mean follow-up of 3.5 years [57]. In a series on 31 patients, Cho et al. reported improvement of pain depending on the intraoperative findings at an average follow-up of 6.3 years: in 11/16 patients without a causative finding and undergoing partial sensory rhizotomy; in 5/7 patients with arterial compression; and in 3/4 patients with venous compression; in 3/4 patients with Teflon adhesions [17]. Bakker et al. reported a series in which they had abandoned neurolysis, because of poor results secondary to facial numbness, with 19 out of 33 patients being pain-free without medication at 12-month follow-up [7].

In a series of 41 patients, by applying a stitched sling retraction for a new vessel, or neurolysis in the case of no intraoperative finding, 30 patients had complete pain relief, and 7 patients had partial pain relief at a mean follow-up of 42 months [53]. In a series of 127 patients, Liu et al. reported 98 patients with BNI II, 22 patients with BNI III and 7 patients with BNI IV with a mean postoperative follow-up of 105.92 months (range 63–167 months) [22]. In the series by Wang et al. comparing 137 reoperated patients,

109 had immediate pain relief, and 89 patients remained pain-free to at least 1 year after follow-up [55].

The frequency of hypesthesia is clearly higher in cohorts from centers performing mechanical intraoperative measures to alter the sensory function of the trigeminal nerve (e.g. combing, or pinching) either routinely, or in patients in whom no clear intraoperative cause was thought to be found [13, 17, 55, 60, 78]. Since long-term outcome with posterior fossa re-exploration is similar regardless of intentional surgical microtrauma, or not, but considering the higher rate of hypesthesia, we suggest that such measures should be avoided.

10.9 No-Contact Techniques

There is a growing interest in the use of noncontact techniques for primary MVD, which can also be applied in posterior fossa re-exploration. Contact of implant material with the nerve predisposes to a risk of recurrence due to compression or adherence, as mentioned above. This was corroborated in a large series showing a higher rate of patients with sustained relief of pain at a follow-up of 15 years by using a noncompressive technique [47].

The same principle has been applied in recurrence cases, with evidence of high efficacy and low rates of recurrence. Matsushima et al. have described on how the adherent Teflon felt to the offending vessel can be fixed to the tentorium using Bio-bond, achieving pain relief in 6 reoperated cases, and observing no recurrence with a mean follow-up of 3 years [59]. Masuoka et al. described the outcome of 50 patients who underwent MVD with a "stitched sling retraction" technique, from which 2 recurrences were noted at a mean follow-up of 5.2 years (range 1.8–6.8 years). None of the patients were reported to undergo another re-exploration [48]. Steinberg et al. reported the outcome of a tentorial sling technique in 45 patients with trigeminal neuralgia at a mean follow-up of 16 months (range 2–36 months), from which 3 patients did develop recurrence of pain. During re-exploration of these patients, all had an intact tentorial sling, although one patient had an ectatic portion of the SCA in contact with the trigeminal nerve, another one had significant adhesions, and the last one presented neither compression nor adhesions of the trigeminal nerve [16]. Patra et al. presented a case of transposition using a vascular clip and creating a small slit in the tentorium in a primary case of TN, achieving complete relief of pain at 6-month follow-up [79]. Other transposition techniques include the use of biological glue and other "sling" techniques with different materials [80].

10.10 Conclusion

Posterior fossa re-exploration is a useful treatment modality for recurrent TN. A tailored approach to address the specific findings associated with recurrence can achieve significant pain relief in the majority of patients without the necessity of direct manipulation of the trigeminal nerve, thus lowering the risk for facial hypesthesia. In the future, it might be worthwhile to explore more "no contact" approaches, including sling techniques, to achieve an even lower risk for recurrence of trigeminal neuralgia.

References

1. Barker FG, Jannetta PJ, Bissonette DJ, Larkins MV, Jho HD. The long-term outcome of microvascular decompression for trigeminal neuralgia. N Engl J Med. 1996;334(17):1077–83.
2. Theodosopoulos PV, Marco E, Applebury C, Lamborn KR, Wilson CB. Predictive model for pain recurrence after posterior fossa surgery for trigeminal neuralgia. Arch Neurol. 2002 Aug;59(8):1297–302.
3. Chen JF, Tu PH, Lee ST. Repeated percutaneous balloon compression for recurrent trigeminal neuralgia: a long-term study. World Neurosurg. 2012;77(2):352–6.
4. Liu G, Du Y, Wang X, Ren Y. Efficacy and safety of repeated percutaneous radiofrequency thermocoagulation for recurrent trigeminal neuralgia. Front Neurol. 2019;18(9):1189.
5. Raygor KP, Wang DD, Ward MM, Barbaro NM, Chang EF. Long-term pain outcomes for recurrent idiopathic trigeminal neuralgia after stereotactic radiosurgery: a prospective comparison of first-time

microvascular decompression and repeat stereotactic radiosurgery. J Neurosurg. 2018;1:1–9.
6. Sarica C, Iorio-Morin C, Aguirre-Padilla DH, Paff M, Villeneuve SA, Vetkas A, Yamamoto K, Samuel N, Milano V, Loh A, Santyr B, Zemmar A, Lozano AM, Hodaie M. Clinical outcomes and complications of peripheral nerve field stimulation in the management of refractory trigeminal pain: a systematic review and meta-analysis. J Neurosurg. 2022;18:1–9.
7. Bakker NA, Van Dijk JM, Immenga S, Wagemakers M, Metzemaekers JD. Repeat microvascular decompression for recurrent idiopathic trigeminal neuralgia. J Neurosurg. 2014;121(4):936–9.
8. Hatipoglu Majernik G, Wolff Fernandes F, Al-Afif S, Heissler HE, Krauss JK. Microsurgical posterior fossa re-exploration for recurrent trigeminal neuralgia after previous microvascular decompression: common grounds-scarring, deformation, and the "piston effect". Acta Neurochir. 2023;165(12):3877–85.
9. Inoue T, Shitara S, Goto Y, Prasetya M, Radcliffe L, Fukushima T. Redo surgery for trigeminal neuralgia: reasons for re-exploration and long-term outcomes. Acta Neurochir. 2021;163(9):2407–16.
10. Jannetta PJ, Bissonette DJ. Management of the failed patient with trigeminal neuralgia. Clin Neurosurg. 1985;32:334–47.
11. Wolff Fernandes F, Krauss JK. Microvascular decompression: a bibliometric analysis of the 100 most cited papers. World Neurosurg. 2022;164:e67–81.
12. Herta J, Schmied T, Loidl TB, Wang WT, Marik W, Winter F, Tomschik M, Ferraz-Leite H, Rössler K, Dorfer C. Microvascular decompression in trigeminal neuralgia: predictors of pain relief, complication avoidance, and lessons learned. Acta Neurochir. 2021;163(12):3321–36.
13. Hussain MA, Konteas A, Sunderland G, Franceschini P, Byrne P, Osman-Farah J, Eldridge P. Re-exploration of microvascular decompression in recurrent trigeminal neuralgia and intraoperative management options. World Neurosurg. 2018;117:e67–74.
14. Mazzucchi E, Brinzeu A, Sindou M. Arachnoiditis as an outcome factor for microvascular decompression in classical trigeminal neuralgia. Acta Neurochir. 2019;161(8):1589–98.
15. Sabourin V, Mazza J, Garzon T, Head J, Ye D, Stefanelli A, Al Saiegh F, Lavergne P, Evans J. Internal neurolysis with and without microvascular decompression for trigeminal neuralgia: case series. World Neurosurg. 2020;143:e70–7.
16. Steinberg JA, Sack J, Wilson B, Weingarten D, Carter B, Khalessi A, Ben-Haim S, Alksne J. Tentorial sling for microvascular decompression in patients with trigeminal neuralgia: a description of operative technique and clinical outcomes. J Neurosurg. 2018;130(4):1315–20.
17. Cho DY, Chang CG, Wang YC, Wang FH, Shen CC, Yang DY. Repeat operations in failed microvascular decompression for trigeminal neuralgia. Neurosurgery. 1994;35(4):665–9.
18. Burchiel KJ, Clarke H, Haglund M, Loeser JD. Long-term efficacy of microvascular decompression of trigeminal neuralgia. J Neurosurg. 1988;69(1):35–8.
19. Sun T, Saito S, Nakai O, Ando T. Long-term results of microvascular decompression for trigeminal neuralgia with reference to probability of recurrence. Acta Neurochir. 1994;126(2–4):144–8.
20. Przybylowski CJ, Cole TS, Baranoski JF, Little AS, Smith KA, Shetter AG. Radiosurgery for multiple sclerosis-related trigeminal neuralgia: retrospective review of long-term outcomes. J Neurosurg. 2018;30:1–8.
21. Li L, Seaman SC, Bathla G, Smith MC, Dundar B, Noeller J, Hitchon PW. Microvascular decompression versus stereotactic radiosurgery for trigeminal neuralgia: a single-institution experience. World Neurosurg. 2020;143:e400–8.
22. Liu J, Wu G, Xiang H, Liu R, Li F, Hei B, Qian W, Song H, Liu Z. Long-term retrospective analysis of microvascular decompression in patients with recurrent trigeminal neuralgia. Front Neurol. 2020a;21(11):584224.
23. Liu R, Deng Z, Zhang L, Liu Y, Wang Z, Yu Y. The long-term outcomes and predictors of microvascular decompression with or without partial sensory rhizotomy for trigeminal neuralgia. J Pain Res. 2020b;5(13):301–12.
24. Pressman E, Hasegawa H, Farooq J, Cohen-Cohen S, Noureldine MHA, Kumar JI, Chen L, Mhaskar R, van Loveren H, Van Gompel JJ, Agazzi S. Teflon versus Ivalon in microvascular decompression for trigeminal neuralgia: a 2-center 10-year comparison. World Neurosurg. 2021;146:e822–8.
25. Chen JF, Lee ST. Comparison of percutaneous trigeminal ganglion compression and microvascular decompression for the management of trigeminal neuralgia. Clin Neurol Neurosurg. 2003;105(3):203–8.
26. Tatli M, Satici O, Kanpolat Y, Sindou M. Various surgical modalities for trigeminal neuralgia: literature study of respective long-term outcomes. Acta Neurochir. 2008;150(3):243–55.
27. Wu J, Xiao Y, Chen B, Zhang R, Dai M, Zhang Y. Efficacy and safety of microvascular decompression versus percutaneous balloon compression in the treatment of trigeminal neuralgia: a systematic review and meta-analysis. Ann Palliat Med. 2022;11(4):1391–400.
28. Zhou Y, Dou NN, Liu XL, Wang H, Zhong J. A comparative review of the outcome following MVD and PBC in patients with trigeminal neuralgia. J Neurol Surg A Cent Eur Neurosurg. 2023;84(5):470–6.
29. Jiao L, Ye H, Lv J, Xie Y, Sun W, Ding G, Cui S. A systematic review of repeat microvascular decompression for recurrent or persistent trigeminal neuralgia. World Neurosurg. 2022;158:226–33.
30. Sindou M, Leston J, Decullier E, Chapuis F. Microvascular decompression for primary trigeminal neuralgia: long-term effectiveness and prognostic factors in a series of 362 consecutive patients with

clear-cut neurovascular conflicts who underwent pure decompression. J Neurosurg. 2007;107(6):1144–53.
31. Van Loveren H, Tew JM, Keller JT, Nurre MA. A 10-year experience in the treatment of trigeminal neuralgia. J Neurosurg. 1982;57(6):757–64.
32. Zorman G, Wilson CB. Outcome following microsurgical vascular decompression or partial sensory rhizotomy in 125 cases of trigeminal neuralgia. Neurology. 1984;34(10):1362–5.
33. Bederson JB, Wilson CB. Evaluation of microvascular decompression and partial sensory rhizotomy in 252 cases of trigeminal neuralgia. J Neurosurg. 1989;71(3):359–67.
34. Klun B. Microvascular decompression and partial sensory rhizotomy in the treatment of trigeminal neuralgia: personal experience with 220 patients. Neurosurgery. 1992;30(1):49–52.
35. Cutbush K, Atkinson RL. Treatment of trigeminal neuralgia by posterior fossa microvascular decompression. Aust N Z J Surg. 1994;64(3):173–6.
36. Sindou MP, Chiha M, Mertens P. Anatomical findings observed during microsurgical approaches of the cerebellopontine angle for vascular decompression in trigeminal neuralgia (350 cases). Stereotact Funct Neurosurg. 1994;63(1–4):203–7.
37. Mendoza N, Illingworth RD. Trigeminal neuralgia treated by microvascular decompression: a long-term follow-up study. Br J Neurosurg. 1995;9(1):13–20.
38. Rath SA, Klein HJ, Richter HP. Findings and long-term results of subsequent operations after failed microvascular decompression for trigeminal neuralgia. Neurosurgery. 1996;39(5):933–8.
39. Liao JJ, Cheng WC, Chang CN, Yang JT, Wei KC, Hsu YH, Lin TK. Reoperation for recurrent trigeminal neuralgia after microvascular decompression. Surg Neurol. 1997;47(6):562–70.
40. Kondo A. Follow-up results of microvascular decompression in trigeminal neuralgia and hemifacial spasm. Neurosurgery. 1997;40(1):46–52.
41. Lee KH, Chang JW, Park YG, Chung SS. Microvascular decompression and percutaneous rhizotomy in trigeminal neuralgia. Stereotact Funct Neurosurg. 1997;68(1–4):196–9.
42. Zhong J, Li ST, Zhu J, Guan HX, Zhou QM, Jiao W, Ying TT, Yang XS, Zhan WC, Hua XM. A clinical analysis on microvascular decompression surgery in a series of 3000 cases. Clin Neurol Neurosurg. 2012;114(7):846–51.
43. Haridas A, Mathewson C, Eljamel S. Long-term results of 405 refractory trigeminal neuralgia surgeries in 256 patients. Zentralbl Neurochir. 2008;69(4):170–4.
44. Jafree DJ, Zakrzewska JM. Long-term pain relief at five years after medical, repeat surgical procedures or no management for recurrence of trigeminal neuralgia after microvascular decompression: analysis of a historical cohort. Br J Neurosurg. 2019;33(1):31–6.
45. Greve T, Tonn JC, Mehrkens JH. Microvascular decompression for trigeminal neuralgia in the elderly: efficacy and safety. J Neurol. 2021;268(2):532–40.
46. Andersen ASS, Heinskou TB, Rochat P, Springborg JB, Noory N, Smilkov EA, Bendtsen L, Maarbjerg S. Microvascular decompression in trigeminal neuralgia—a prospective study of 115 patients. J Headache Pain. 2022;23(1):145.
47. Sindou M, Leston JM, Decullier E, Chapuis F. Microvascular decompression for trigeminal neuralgia: the importance of a noncompressive technique—Kaplan-Meier analysis in a consecutive series of 330 patients. Neurosurgery. 2008;63(4 Suppl 2):341–51.
48. Masuoka J, Matsushima T, Inoue K, Nakahara Y, Takase Y, Kawashima M. Outcome of microvascular decompression for trigeminal neuralgia treated with the stitched sling retraction technique. Neurosurg Rev. 2015;38(2):361–5.
49. Broggi G, Ferroli P, Franzini A, Servello D, Dones I. Microvascular decompression for trigeminal neuralgia: comments on a series of 250 cases, including 10 patients with multiple sclerosis. J Neurol Neurosurg Psychiatry. 2000;68(1):59–64.
50. Hatipoglu Majernik G, Al-Afif S, Heissler HE, Krauss JK. Operative findings and outcome of microvascular decompression/adhesiolysis for trigeminal neuralgia in multiple sclerosis without demyelinating brain stem lesions. Clin Neurol Neurosurg. 2021 Jan;200:106376.
51. Sindou M, Howeidy T, Acevedo G. Anatomical observations during microvascular decompression for idiopathic trigeminal neuralgia (with correlations between topography of pain and site of the neurovascular conflict). Prospective study in a series of 579 patients. Acta Neurochir. 2002;144(1):1–13.
52. Capelle HH, Brandis A, Tschan CA, Krauss JK. Treatment of recurrent trigeminal neuralgia due to Teflon granuloma. J Headache Pain. 2010;11(4):339–44.
53. Cheng J, Meng J, Lei D, Hui X. Repeat microvascular decompression for patients with persistent or recurrent trigeminal neuralgia: prognostic factors and long-term outcomes. Medicine (Baltimore). 2019;98(18):e15167.
54. Sun T, Wang W, Huang Q, He L, Su Y, Li N, Liu J, Yang C. Teflon granuloma: a common cause of recurrent trigeminal neuralgia. World Neurosurg. 2022;158:e612–7.
55. Wang B, Zhang L, Yu Y. Treatment of redo-microvascular decompression or internal neurolysis plus microvascular decompression for recurrent trigeminal neuralgia: a review of long-term effectiveness and safety. J Int Med Res. 2022;50(3):3000605221080721.
56. Zhong J. Identification of the leverage point in the offending artery. Acta Neurochir. 2024;166(1):10.
57. Kureshi SA, Wilkins RH. Posterior fossa reexploration for persistent or recurrent trigeminal neuralgia or hemifacial spasm: surgical findings and therapeutic implications. Neurosurgery. 1998;43(5):1111–7.

58. Chen J, Lee S, Lui T, Yeh Y, Chen T, Tzaan W. Teflon granuloma after microvascular decompression for trigeminal neuralgia. Surg Neurol. 2000;53(3):281–7.
59. Matsushima T, Yamaguchi T, Inoue TK, Matsukado K, Fukui M. Recurrent trigeminal neuralgia after microvascular decompression using an interposing technique. Teflon felt adhesion and the sling retraction technique. Acta Neurochir. 2000;142(5):557–61.
60. Amador N, Pollock BE. Repeat posterior fossa exploration for patients with persistent or recurrent idiopathic trigeminal neuralgia. J Neurosurg. 2008;108(5):916–20.
61. Gu W, Zhao W. Microvascular decompression for recurrent trigeminal neuralgia. J Clin Neurosci. 2014;21(9):1549–53.
62. Yang DB, Jiang DY, Chen HC, Wang ZM. Second microvascular decompression for trigeminal neuralgia in recurrent cases after microvascular decompression. J Craniofac Surg. 2015;26(2):491–4.
63. Feng BH, Wang XH, Li ST. Posterior fossa re-exploration for recurrent trigeminal neuralgia: operative findings and surgical techniques. J Craniofac Surg. 2018;29:1284–6.
64. Huang Z, Pu B, Li F, Liu K, Hua C, Li C, Zhao C, Li J, Li X. Analysis of failed microvascular decompression in patients with trigeminal neuralgia. J Neurol Surg B Skull Base. 2020;81(5):567–71.
65. McLaughlin MR, Jannetta PJ, Clyde BL, Subach BR, Comey CH, Resnick DK. Microvascular decompression of cranial nerves: lessons learned after 4400 operations. J Neurosurg. 1999;90(1):1–8.
66. Zhong J, Zhu J, Sun H, Dou NN, Wang YN, Ying TT, Xia L, Liu MX, Tao BB, Li ST. Microvascular decompression surgery: surgical principles and technical nuances based on 4000 cases. Neurol Res. 2014;36(10):882–93.
67. Lee SH, Levy EI, Scarrow AM, Kassam A, Jannetta PJ. Recurrent trigeminal neuralgia attributable to veins after microvascular decompression. Neurosurgery. 2000;46(2):356–62.
68. Soni P, Potter T, Soni PP, Estemalik E, Recinos PF, Kshettry VR. Outcomes of microvascular decompression for trigeminal neuralgia with purely venous compression: a systematic review and meta-analysis. Clin Neurol Neurosurg. 2020;198:106230.
69. Premsagar IC, Moss T, Coakham HB. Teflon-induced granuloma following treatment of trigeminal neuralgia by microvascular decompression. Report of two cases. J Neurosurg. 1997;87(3):454–7.
70. Wolff Fernandes F, Schmeitz CD, Hartmann C, Krauss JK. Recurrence of trigeminal neuralgia after microvascular decompression: a systematical histopathological evaluation of Teflon granuloma. J Neurosurg (in press). 2025.
71. Sindou M, Brinzeu A. Trigeminal Neuralgias: A Neurosurgical Illustrated guide. Cham: Springer; 2023.
72. Bendtsen L, Zakrzewska JM, Abbott J, Braschinsky M, Di Stefano G, Donnet A, Eide PK, Leal PRL, Maarbjerg S, May A, Nurmikko T, Obermann M, Jensen TS, Cruccu G. European academy of neurology guideline on trigeminal neuralgia. Eur J Neurol. 2019;26(6):831–49.
73. Hatipoglu Majernik G, Wolff Fernandes F, Al-Afif S, Heissler HE, Palmaers T, Atallah O, Scheinichen D, Krauss JK. Routine postoperative admission to the neurocritical intensive care unit after microvascular decompression: necessary or can it be abandoned? Neurosurg Rev. 2022;46(1):12.
74. Flor H, Rasche D, Islamian AP, Rolko C, Yilmaz P, Ruppolt M, Capelle HH, Tronnier V, Krauss JK. Subtle sensory abnormalities detected by quantitative sensory testing in patients with trigeminal neuralgia. Pain Physician. 2016;19(7):507–18.
75. Hatipoglu Majernik G, Al-Afif S, Heissler HE, Cassini Ascencao L, Krauss JK. Microvascular decompression: is routine postoperative CT imaging necessary? Acta Neurochir. 2020;162(5):1095–9.
76. Pirayesh Islamian A, Lütjens G, Krauss JK. Microvascular decompression of the eighth cranial nerve for unilateral pulsatile tinnitus. Clin Neurol Neurosurg. 2014;117:102–6.
77. Younes WM, Capelle HH, Krauss JK. Microvascular decompression of the anterior inferior cerebellar artery for intermediate nerve neuralgia. Stereotact Funct Neurosurg. 2010;88(3):193–5.
78. Zheng W, Dong X, Wang D, Hu Q, Du Q. Long time efficacy and safety of microvascular decompression combined with internal neurolysis for recurrent trigeminal neuralgia. J Korean Neurosurg Soc. 2021;64(6):966–74.
79. Patra DP, Turcotte EL, Krishna C, Zimmerman RS, Batjer HH, Bendok BR. Microvascular decompression technique for trigeminal neuralgia using a vascular clip. World Neurosurg. 2021;154:1.
80. Ohta M, Komatsu F, Abe H, Sakamoto S, Tsugu H, Oshiro S, Fukushima T. Complication caused by use of fibrin glue in vessel transposition for trigeminal neuralgia. Neurol Med Chir (Tokyo). 2008;48(1):30–2.

11 Atypical Trigeminal Neuralgias: Neurosurgical Management

Marc Sindou and Andrei Brinzeu

11.1 Introduction

According to the International Headache Society (IHS), **trigeminal neuralgia (TN)** is defined as "a disorder characterized by recurrent unilateral brief electric shock-like pains, abrupt in onset and termination, limited to the distribution of one or more division(s) of the trigeminal nerve and triggered by innocuous stimuli. It may develop without apparent cause or be a result of another disorder." [1].

Easy in the typical form, **the diagnosis can be difficult with atypical presentations**. The choice of effective medication for these patients while attempting to limit side effects and, when the neuralgia becomes refractory, the decision for the appropriate surgical method are puzzling.

The **aim of this chapter** is to define the frame of these particular clinical presentations and propose trails to help find solutions for their therapeutic management.

M. Sindou (✉)
Department of Neurosurgery, University of Lyon, Lyon, France

A. Brinzeu
Neuroscience Research Center, Department of Neurosciences, University of Medicine "Victor Babes", Timisoara, Romania

11.2 Definitions and Clinical Presentations

The diagnosis of TN is clinical. Classification requires imaging.

Trigeminal neuralgia can reveal an underlying pathology and thus corresponds to **"secondary"** neuralgia. When considered **"primary,"** TN is often due to vascular compression with structural alteration(s) of the root; in this eventuality it is said to be **"classical"** [2]. When no etiology is found, the neuralgia is termed **"idiopathic"** [3].

The incidence of primary TNs is 4–13 new cases per year per 100,000 population according to reports [4]. Primary TN is rather a disease of middle age and senescence, with pain occurring three out of four times after the age of 50; late onset after age 70 is not uncommon. The female predominance is constant in all the series with a prevalence ratio from 2:3 to 3:5 according to reports.

11.3 Classification on Presumed Etiology [2]

1. ***Secondary Trigeminal Neuralgia***

   Trigeminal neuralgia caused by an underlying disease. Clinical examination often shows sensory changes in a significant proportion of these patients.

S.-T. Li et al. (eds.), *Microvascular Decompression Surgery*,
https://doi.org/10.1007/978-981-96-0767-9_11

Diagnostic criteria

(a) *Recurrent paroxysms of unilateral facial pain, either purely paroxysmal or associated with concomitant continuous or near-continuous pain.*

(b) *Underlying disease demonstrated and known to be able to cause neuralgia.*

2. ***Classical Trigeminal Neuralgia***

Trigeminal neuralgia developing without apparent cause other than neurovascular compression.

Diagnostic criteria

(a) *Recurrent paroxysms of unilateral facial pain [Classical TN may be purely paroxysmal or with concomitant continuous pain].*

(b) *Demonstration on MRI (or during surgery) of neurovascular compression (not simply contact) with morphological changes in the trigeminal nerve root.*

3. ***Idiopathic Trigeminal Neuralgia***

Trigeminal neuralgia for which investigations do not show significant abnormalities.

Diagnostic criteria

(a) *Recurrent paroxysms of unilateral facial pain, either purely paroxysmal or associated with concomitant continuous or near-continuous pain.*

(b) *Neither Classical trigeminal neuralgia nor Secondary trigeminal neuralgia has been confirmed by adequate investigation including electrophysiological tests and MRI.*

(c) *Not better accounted for another ICHD-3 diagnosis (International Classification of Headache Disorders).*

11.3.1 The Atypical Trigeminal Neuralgia(s) [= Trigeminal Neuralgias with Concomitant Continuous Pain]

Trigeminal neuralgias can take an atypical presentation, characterized by the association to paroxysmal pain of a permanent background of deep aching or burning pain. The paroxysmal component can be on the back row or even be absent, especially if the patient is under anticonvulsant medications. This presentation has been termed by the ICHD (International Classification of Headache Disorders): "Trigeminal neuralgia with concomitant continuous pain" [1].

If the paroxysmal component is missing, it can be difficult to establish relation of the pain with the frame of TN. It is therefore essential to investigate by questioning the existence of paroxysms at the onset of the disease, before anticonvulsants were administered. In the most difficult situations in which the diagnosis would remain doubtful, anticonvulsant drugs can be legitimately withdrawn; the test usually results in the reappearance of the paroxysmal component (Fig. 11.1).

Patients with a continuous background of pain may have some degree of sensory loss, more often than those that presented with paroxysmal attacks solely, as pointed out by a quantitative sensory testing study [5]. This hypoesthesia—somewhat misleading—must be verified by several examinations as it could be related to the proximity of the last painful attack.

The incidence of atypical trigeminal neuralgia is variously evaluated according to the reports, some from neurosurgical origin others not. In our global "surgical" series of more than 6000 patients operated on over a 25 year-period, at the time they were referred for surgery (from 1 to 36 years after onset of the disease, 6.4 years on average), 35% of them presented with an atypical form. It has been suggested by Burchiel that along the natural history of all neuralgias one encounters more and more a continuous background of pain [6]. Also Maarbjerg found that 49% of his 158 patients' series had a concomitant background of pain with a significant difference in the response to sodium channel blockers [7]. However, this has not been verified in a more recent series of 200 patients under medical treatment alone [8].

The rather high frequency of neuralgias with an atypical clinical presentation when the patients are seen after a long evolution, as those often referred to the surgeon, is not difficult to understand. A long evolution of the neuralgia may induce chronic damage to the nerve therefore

Fig. 11.1 Diagnosis of Atypical Trigeminal Neuralgia, from Unilateral Oro-Facial pain to Trigeminal Neuralgia

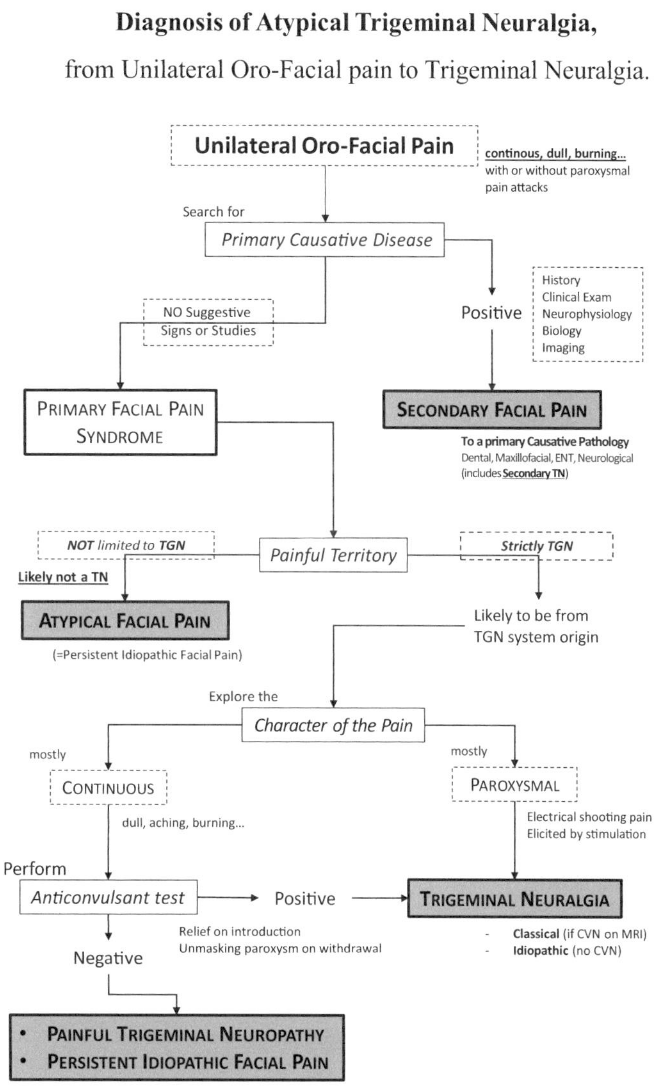

contributing to a continuous background of the pain and reduction of the intermittent attacks. In those patients the interview should try to retrospectively find out paroxysms, as well as the provoked character of the pains at the onset of the condition. Difficulty of diagnosis may even justify halting the treatment and wait for the reappearance of the paroxysmal component that may not manifest under carbamazepine or equivalents.

Terminology remains a matter of debate. William Sweet from Harvard University, the reference neurosurgeon in the 1970s/1980s [9] and more recently the IHS Committee [1] distinguished Classical TNs in Typical and Atypical on their clinical characteristics, the first being "purely paroxysmal," the second « with concomitant continuous pain.»

Burchiel in 2003 introduced an alternative classification system for facial pain [10] Trigeminal neuralgias were divided into Type 1 and Type2. In Type 1, patients presented predominantly (>50%) with pain that was episodic, lancinating, "electric," triggerable, subject to pain-free intervals and generally responsive to anticonvulsant therapy, while in Type 2, patients presented with more constant (>50%) dull, aching, burning pain, without free intervals and fundamentally nonresponsive to anticonvulsant therapy. For Burchiel atypical facial pain was reserved (as in the past) for patients with proven psychogenic pain. The difficulty of this system is in the quantification of the degree of atypical pain. It is hard to choose between patients with 50% or less atypical signs. According to Maarbjerg, in this system some patients with "Persistent idiopathic facial pain" may end up being classified as Type 2 trigeminal neuralgia, whereas in other classification systems they would not be included in the neuralgia group [11, 12]. However, the Burchiel's classification is widely used in the neurosurgical community and particularly so in the series analyzing outcome after surgical treatment.

11.3.2 Atypical Trigeminal Neuralgia(s): Difficulties for Diagnosis (Table 11.1)

Although not frequent, but because atypical in their clinical presentation, **Trigeminal neuralgias with autonomic involvement** have to be mentioned. Autonomic symptoms such as nasal congestion, lacrimation, and redness of the eye may be present especially in the neuralgia involving the ophthalmic division; their presence does not preclude the diagnosis of trigeminal neuralgia. Recommended action is to use a carbamazepine test to distinguish between trigeminal neuralgia and cluster headache.

Table 11.1 Differential Characteristics of the main various Facial Pain Syndromes

Facial pain syndrome Characteristics	Trigeminal neuralgias	Trigeminal autonomic cephalalgias (cluster headache)	Painful trigeminal neuropathies (Neuropathic pain)	Persistent idiopathic facial pain (atypical facial pain)
Gender	Slight female predominance	Major male predominance	Any gender	Female predominance
Age	> 50	30–50	Any age	Any age
Topography	Strictly unilateral* Trigeminal root divisions	Strictly unilateral* Territory of the external carotid (retro-orbital)	Peripheral territory Or Trigeminal root divisions	Deep in the – Maxillary – Frontal – Dental Regions Unsystematized diffuse facial,
Pain characteristics	Paroxysmal: Shooting, electric, shock-like In atypical presentation: – Concomitant continuous pain – In addition to paroxysmal pain	Throbbing, burning, Often accompanied by vasomotor disturbances: Tearing, eye redness, Claude Bernard Horner sign	Burning continuous background pain, often associated with paresthesias/ dysesthesias	Dull, aching, nagging
Rhythm	Attack of pain for a few seconds to several minutes Refractory period	Attack lasts from one to several hours Period of several weeks	Steady pain	Daily >2 h/day >3 months
Clinical evaluation	Normal in the typical form	Dysautonomic signs in the face	Hypoesthesia, allodynia	Normal
Exploratory studies	Potential NVC in classical TN	Wise to ask for MRI	Depending on the damaging causal agent	Negative
Response to pharmacotherapy	Responds to anticonvulsants (carbamazepine)	Responds to triptans	No specific medication	Does not respond directly to anything (in particular not anticonvulsants)

*can be on both sides but not synchronously

A particularly difficult situation is the one encountered with the **patients who previously had trigeminal surgery** and still suffer from a (rather marked) background of continuous pain, associated with more or less of paroxysmal attacks. Recurrence is very common after neurolytic or destructive surgery on the peripheral branches of the trigeminal nerve. Also, the lesioning techniques directed to the trigeminal root or ganglion whether percutaneous or radio-surgical may produce more or less significant painful hypoesthesia in the territory of the targeted fibers, as well as some degree of paresthesia and/or dysesthesias. At least a part of those disturbances is likely to fall within the frame of neuropathic pain, known to be difficult to control. The differential diagnosis between neuropathic pain and a remaining neuralgic component is essentially based on clinical criteria; it should also take into account the sensitivity to anticonvulsants, and requires new neurophysiological investigations and fine imaging.

Perhaps the most difficult problem when confronted to atypical trigeminal neuralgia is its **differentiation from the so-called atypical facial pain condition.** Their distinction is therapeutically crucial. "Atypical facial pain" **termed by the IHS as "persistent idiopathic facial pain"** is not significantly influenced by the anticonvulsant drugs [1]. These patients should not be treated surgically. As a matter of fact, "persistent idiopathic facial pain" is a totally different entity from atypical trigeminal neuralgia, and is generally considered of psychological origin. The differential diagnosis between atypical trigeminal neuralgia and atypical facial pain can be very difficult to the point that Sweet qualified the later «La bête noire du neurochirurgien» in french in his book "Pain and the Neurosurgeon: a forty-year experience"[13].

11.3.3 Atypical Trigeminal Neuralgia and Neurovascular Conflicts

Differences between typical and atypical TNs, in etiology and long-term outcome, have not yet been definitively put in evidence and remain controversial.

Miller et al. reported that in patients with Type 1 presentation, neuralgia was more often associated with arterial compression while venous compression or no compression at all was more frequent in Type 2 patients. Type 1; patients also were less likely to recur after microvascular decompression than Type 2 patients [14].

In our series of microvascular decompression which enrolled 362 patients with neurovascular conflicts, and which included the cases with atypical elements in their clinical presentation—while less frequent (34.5%) than those with a purely typical form—the group with atypical TN did not fare worse after neurovascular decompression than the one with typical presentation [15].

However, in Maarbjerg et al.'s study, correlation of neurovascular conflict with typical or atypical presentation could not be made [11, 12].

The comment can therefore be made that the distinction between typical and atypical neuralgias is not sufficient to define distinct clinical entities, but that—in concordance to Burchiel and Miller's views—when the continuous background of pain predominates over paroxysmal attacks, outcome is poorer, therefore arguing for a separate clinical and perhaps pathophysiological entity of the Type 2 neuralgia. This would be enforced by the decreased likelihood of an active vascular compression. However, this appears to be accounted for in the IHS classification by the idiopathic trigeminal neuralgia diagnosis which indeed has poorer outcome upon vascular decompression. In order to clearly define these entities further studies are needed in imaging in order to provide methods to differentiate between active and insignificant neurovascular conflicts as well as statistical analysis on clusters of patients to make the distinction between the proposed clinical entities [16, 17].

To be recalled, standard imaging is most often able to rule out secondary neuralgias and—if negative—to orientate the diagnosis toward the primary nature of the neuralgia. Standard imaging is not sufficient to study the fine anatomy of the nerves and vascular structures. To detect and-characterize NVCs, which differentiate Classical TN from Idiopathic TN, a high-resolution MRI is needed. If available, a 3-Tesla machine is preferred; otherwise, a 1.5-Tesla machine is mostly sufficient. Optimal reliability necessitates the association of the three following sequences. The high-resolution 3D-T2 sequence gives fine images with good contrast between the cerebrospinal fluid (in hypersignal) and the vascular and nerve structures. The 3D-time-of-flight-angiography (3D-TOF-angiography) sequence visualizes the high flux vessels, i.e., principally the arteries. The 3D-T1 sequence with gadolinium injection depicts (in hypersignal) all the vascular structures, i.e., not only the arteries but also the veins [18–20]. The diffusion-tensor imaging (DTI) methodology, which enables the analysis of the white matter integrity by means of in vivo measurements of molecular diffusivity, may be indicated to detect alteration of the neural tissue at the site of a suspected compressive vessel [21].

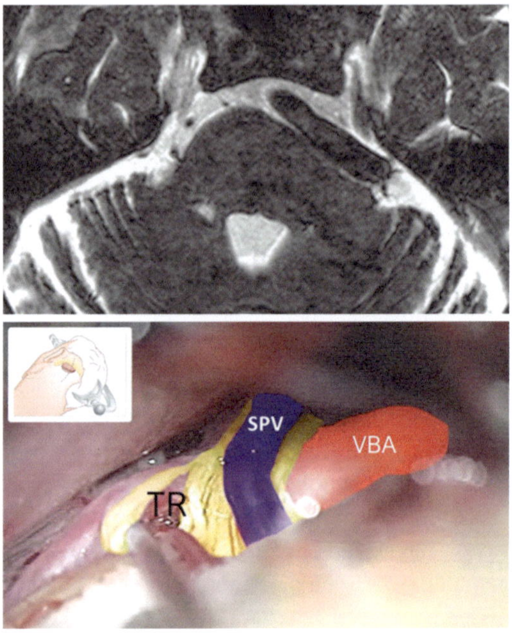

Fig. 11.2 Left classical, atypical, trigeminal neuralgia due to severe compression and stretching of the trigeminal root (TR) by a megadolicho-VertebroBasilar Artery (VBA), as shown on corresponding high-resolution T2-MRI. Note the superior petrosal vein (SPV) parallel to the root

11.4 Anatomical Factors Potentially Favoring Atypical Presentation

Outside iatrogenic causes adding to the paroxysmal component of the neuralgia a background of continuous pain, to our knowledge there are no published studies searching for potential factor(s) able to definitively confer it an atypical clinical presentation, with perhaps the exception of a long evolution over time. However, on approximately 6000 patients' experience of dealing with their TN, in spite of no specific statistical cluster analysis (that we deeply regret), we estimate that some anatomical factors play a role in modifying the neuralgia toward an atypical clinical presentation, more or less dominated by a "concomitant continuous painful component" according to the IHS definition.

11.4.1 Megadolicho-Vertebro-Basilar Artery

The biggest compressions exerted by arteries (that represented 93% of the encountered NVCs in our series) were those by the vertebro-basilar (VB) system; its arteries being elongated, of huge caliber, and additionally with atheromatous walls. Megadolicho-VB arteries implicated in the 579 enrolled patients for the study amounted at 3.5% of the cases [22].

If a "clean" and safe decompression appears to not be possible, one can have recourse to partial rhizotomy, limited to the fascicles corresponding to the pain territory (Fig. 11.2).

11.4.2 Vein with Print on the Root

In our series of classical TNs who underwent MVD, the incidence of venous contact/compression was as high as 38% [22]. In 8.9% a vein was the sole compressive vessel, most often the Inferior Transverse Vein, located at exit of the root from the porus of the trigeminal cave (Fig. 11.3). In 29.1% the venous compression was associated to an arterial compression (Fig. 11.4). In approximately half of the 38%

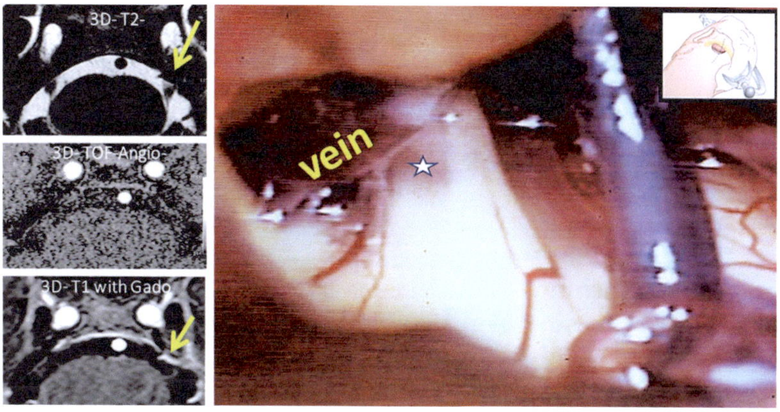

Fig. 11.3 Left classical, atypical, trigeminal neuralgia due to pure venous neurovascular conflict, as demonstarted on the axial section of the T1 + Gadolinium MRI sequence (compared to the TOF-Angio sequence). The conflicting vessel is the inferior transverse pontine vein, belonging to the deep superior petrosal venous system (operative view). The venous compression created a focal demyelination, manifested by a grayish aspect in the root (star). Decompression was achieved by coagulation and suppression of the compressive vein

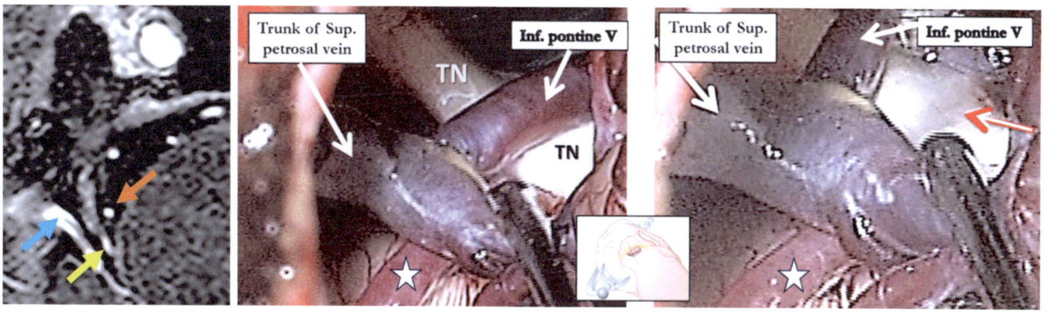

Fig. 11.4 Exposure through a right infratentorial–supracerebellar approach, inside the cerebello-mesencephalic fissure, of the superior petrosal venous trunk which drains the superior petrosal vein with its pontine affluent to the superior petrosal sinus. The trigeminal nerve root (TN) is squeezed between the inferior pontine vein, dorsally, and the superior cerebellar artery with its two division branches (star), ventrally, the later pushing down the root onto the inferior pontine vein. See on the right image, under retraction of the inferior pontine vein, the print of the vein on the root, marked by a focal greyish discoloration at the conflict site, of the highest grade III of our compression classification (red/yellow arrow). Decompression was performed by liberating the root from the venous compression and by pushing upward the superior cerebellar artery with a plate of Teflon to maintain it apart (not shown). On the left image, MRI with T1+ Gado sequence shows the mixed arterial/venous conflict, with the superior petrosal venous trunk (blue arrow), the inferior transverse vein dorsally to the root (yellow arrow), and the superior cerebellar artery ventrally (orange arrow)

(17.6%), the vein exerted a marked compression on the root. In our study, venous compressions were not only at TREZ (27%), but also at the mid-cisternal portion of the root (40%) or the porus (33%) [23]. This large distribution of locations justifies a systematic exploration of the entire root, from brainstem to trigeminal cave.

Certainty about the responsibility of a vein as a compressive vessel is often difficult, and testing its compressive effect (i.e., mobilizing it) can be hazardous. Our criteria for retaining a vein as a compressive factor are the following:

1. On imaging including T2, TOF–Angio, and T1 + Gadolinium—sequence, vein achieving a cross-compression rather than having a parallel course;

2. Upon intraoperative exploration, vein making a print, especially if there is a grayish discoloration of the root at level of the compression. At porus, exploration is often confronted to veins stuck to the root by arachnoid adhesions, that must be dissected free.

11.4.3 Angulation/Stretching of the Root on Crossing over the Upper Petrous Ridge

The shape of the petrous ridge, namely its sharpness at porus of Meckel cave, and angulation of the TGN at crossing over the upper ridge can be an alternative or a supplementary factor that may cause or contribute to the neuralgia (Fig. 11.5).

In a study on 42 patients, the averaged bony angle of the petrous ridge was found to be more acute on the neuralgic (86^0) than on the asymptomatic side (90^0) ($p = 0.06$), and highly significantly sharper (86^0) than that of the control group (98^0) ($p = 0.004$) [16, 17]. In same study, in patients with grade II or III of compression the angle of the nerve on crossing over the upper ridge was found at 140^0 on average on the side of the neuralgia vs. 149^0 on the asymptomatic side ($p = 0.003$).

More generally, angulation with stretching of the root on crossing over the petrous ridge is frequently observed in elder patients with important global atrophy, corresponding to a so-called **sagging phenomenon** of brainstem and cerebellum in the posterior fossa (Fig. 11.6). This anatomical/imaging phenomenon is so that those structures are submitted to ptosis with traction of the TGNs on the petrous ridge. At the point of the angulation, the root— most often atrophic—is ribbon-shaped, with a grayish aspect likely to correspond to local demyelination [16, 17]. Such a mechanism encountered in classical TNs can be evocated, also and even more, to explain a number of so-called idiopathic TNs, especially in aged patients. Those patients should not undergo open MVD surgery.

11.4.4 Role of the (Small) Size of the Cerebello-Pontine Angle Cistern

Studies based on volumetric measurements showed that patients with TN tended to have a smaller CPA cistern than normal subjects, and that cistern was smaller on the affected side rather than on the contralateral side. [24–29]. Also, Parise et al. showed that in patients suffering from TN, nerves were shorter on the affected side

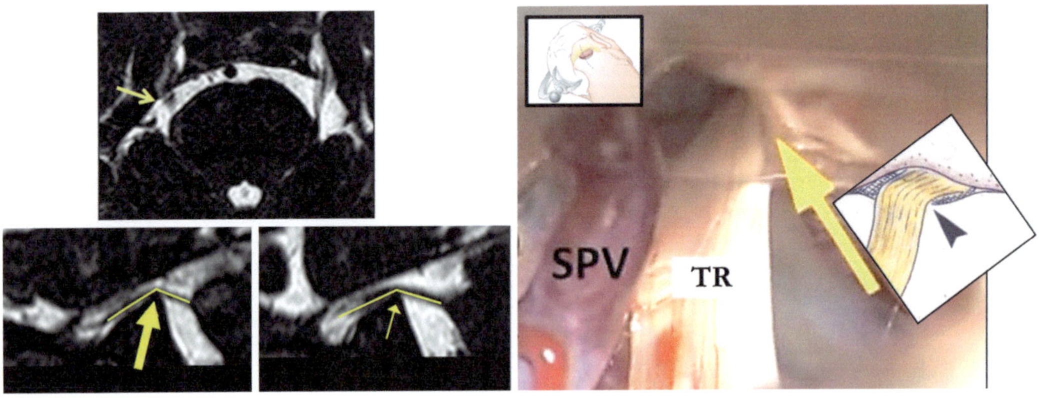

Fig. 11.5 Illustrative case of a right trigeminal neuralgia linked to an angulation/stretching of the trigeminal root (TR) on crossing over the petrous ridge at exit of root from porus of the trigeminal cave (bigger arrow). Note on MRI the more marked angulation of the root on the right side at crossing over the petrous ridge (yellow arrow). Also note on the operative view the ribbon-shaped and the grayish aspect (= demyelination) of the root at level of the angulation (arrow). In this case the Superior Petrosal Vein (SPV), coursing parallel to the root, was not considered conflicting the root

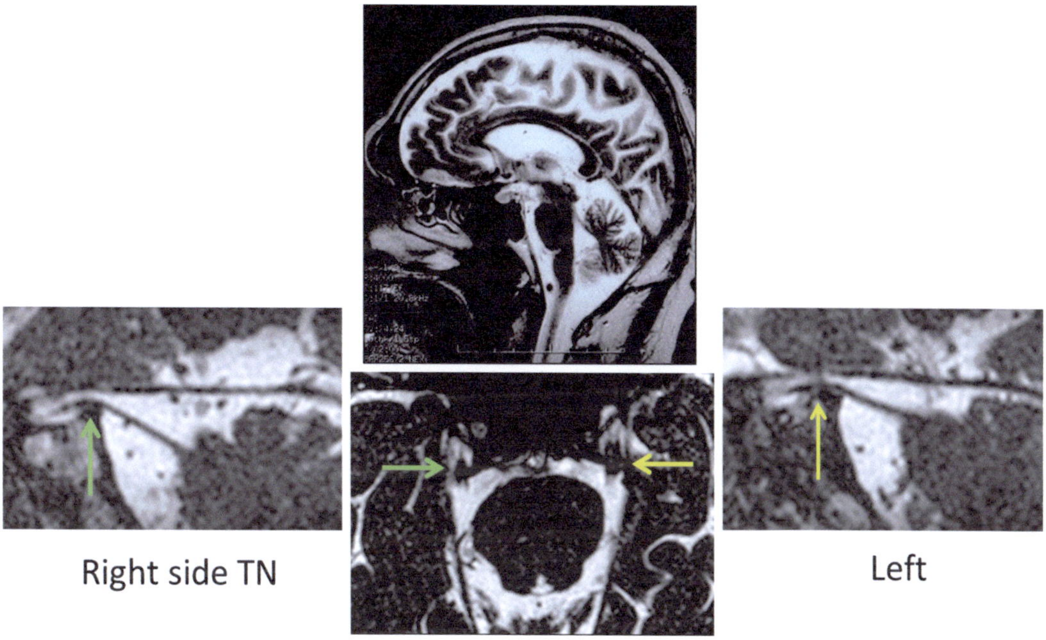

Fig. 11.6 Stretched trigeminal roots with angulation on crossing over the upper petrous ridge (arrows) as often encountered in patients with important atrophic brain and cerebellum, well visible on the MRI pictures. Such "Sagging phenomenon" was often noticed by the senior author on the occasion of posterior fossa exploration in elder patients suffering from trigeminal neuralgia. A grayish aspect of the nerve at the point of angulation, corresponding to local demyelination, was frequently observed in those patients. Hypothesis is that the TGNs undergo traction by the gravity of the brainstem and cerebellum. This phenomenon might be a factor influencing the pathogenesis of the neuralgia, and also could explain the eventual failure or incomplete effect of the MVD procedure, even when a neurovascular conflict is found, especially in elder patients

[27]. In brief, cisterns of small capacity with subsequently trigeminal root more or less squeezed in between pons, cerebellum, and petrous pyramid favorize impaction of vessel(s) into the root. This corresponds to the concept of the so-called crowded posterior fossa (Fig. 11.7).

11.4.5 Presence of Local "Arachnoiditis"

The presence of thickened arachnoid membranes responsible for adhesions and coalescence between nerve and neighboring vessels is not so uncommon finding in patients with classical TN (Figs. 11.8). Such local "arachnoiditis" was found in 13% of the patients in a series of 375 patients who were operated on for MVD [30]. In these 13%, the clinical presentation of the neuralgia was typical in 59% of the patients and atypical in 31%, which is 10% higher than the percentage of the whole series [31]. In the group with local arachnoiditis the outcome was poorer, with a probability of being pain free at 15 years of follow-up of 42%, versus 80% for the whole series. However, the pain free probability was of 75.2% when the NVC was of a high grade of compression vs only of 33% when the NVC was of a low grade [30].

Unfortunately, the present state of imaging technology cannot reliably predict focal arachnoiditis, and therefore help to forecast pejorative prognosis.

11.4.6 Presence of a Global Atrophy of the Root, and the Role of Age

In many patients suffering from primary trigeminal neuralgia, especially elder patients, the

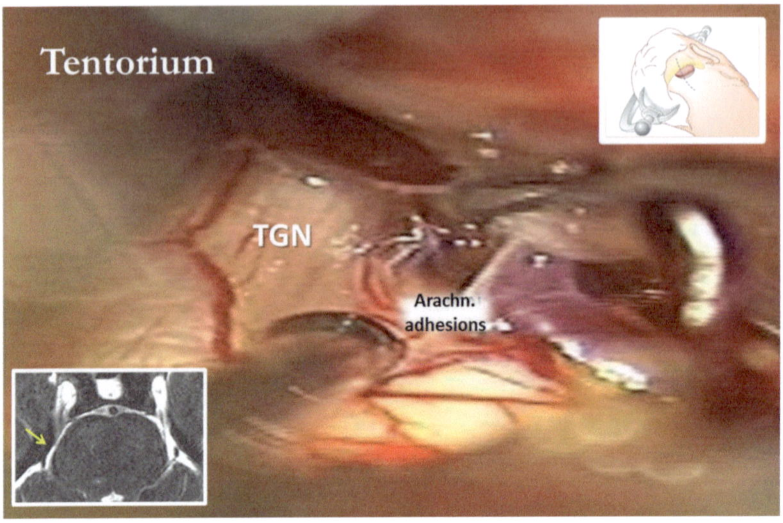

Fig. 11.7 Illustrative case of small size of the cerebellopontine angle cistern on the right side in a patient affected with a right trigeminal neuralgia. Its reduced capacity, as can be noticed in the MRI compared to the contralateral side, by being responsible for a squeezed TGN, was considered likely to play a role in the genesis of the neuralgia. Pain was relieved after decompressive craniectomy with duroplasty enlargement of the posterior fossa, freeing the TGN from the arachnoid adhesions, and additional sacrifice of the stuck vein

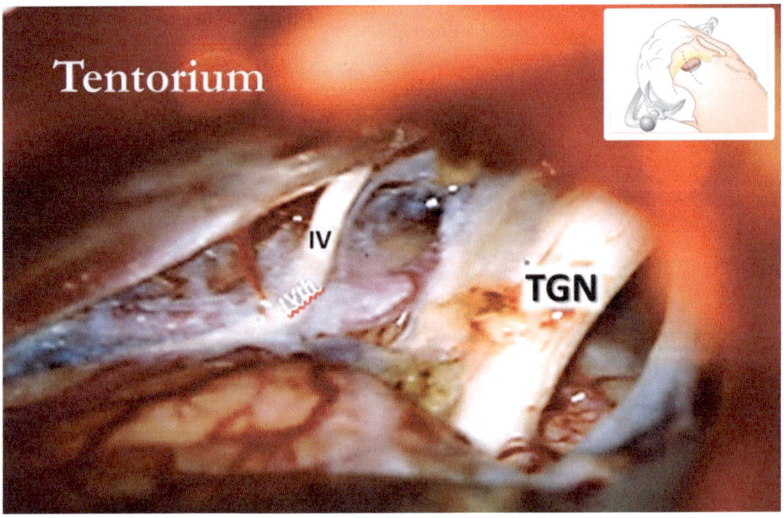

Fig. 11.8 Intraoperative image illustrating a case of strong local arachnoiditis. The arachnoid membrane was thick, hard at dissection, and adhesive to the trigeminal nerve root (TGN), and also to the trochlear nerve (IV)

trigeminal root (TR) was found **globally atrophic**, whether root was with or without vascular compression, that is in 42% of our surgically-explored patients (Fig. 11.9). Atrophy was marked to severe (i.e., equal or more than half of what would be considered a normal diameter in approximately half of those [22]. Global atrophy can be easily seen on T2-sequence of high-resolution MRI. At surgery, roots may present with a grayish aspect testifying a more or less degree of demyelination compared with healthy TGNs. We interpretate such global atrophy as a stigma of neuropathic alteration of the whole root.

In a statistical correlative study on the long-term outcome (15 years) following MVD, the influence of such global atrophy of the root on pain relief was evaluated [31]. Although probability of relief was lesser in the group with a

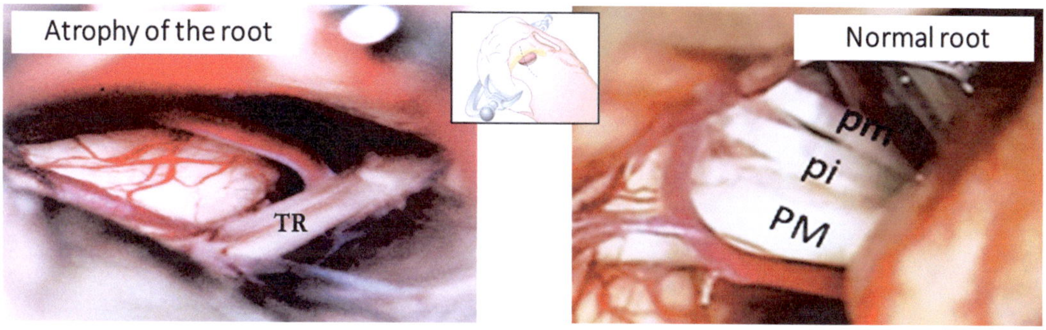

Fig. 11.9 In many patients suffering from trigeminal neuralgia, especially elder patients, the trigeminal root (TR) is frequently seen with global atrophy, whether root is w/ or w/o vascular compression. Left operative image illustrates a globally atrophic TR; the elongated superior cerebellar artery in a superomedial situation does not seem to be compressive for the root. For comparison purpose, right image shows a healthy trigeminal root in the right cerebellopontine angle cistern. *PM* pars major, *pi* pars intermediaris, *pm* pars minor

severely atrophic root, difference did not reveal statistically significant ($p = 0.36$).

Study of the **influence of age** on probability of long-term outcome after MVD showed that the group of the elder patients, i.e., those above 70 years of age (more propitious to harbor root atrophy), have not a lower rate of pain relief than the younger group [31].

11.5 Available Methods

When confronted to an atypical clinical presentation, because—classically— relief is more difficult to obtain than in the typical presentation, pros-and cons-of the considered surgical method have to be critically weighted.

Below, we provide a few (simple) recommendations based on our experience in managing trigeminal neuralgia and its neurosurgical treatment.

11.5.1 MVD

- Keyhole approach should be **infratentorial-supracerebellar** to minimize stretching of the VIIth-VIIth nerve complex and so avoid cochlear/vestibular disturbances.
- The veins of the superior petrosal system, by nature satellite of the trigeminal root at the upper part of the cerebello-pontine angle cistern, should be spared as much as possible to prevent from venous infarction.
- Exploration of the TGN should be from brainstem to trigeminal porus of Meckel cave, as NVCs are not always at TREZ (45%); they can be located more peripherally at midportion of root (40%) or even at porus (15%).
- Multiple conflicts in same patient should be systematically searched for; they have been found in our series in as many as 36% of the patients.
- MVD should not be "neo-compressive"; transposition obtains better long-term relief than interposition of foreign material touching the root (Fig. 11.10). Teflon in contact with the root (the most often used material, considered rather well-tolerated) may not only exert a more or less degree of compression but also be at the origin of granuloma formation (rarely). Importantly Teflon fibers, when in contact with the nerve, tend to generate adhesions, and to an even more aggressive degree incorporate its constituting fibers to the nerve parenchyma itself, as can be observed on the occasion of redoing decompression.

11.5.2 Percutaneous Lesioning-Techniques

They are all performed percutaneously through the Foramen Ovale, via a transjugal then pterygomaxillary trajectory (so-called Hartel route).

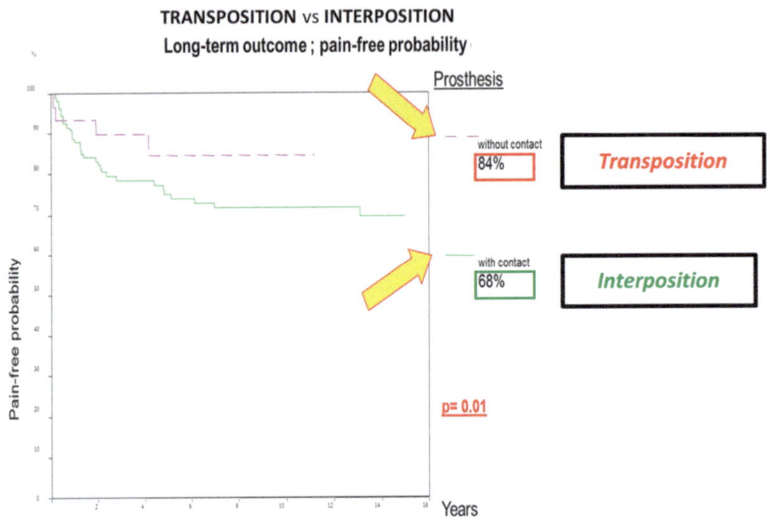

Fig. 11.10 Decompression should be non-neocompressive. Goal is to maintain the conflicting vessel apart of the compressed root. This can be achieved by transposition of the vessel or by interposition of material inserted in between the root and the vessel. Kaplan-Meier statistical analysis shows higher probability of better long-term (10 years) outcome when the transposition method can be performed ($p = 0.01$)

11.5.2.1 RF-Thermorhizotomy

- Target should preferably be in the so-called **Triangular Plexus** part of the retro-gasserian portion of the trigeminal system. Reasons are the following:
  - This location (on the axons arising from the dorsal root ganglion) is the logical one to obtain effect on the pathological site of the TGN, through axonal degeneration of the afferent fibers to brainstem;
  - The triangular plexus has a marked somatotopy corresponding to the three territories of the root distribution;
  - Sparing the body-cells of the trigeminal ganglion itself is a better protection from corneal ulcer complications [32].
- The RF-thermorhizotomy operation needs participation of the patient during the various awake-steps of the procedure, and a close cooperation with the anesthesiologist [33].
- Regarding outcome, the lesser the postoperative (bothering) hypoesthesia, the higher the rate of pain recurrence. Therefore, the benefit/risk ratio linked to a more or less pronounced thermo-lesion should be discussed with the patient, formalized in the form of a "contract," and written down in the signed informed consent.

11.5.2.2 Balloon Compression

- The Balloon compression technique, which is performed under general anesthesia, is rather comfortable for the patient, but has no topographic selectivity in relation with the painful territory.
- The important criteria (not always easy to obtain) to confirm the appropriate location of the inflated balloon **inside the Meckel cave** is its pear-shape after being filled with contrast-medium.
- Balloon compression has the advantage to expose to a low rate of corneal anesthesia, so that the procedure can be preferred to RF-thermorhizotomy, especially when neuralgia involves the V2 and/or the V1 territory(ies).

11.5.2.3 Glycerol Neurolysis

- This method is widely used due to its simplicity and low cost. The glycerol is injected **within the trigeminal cistern** under X-ray guidance. Inconvenience is that the diffusion of the neurolytic agent to the neighboring subarachnoid spaces is not totally under control, which may lead to harmful side effects.

11.5.3 Stereotactic Radiosurgery

- Stereotactic Radio-Surgery (SRS) is a less-invasive surgical technique for treating trigeminal neuralgias. Consensus is that the irradiation (done by definition in a single session) be at the high dose of 80–90 grays.
- Safest target is the retrogasserian mid-portion of the root, compared to the TREZ (Trigeminal Root Entry Zone), a zone at risk for brainstem integrity.
- For certain teams the creation of hypoesthesia is not necessary to obtain a valuable pain relief, for others on the contrary the duration of the pain sedation is correlated with the existence of a postoperative hypoesthesia and consequently with a certain degree of dysesthesias.
- SRS usually takes some months to become effective. However, this inconvenience is not a major problem for most patients with the exception of those referred in painful condition.
- The efficacy of SRS on the atypical form of TN, namely its continuous component has not yet been specifically evaluated.

11.5.4 Open Partial Rhizotomies

There are mainly two types of open partial rhizotomies:

1. The Sub-temporal Trigeminal Retrogasserian Neurotomy (as described by Frazier),
2. The Juxta-pontine Trigeminal Rhizotomy (as described by Dandy).

Although interruptive by definition, they keep a place in the neurosurgical armamentarium, especially for refractory secondary TNs, particularly those encountered in tumor cases.

Juxta-pontine rhizotomy may be the solution for TNs due to compression of the TGN by a huge megadolicho-Vertebro-Basilar Artery, when conservative decompression cannot be effectively performed.

11.6 Outcome After Surgery for Atypical Trigeminal Neuralgias

11.6.1 Outcome After MVD

In our various articles published along time [3, 15, 22, 31, 34, 35], the neuralgia was estimated relieved if the patient had no pain or only sporadic pain episodes that did not require treatment, i.e., BNI I or II, respectively (Fig. 11.11).

In our 356 patients with a long-term follow-up and studied with a Kaplan-Meir statistical analysis, probability of cure was 81.2% at 1 year and 73.4% at 15 years [31]. This data is consistent with recent literature reviews [36, 37]. In our own experience, the long-term outcome was similar whether the clinical presentation was typical or atypical, provided the permanent background of pain be not of iatrogenic origin [15] (Fig. 11.12). However, the background of pain needed a certain delay (several months) to disappear. However, this similarity in effect is not a finding shared by a majority of authors.

Importantly, the outcome was found dependent on the grade of the conflict. Grade I compression patients fared worst with a 65% of probability to benefit pain relief at 15 years, whereas grade II and Grade III showed a probability of cure at 15 years of 75% and 85%, respectively [31] (Fig. 11.13).

Regarding results in patients in whom implication of a venous compression was retained [34], the probability to be pain-free at 10 years after decompression of venous NVCs was quasi-similar between arterial and venous NVCs. NVCs with high degree of compression by the vein, like those with arteries, had better outcome (Fig. 11.13).

Also to be noted, the presence of severe local arachnoiditis had a significant negative role on the long-term prognosis ($p = 0.002$) [30, 34] (Fig. 11.14).

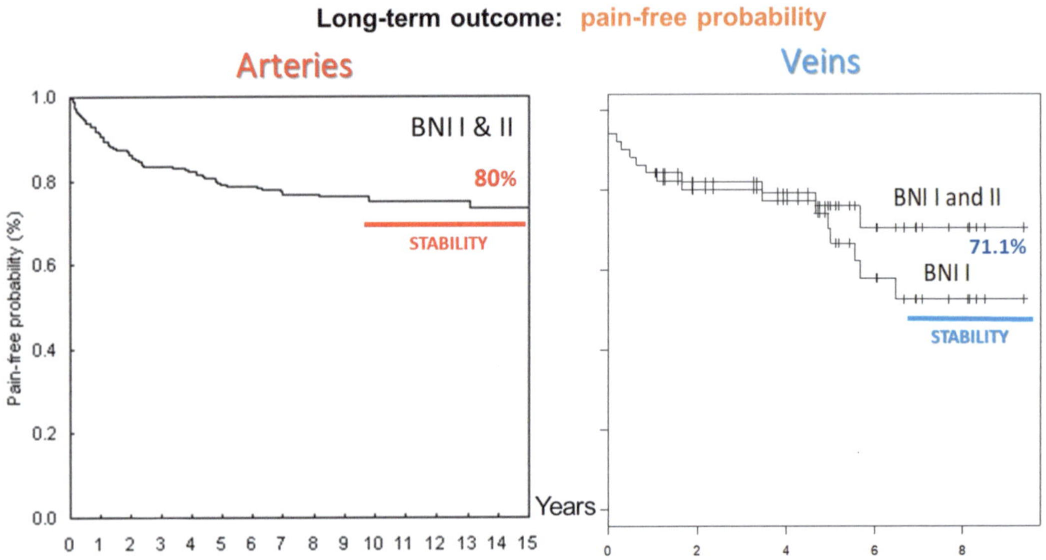

Fig. 11.11 Comparison of probability of long-term outcome after MVD between the groups of classical trigeminal neuralgias due to arterial vs. venous Neuro-Vascular Conflicts (NVCs). Probability of being pain-free (BNI I or II) for the arterial group was of 80%. At 8 years the probability of pain relief (BNI I or II) for the group with venous NVCs was of 71.1%. Data from a personal series of 1800 patients treated with MVD. Note the relative stability of the curves after 4 years of follow-up

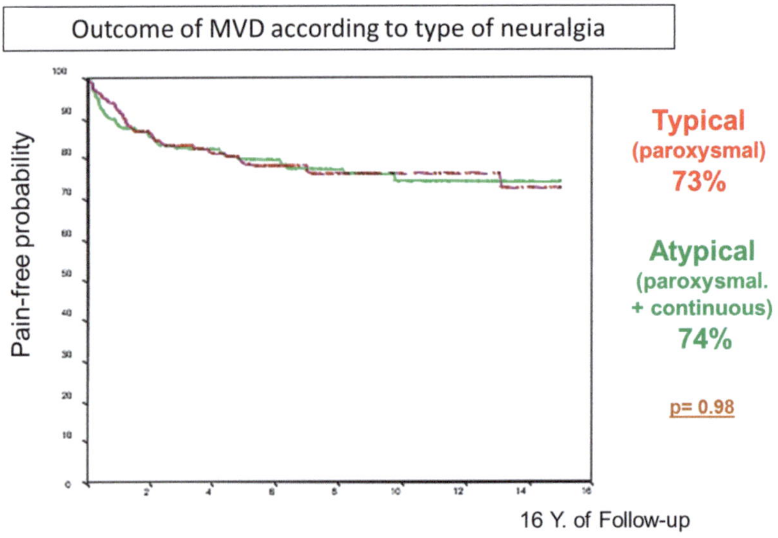

Fig. 11.12 Long-term (15 years) probability for MVD to obtain pain relief (BNI I or II) in classical trigeminal neuralgia according to clinical presentation: typical (i.e., with pure paroxysmal crises) or atypical (i.e., paroxysms associated with a background of continuous pain). Comparative study shows same effectiveness in both presentations ($p = 0.98$). However in the group of patients with atypical presentation, disappearance of the continuous pain component most often needed a delay of several months to a few years

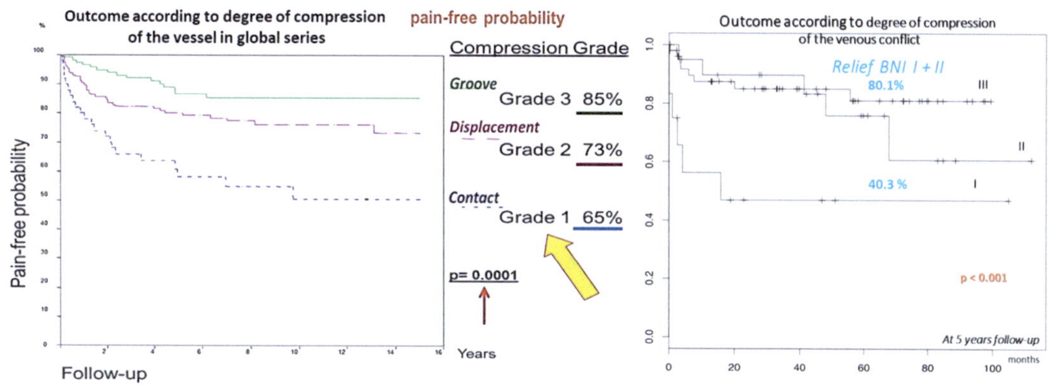

Fig. 11.13 Long-term (15 years) probability of MVD efficacy (BNI I or II) according to the grade of compression of the conflicting vessel (as estimated at surgery) in our overall series of classical TNs. Probability is significantly better for the higher grades of compression ($P = 0.0001$). Note that probability of obtaining relief was only of 65% for the group of patients having grade I of root compression (i.e., simple contact). This raises the hypothesis of other (or additional) factor in the genesis of the neuralgia when vessel is only in simple contact. Considering the group harboring a venous conflict, statistical study of probability of MVD to obtain pain relief (BNI I or II) according to the degree of compression by the venous conflict is of 80.1% for grade III of compression (i.e., major compression) vs. only 40.3% for grade I (i.e., only contact of the vessel to the root).Values are quite similar to the ones observed with the arterial NVCs

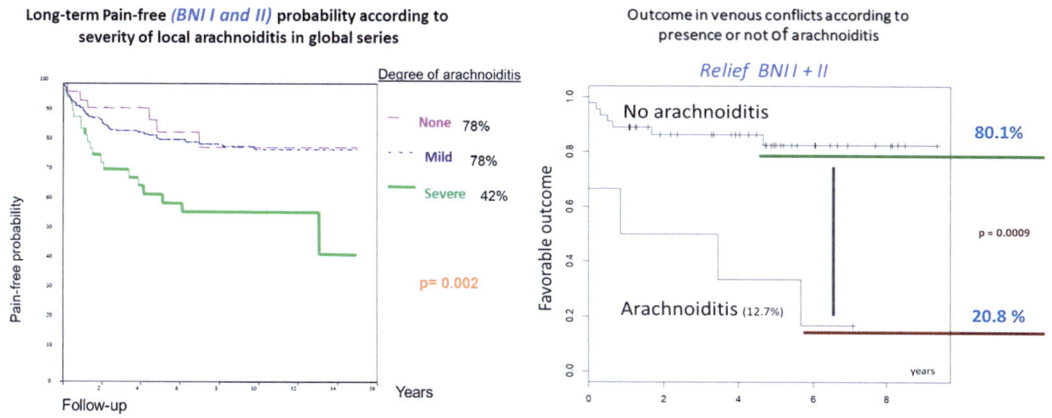

Fig. 11.14 Long-term (15 years) probability of pain relief (BNI I or II) in classical trigeminal neuralgia after MVD according to the presence or not of an associated local arachnoiditis and its severity. A marked arachnoiditis manifested by a focally thickened membrane with adhesion to the root constitutes a significant pejorative prognostic factor ($p = 0.002$). Statistical study of probability of MVD to obtain pain relief (BNI I or II) according to the absence or the presence of local arachnoiditis associated to the venous conflict shows a high probability of pain relief (80.1%) in its absence, and a low probability (20.89%) in its presence ($p = 0.0009$). Presence of a marked arachnoiditis when dealing with a potentially venous conflict is a pejorative factor, similarly to what was observed in the group of arterial conflicts associated with arachnoiditis

11.6.2 Outcome After Percutaneous-Lesioning Surgery or SRS

The lesioning techniques or the SRS, whatever their modality, are effective on pain transmission; but they generate more or less side effects, of which numbness, paresthesia, and dysesthesias are the dominant component, and corneal anesthesia with keratitis a subsequent risk.

Only the paroxysmal components of the pain can be valuably relieved by those techniques.

The lesser the postoperative hypoesthesia, the higher the risk of recurrence. The stronger the hypoesthesia, the more risk of bothering paresthesia, dysesthesias, and secondary anesthesia dolorosa [38].

In the atypical form of the TNs, the background of continuous pain component is not particularly influenced by the lesioning techniques. The possibility of aggravating it should be taken into consideration.

11.7 Decision-Making for Indications and Conclusions

According to the International Headache Society (IHS) definition, "Atypical Trigeminal Neuralgia" is "Trigeminal Neuralgia with Concomitant Continuous Pain" [1]. Establishing the character of Primary TN obeys these succesive steps:

First is the elimination of a causal disease by a complete clinical examination, oriented laboratory investigations (biology, neurophysiology…), and in particular imaging. Positivity of these may lead to the diagnosis of *secondary TN* and a specific treatment.

When the neuralgia is considered primary, high-resolution imaging is required to differentiate between *classical TN*—by definition linked to the presence of a neurovascular conflict (NVC) [2]—and *Idiopathic TN*.

The consensus is that the first surgical option for classical TN should be micro-vascular decompression (MVD), especially if the conflict appears to be severe (i.e., of high degree) (Fig. 11.15). Otherwise, the first option should be percutaneous lesioning or SRS, as for idiopathic TN. Provided the background of pain is not of iatrogenic origin it can be alleviated if not totally suppressed by MVD, generally after a certain delay.

The main diagnostic problem is to differentiate atypical TN form *persistent idiopathic facial pain*. This diagnostic problem is even more important when taking into account the fact that these latter patients should not be operated on. Diagnosis is particularly difficult when the paroxysmal component of the atypical TN is not predominant or has been masked by the anticonvulsant medications.

Concerning the putative mechanisms of the atypical component of the TNs—considered neu-

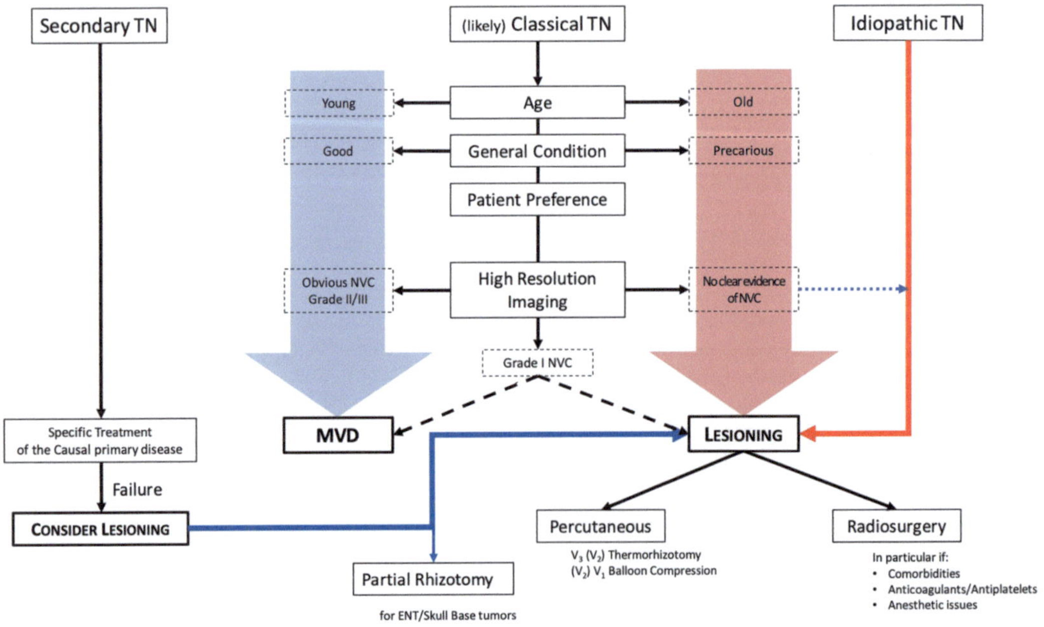

Fig. 11.15 Decision-making to choose neurosurgical procedures for Atypical Trigeminal Neuralgias

ropathic—an often-admitted interpretation is the long duration of the pathological condition, a situation often encountered by neurosurgeons when patients are referred for surgery.

Although not fully studied, a number of anatomical conditions observed in the frame of classical or idiopathic TN could play a role in the atypical clinical presentation. Among these are focal arachnoiditis, angulation/stretching of the root over the petrous ridge on exit from the Meckel Cave.

Further research on the mechanisms of the neuralgia—in particular through imaging—and into ways of distinguishing subtypes of patients through cluster analyses would aid in the better management of these patients.

References

1. IHS C. Headache classification Committee of the International Headache Society (IHS) the international classification of headache disorders, 3rd edition. Cephalalgia. 2018;38(1):1–211.
2. Cruccu G, Finnerup NB, Jensen TS, Scholz J, Sindou M, Svensson P, Treede RD, Zakrzewska JM, Nurmikko T. Trigeminal neuralgia: new classification and diagnostic grading for practice and research. Neurology. 2016;87(2):220–8.
3. Bendtsen L, Zakrzewska JM, Abbott J, Braschinsky M, Di Stefano G, Donnet A, Eide PK, Leal PRL, Maarbjerg S, May A, Nurmikko T, Obermann M, Jensen TS, Cruccu G. European academy of neurology guideline on trigeminal neuralgia. Eur J Neurol. 2019;26(6):831–49.
4. Laurent B, Keravel Y, Sindou M. Clinical aspects of trigeminal neuralgia. Neurochirurgie. 2009;55(2):181–4.
5. Younis S, Maarbjerg S, Reimer M, Wolfram F, Olesen J, Baron R, Bendtsen L. Quantitative sensory testing in classical trigeminal neuralgia-a blinded study in patients with and without concomitant persistent pain. Pain. 2016;157(7):1407–14.
6. Burchiel KJ, Slavin KV. On the natural history of trigeminal neuralgia. Neurosurgery. 2000;46(1):152–154; discussion 154-155.
7. Maarbjerg S, Gozalov A, Olesen J, Bendtsen L. Concomitant persistent pain in classical trigeminal neuralgia—evidence for different subtypes. Headache. 2014;54(7):1173–83.
8. Di Stefano G, La Cesa S, Truini A, Cruccu G. Natural history and outcome of 200 outpatients with classical trigeminal neuralgia treated with carbamazepine or oxcarbazepine in a tertiary Centre for neuropathic pain. J Headache Pain. 2014;15(1):34.
9. Gybels JM, Sweet WH. Neurosurgical treatment of persistent pain. Physiological and pathological mechanisms of human pain. Pain Headache. 1989;11:1–402.
10. Burchiel KJ. A new classification for facial pain. Neurosurgery. 2003;53(5):1164–1166; discussion 1166-1167.
11. Maarbjerg S, Wolfram F, Gozalov A, Olesen J, Bendtsen L. Association between neurovascular contact and clinical characteristics in classical trigeminal neuralgia: a prospective clinical study using 3.0 tesla MRI. Cephalalgia. 2015a;35(12):1077–84.
12. Maarbjerg S, Wolfram F, Gozalov A, Olesen J, Bendtsen L. Significance of neurovascular contact in classical trigeminal neuralgia. Brain. 2015b;138(Pt 2):311–9.
13. White JC, Sweet WH. Pain and the neurosurgeon; a forty-year experience. Springfield: C. C. Thomas; 1969.
14. Miller JP, Magill ST, Acar F, Burchiel KJ. Predictors of long-term success after microvascular decompression for trigeminal neuralgia. J Neurosurg. 2009;110(4):620–6.
15. Sindou M, Leston J, Howeidy T, Decullier E, Chapuis F. Micro-vascular decompression for primary trigeminal neuralgia (typical or atypical). Long-term effectiveness on pain; prospective study with survival analysis in a consecutive series of 362 patients. Acta Neurochir. 2006;148(12):1235–45. discussion 1245
16. Brinzeu A, Dumot C, Sindou M. Role of the petrous ridge and angulation of the trigeminal nerve in the pathogenesis of trigeminal neuralgia, with implications for microvascular decompression. Acta Neurochir. 2018a;160(5):971–6.
17. Brinzeu A, Drogba L, Sindou M. Reliability of MRI for predicting characteristics of neurovascular conflicts in trigeminal neuralgia: implications for surgical decision-making. J Neurosurg. 2018b;130:611–21.
18. Leal PR, Hermier M, Froment JC, Souza MA, Cristino-Filho G, Sindou M. Preoperative demonstration of the neurovascular compression characteristics with special emphasis on the degree of compression, using high-resolution magnetic resonance imaging: a prospective study, with comparison to surgical findings in 100 consecutive patients who underwent microvascular decompression for trigeminal neuralgia. Acta Neurochir. 2010;152(5):817–25.
19. Leal PR, Hermier M, Souza MA, Cristino-Filho G, Froment JC, Sindou M. Visualization of vascular compression of the trigeminal nerve with high-resolution 3T MRI: a prospective study comparing preoperative imaging analysis to surgical findings in 40 consecutive patients who underwent microvascular decompression for trigeminal neuralgia. Neurosurgery. 2011a;69(1):15–25. discussion 26.
20. Leal PR, Barbier C, Hermier M, Souza MA, Cristino-Filho G, Sindou M. Atrophic changes in the trigeminal nerves of patients with trigeminal neuralgia due to neurovascular compression and their association with the severity of compression and clinical outcomes. J Neurosurg. 2014;120:1484–95.

21. Leal PR, Roch JA, Hermier M, Souza MA, Cristino-Filho G, Sindou M. Structural abnormalities of the trigeminal root revealed by diffusion tensor imaging in patients with trigeminal neuralgia caused by neurovascular compression: a prospective, double-blind, controlled study. Pain. 2011b;152:2357–64.
22. Sindou M, Howeidy T, Acevedo G. Anatomical observations during microvascular decompression for idiopathic trigeminal neuralgia (with correlations between topography of pain and site of the neurovascular conflict). Prospective study in a series of 579 patients. Acta Neurochir. 2002;144(1):1–12; discussion 12-13.
23. Dumot C, Sindou M. Trigeminal neuralgia due to neurovascular conflicts from venous origin: an anatomical-surgical study (consecutive series of 124 operated cases). Acta Neurochir. 2015;157(3):455–66.
24. Ha SM, Kim SH, Yoo EH, Han IB, Shin DA, Cho KG, Chung SS, Park YS. Patients with idiopathic trigeminal neuralgia have a sharper-than-normal trigeminal-pontine angle and trigeminal nerve atrophy. Acta Neurochir. 2012;154(9):1627–33.
25. Horínek D, Brezová V, Nimsky C, Belsan T, Martinkovic L, Masopust V, Vrána J, Kozler P, Plas J, Krýsl D, Varjassyová A, Ghaly Y, Benes V. The MRI volumetry of the posterior fossa and its substructures in trigeminal neuralgia: a validated study. Acta Neurochir. 2009;151(6):669–75.
26. Mueller HR, Levy A. On the pathogenesis of trigeminal neuralgia. Study of mechanical factors by means of craniometry. Acta Neurochir. 1963;11:385–97.
27. Parise M, Acioly MA, Ribeiro CT, Vincent M, Gasparetto EL. The role of the cerebellopontine angle cistern area and trigeminal nerve length in the pathogenesis of trigeminal neuralgia: a prospective case-control study. Acta Neurochir. 2013;155(5):863–8.
28. Parise M, Ribeiro CT, Vincent M, Gasparetto E. Small cerebellopontine angle cisterns inpatients with trigeminal neuralgia. J Neurosurg. 2010;112(4):900–1. author reply 901
29. Rasche D, Kress B, Stippich C, Nennig E, Sartor K, Tronnier VM. Volumetric measurement of the pontomesencephalic cistern in patients with trigeminal neuralgia and healthy controls. Neurosurgery. 2006;59(3):614–620; discussion 614-620.
30. Mazzucchi E, Brinzeu A, Sindou M. Arachnoiditis as an outcome factor for microvascular decompression in classical trigeminal neuralgia. Acta Neurochir. 2019;161(8):1589–98.
31. Sindou M, Leston J, Decullier E, Chapuis F. Microvascular decompression for primary trigeminal neuralgia: long-term effectiveness and prognostic factors in a series of 362 consecutive patients with clear-cut neurovascular conflicts who underwent pure decompression. J Neurosurg. 2007;107(6):1144–53.
32. Sindou M, Keravel Y. Percutaneous thermocoagulation of the trigeminal root. A new neurosurgical treatment of essential facial neuralgia. Nouv Press Med. 1976;5(25):1583–4.
33. Sindou MP. Neurophysiological navigation in the trigeminal nerve: use of masticatory responses and facial motor responses evoked by electrical stimulationof the trigeminal rootlets for RF-thermorhizotomy guidance. Stereotact Funct Neurosurg. 1999;73(1–4):117–21.
34. Dumot C, Brinzeu A, Berthiller J, Sindou M. Trigeminal neuralgia due to venous neurovascular conflicts: outcome after microvascular decompression in a series of 55 consecutive patients. Acta Neurochir. 2017;159(2):237–49.
35. Sindou M, Leston JM, Decullier E, Chapuis F. Microvascular decompression for trigeminal neuralgia: the importance of a noncompressive technique—Kaplan-Meier analysis in a consecutive series of 330 patients. Neurosurgery. 2008;63(4 Suppl 2):341–350; discussion 350-341.
36. Sindou M, Brinzeu A. Névralgie du trijumeau et neurochirurgie. EMC Neurologie; 2018.
37. Sindou M, Brinzeu A, Laurent B. Aspects cliniques et thérapeutiques des névralgies des nerfs trijumeau et glossopharyngien. EMC Neurologie; 2021.
38. Sindou M, Brinzeu A. Trigeminal neuralgias: a neurosurgical illustrated guide. Cham: Springer; 2023.

12 Percutaneous Balloon Compression for Trigeminal Neuralgia Treatment: Rationale & Technique

Jun Zhong

While microvascular decompression (MVD) remains the primary treatment for hemifacial spasm, a variety of therapeutic approaches have been used to manage trigeminal neuralgia thus far. Among these, percutaneous balloon compression (PBC) has surged in popularity recently. However, it is essential to comprehend the strategic rationale underlying a treatment modality in relation to the pathogenesis before implementing tactical measures.

12.1 Rationale

12.1.1 The Nature of Trigeminal Neuralgia Attacks

Typically, upon receiving a nociceptive stimulus, the orofacial receptor generates an action potential that propagates along the trigeminal nerve fibers to reach the Gasserian ganglion, which acts as a crucial intermediary hub for energy supply, signal amplification and transmission efficiency. From there, it progresses through brainstem nuclei towards the cortex where this stimulation is processed and interpreted. In patients suffering from trigeminal neuralgia, the brain perceives a disordered impulse initiated from the nerve root rather than the receptor [1]. This ectopic action potential can be ignited by a precise compression characterized by specific combinations of amplitude and frequency that correspond to the individual's blood pressure and heart beat rate, respectively. This appropriate impact can arise not only from vascular structures but also from various sources such as neoplasms or even Teflon felts implanted during a previous operation, or it may have no identifiable cause for those with idiopathic trigeminal neuralgia. As an etiological treatment, microvascular decompression effectively manages the majority of classical trigeminal neuralgia cases but requires craniectomy [2]. Conversely, percutaneous balloon compression, without addressing the underlying cause, efficiently inhibits the generation and propagation of ectopic action potentials by blocking energy supply from the ganglion (Fig. 12.1).

J. Zhong (✉)
Department of Neurosurgery, XinHua Hospital, Shanghai JiaoTong University School of Medicine, Shanghai, China
e-mail: ZhongMDPhD@sjtu.edu.cn

S.-T. Li et al. (eds.), *Microvascular Decompression Surgery*,
https://doi.org/10.1007/978-981-96-0767-9_12

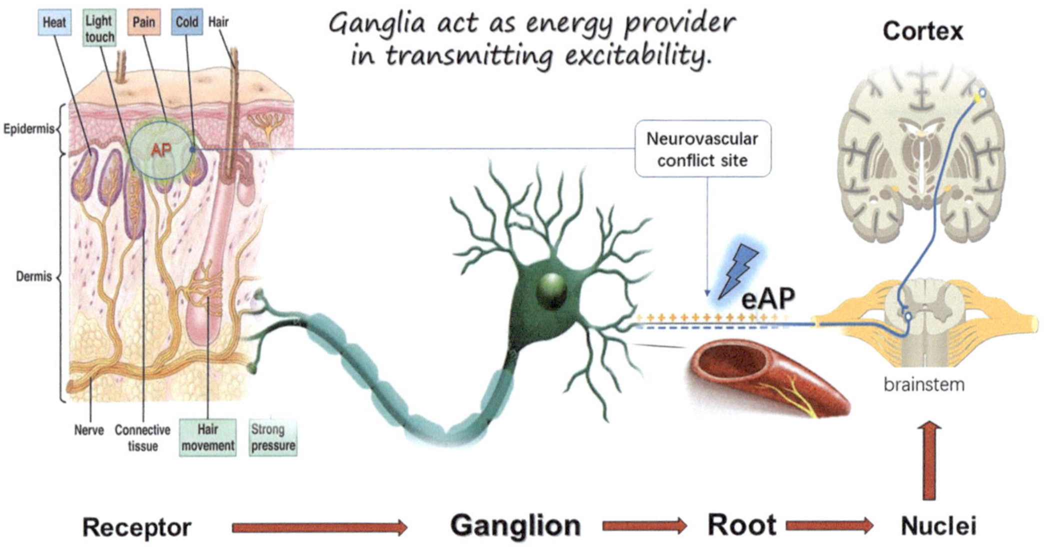

Fig. 12.1 The essence of trigeminal neuralgia. Normally, the orofacial receptor generates an action potential (AP) in response to a nociceptive stimulus, which then propagates through nerve fibers to the semilunar ganglion and further advances to the cortex via brainstem nuclei, ultimately leading to perception of the stimulation. In patients with trigeminal neuralgia, the brain perceives a disordered impulse (eAP) that originates from the nerve root rather than the receptor, often due to vascular compression. The Gasserian ganglion acts as an energy provider in transmitting excitability

12.1.2 Operational Mechanism of PBC

It has been commonly believed that the balloon compression preferentially injured the medium and large myelinated nerves and led to disruption of the ephaptic transmission of pain [3, 4]. However, the plausibility of "ephaptic theory" is questionable, as bioelectricity does not exhibit short-circuiting behavior akin to physical electricity. Considering that these myelinated sensory axons primarily transmit touch and vibration sensations rather than pain, the sole impairment of myelinated nerve fibers does not offer a straightforward explanation for pain alleviation. We postulate that the primary mechanism underlying PBC involves the impairment of pain-sensing neuron cell bodies (somata) in ganglia, rather than axons in rootlets [5]. The former pertains to the non-renewable central nervous system, whereas the latter denotes peripheral nerves with regenerative potential following damage. As generation and conduction of action potentials rely on energy provided from ganglia, PBC virtually "powers off" the trigeminus. This could potentially explain the higher immediate pain relief rate associated with PBC compared to MVD, as not all cases are attributed to vascular compression [6]. Given the structural disparity between thin unmyelinated nociceptive and thick myelinated tactile nerves, a precise compression may hold the potential to selectively induce damage to vulnerable pain-sensing neurons while sparing other neuronal populations. However, the Gasserian ganglion only occupies a small portion of Meckel's cave, with most of the space taken up by the rootlets [7]. When a balloon inflates within the cave, both the axons

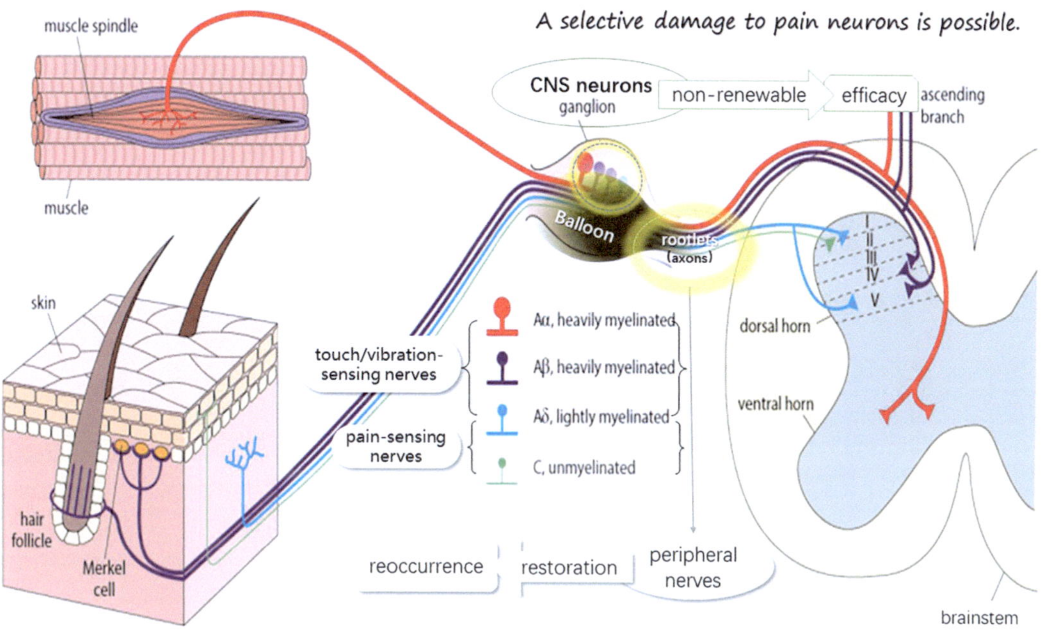

Fig. 12.2 The working mechanism of PBC. The pain nerves are typically smaller and lack myelin, while the tactile and vibration nerves are larger and possess myelin. Therefore, selective damage to vulnerable nociceptive neurons may potentially occur through balloon inflation in Meckel's cave. The ganglion (neurons) and rootlets (axons) belong to the central nervous system (CNS) and peripheral nerves, respectively. While the former is nonrenewable, the latter can regenerate when damaged. Therefore, it is advisable to focus pressure on the anterior semilunar ganglion during balloon inflation within the cave. The early postoperative outcome of being pain-free and numbness arises from the lesion of the pain neurons and all the axons, while the long-term effect of non-reoccurrence and sensory improvement is attributed to the permanent destruction of pain neurons and restoration of peripheral nerves

and neuron somata experience compression, with the highest pressure occurring at the narrowest zone where nerve fibers cross through the porus. This explains the early effect of PBC: painlessness and numbness [8]. However, as time goes on and peripheral nerve fibers gradually regenerate, the numbness improves while the pain tends to reoccur. Accordingly, if the pressure is focused on the anterior semilunar ganglion rather than the posterior majority of rootlets, a favorable long-term outcome of pain relief and sensory restoration without recurrence could be anticipated (Fig. 12.2). In contrast to other percutaneous procedures, which exhibit limited efficacy due to the gradual attenuation of glycerol concentration or thermocoagulation power from the center to the fringe, this mechanical intervention achieves comprehensive compression of the entire Gassarian ganglion by harnessing the counterattack force generated through balloon inflation within the cave [9]. Therefore, we propose a prompt and precise balloon inflation within Meckel's cave with bottom bolstering to effectively compress the semilunar ganglion for enhanced long-term efficacy without inducing significant hypoesthesia [10] (Fig. 12.3).

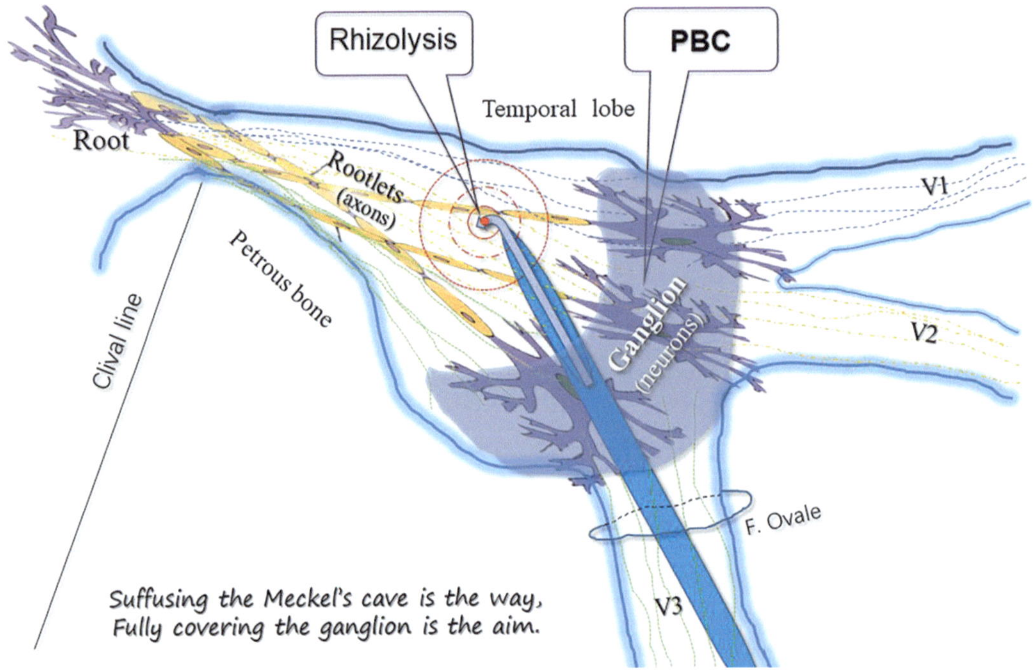

Fig. 12.3 Comparison of various percutaneous processes. Meckel's cave consists of ganglion (dark semilune, the minority) and rootlets (dotted lines, the majority). Three branches of trigeminus (V1, V2, V3) converge into the ganglion and then radiate rootlets entering brainstem via the root. The ganglion refers to the non-regenerable central nerve system (neurons), which play crucial role in the activation of action potential, protein synthesis and energy provision. Conversely, the rootlets (axons) denote renewable peripheral nerve fibers responsible for impulse transmission. Accordingly, the ablation should prioritize targeting the ganglion rather than the rootlets in order to prevent recurrences. The influence of other rhizolyses is effectively constrained by gradually decreasing glycerol concentration or thermocoagulation power from the center to the fringe (concentric circles). Meanwhile, a fully inflated balloon in the cave can evenly distribute pressure over the ganglion, resulting in a favorable outcome without relapse

12.2 Technique

12.2.1 Anatomical Comprehension

The operator must possess adequate qualifications to demonstrate a thorough understanding of the local anatomy and operating principles before commencing PBC. If the operator is capable of comprehending the spatial existence of Meckel's cave through observed projection and perceived resistance feedback, then the process becomes effortlessly manageable. When a balloon is inflated inside Meckel's cave precisely, a pear-shaped opacity becomes evident in the lateral radiograph. The pear projection outlines the contents in the cavity: a rounded bottom facing the semilunar ganglion, a body embracing the rootlets, a head indicating the trigeminal root coming over the porus (neck) and a stalk referring to the catheter tip. Considering the ultimate objective is to reach the bottom of the pear, it would be advantageous to envision a concealed banana within (Fig. 12.4).

12.2.2 Setup and Position

The procedure is performed under general anesthesia with endotracheal intubation, and continuous monitoring of arterial blood pressure, heart rate, and ECG should be maintained throughout the operation. Overreliance on complex imaging techniques such as 3D-CT navigation to locate the foramen ovale is unwise, as they may assist

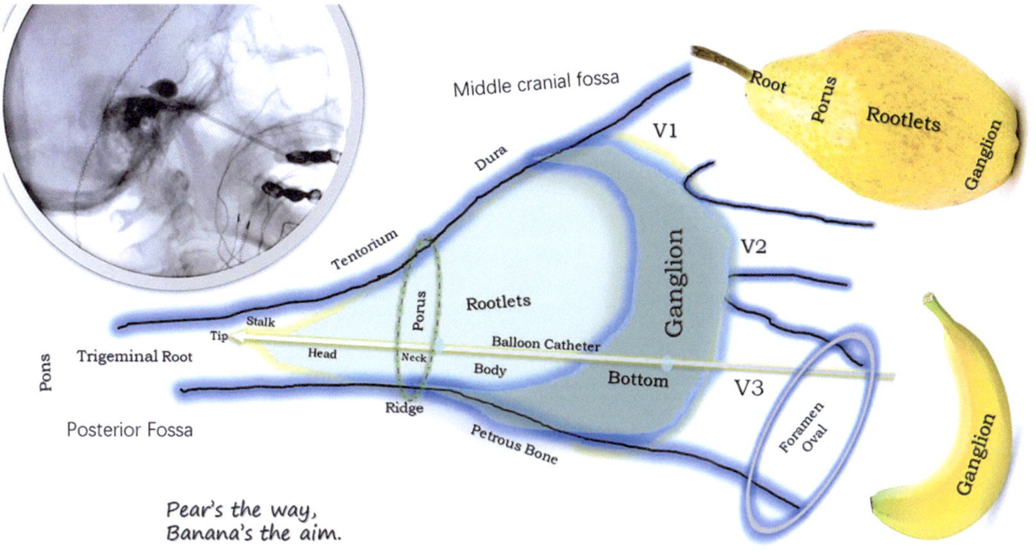

Fig. 12.4 Anatomical comprehension of Meckel's cave in fluoroscopy. When a balloon inflates within Meckel's cave, the lateral radiograph shows a pear-shaped opacity (insert top left). This pear projection delineates various components in the cavity: a rounded bottom facing the semilunar ganglion, a body encompassing the rootlets, a head indicating the trigeminal root through the porus (neck), and a stalk representing the catheter tip. The envisioning of an underlying banana is beneficial as the actual target resides at the base of this pear-shaped structure

beginners in finding it but do not guarantee access to Meckel's cave, which is the core objective of PBC. Normally, a lateral C-arm fluoroscopy provides sufficient guidance in this regard. The patient is positioned supine with his or her head in a neutral position and slight extension of the neck. To achieve well-defined and precise anatomical landmarks in radiographs, it is crucial to maintain stable positioning of the patient's head in a positive normotopia, thereby ensuring superimposition of bilateral acoustic meatus and mandibular condyles throughout the procedure.

12.2.3 Entry Point of the Face

A proper puncture angle is crucial for successful balloon transportation, highlighting the importance of accurately identifying the entry point on the face, which should align with the line connecting the porus and foramen oval. The cutaneous entry point is usually located 2.0–3.0 cm laterally to the commissure of the lips, where a palpable depression indicates the anatomical pathway for the needle between the maxilla and mandible. Basically, a 15-gauge needle with a non-cutting obturator is adopted and an 11# blade is required to make a small incision in the skin before puncturing.

12.2.4 Cannulating

The needle is advanced towards the ipsilateral pupil on the coronal plane and directed to the infra 1/3 of the line between the posterior clinoid and mandibular condyle on the sagittal plane under lateral fluoroscopy, stopping when its tip reaches the foramen oval. Before removing the obturator, ensure that the cannula is stably positioned to prevent potential balloon laceration caused by its sharp mouth rim during the later catheter passage (Fig. 12.5).

12.2.5 Puncturing and Penetrating

To circumvent the interlayer of catheter entry, it is recommended to initially puncture the wall of

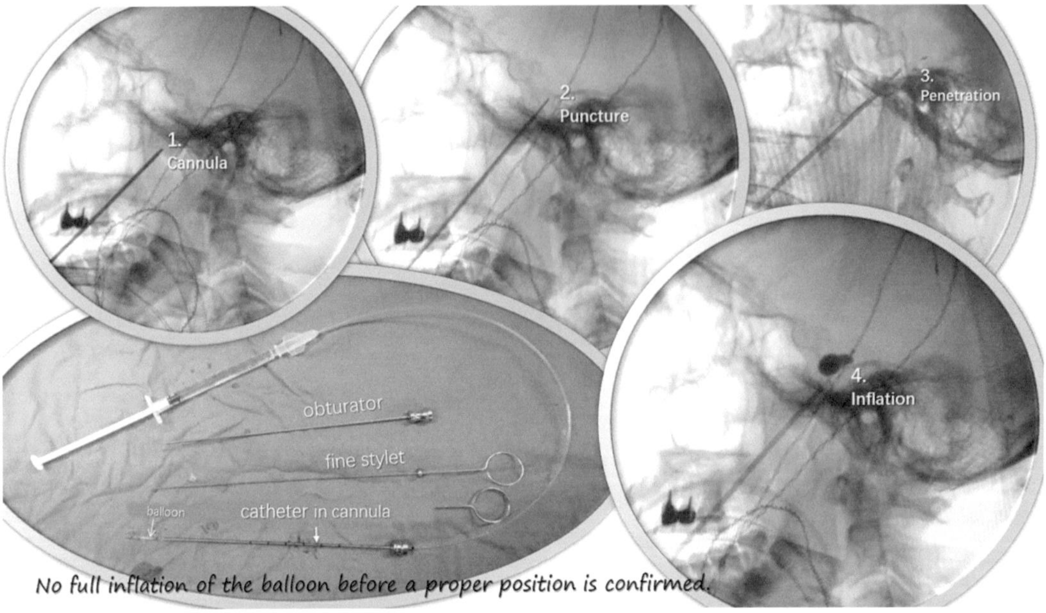

Fig. 12.5 The puncture and penetration procedures. Upon the needle engaging with the foramen ovale (1), the obturator is withdrawn from the cannula and a fine stylet is utilized to puncture the wall of Meckel's cave (2). Then, a catheter containing a guide wire is introduced and advanced through the trigeminus in the cave until its tip points downwards (3). Next, the wire is retracted and the balloon is gently inflated with contrast medium to generate a pear-shaped opacity image under lateral fluoroscopy (4). The advance puncturing ushers the catheter into the cavity and prevents misdirection. During catheter penetrating, damping feedback and downward tip presentation ensure accurate positioning

Meckel's cave using a fine stylet. The distal end of the cannula should be elevated to guide catheter insertion and prevent breaching the ceiling and invading the subdural space upwards. The catheter should produce a noticeable sensory response when entering the trigeminal nerve within the cave. If not, it should be withdrawn and reinserted in a different direction. During position adjustment, the balloon should be deflated adequately to reduce the risk of lacerations when it is extruded through the sharp mouth rim of the cannula. Inflation should only be implemented after achieving proper positioning (Fig. 12.5).

12.2.6 Tentative Inflations

It is recommended to advance the catheter slightly further until its tip is visibly directed downwards, as this image only appears when the catheter has passed through the porus and traversed over the petrosal ridge into the posterior fossa. This serves as evidence to confirm that the balloon is precisely positioned within Meckel's cave. To double check, a cautious and tentative injection is administered to anticipate the formation of a small inverted pear shape. Subsequently, the balloon is deflated and the catheter is slightly retracted prior to gradual reinflation of the balloon. If a neck begins to appear, inflation should be continued until a base becomes visible (Fig. 12.5).

12.2.7 Compression of the Ganglion

The shape and position of the balloon are assessed by referencing nearby anatomical landmarks such as the clivus, sella, and petrous bones. If necessary, it should be deflated and repositioned until achieving a pear-shaped configuration [11, 12]. The primary focus of treatment lies in the

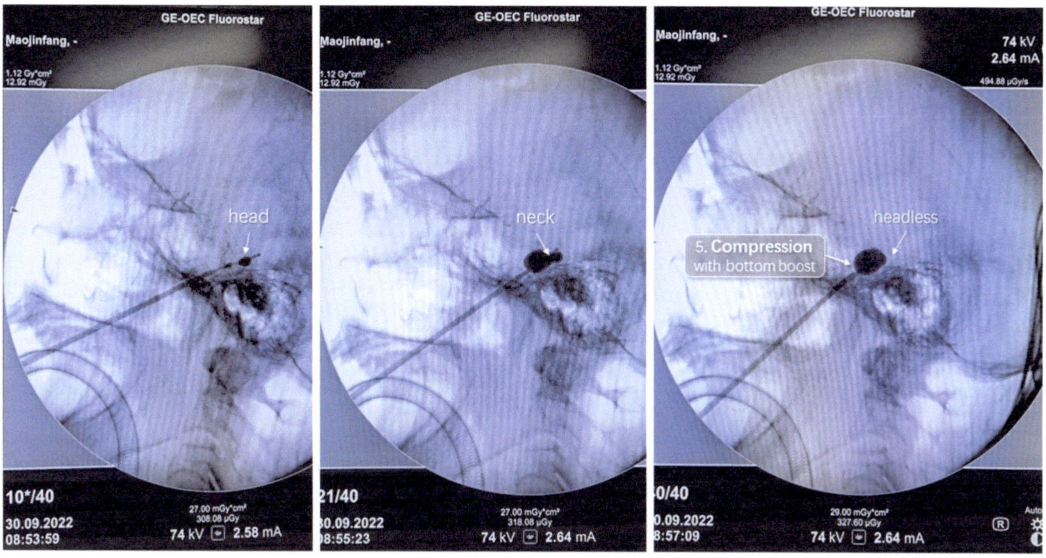

An inverted pear A slim pear A headless pear

The head shows balloon position, not compression target.

Fig. 12.6 A bottom-boosted compression. The small head and neck size allows for using less contrast agent to clearly outline the balloon's fluoroscopic shape. The presence of a tiny inverted pear shape indicates that the catheter has successfully passed through Gessarian ganglion into the root via the porus. Then, the balloon should be deflated to facilitate a slight retraction of the catheter, followed by a gradual reinflation to achieve the desired pear-shaped configuration. The pressure on the ganglion may be less when exerted by a slender pear with an elongated neck compared to a plump pear with a larger base, even if injected with the same volume. Therefore, once the precise positioning of the balloon within the cave is confirmed, it is advisable to pursue a headless pear

Table 12.1 An operational algorithm of PBC

Steps	Actions	Interpretations
1	Cannula	Engaging with foramen ovale
2	Puncture	Piercing the wall of Meckel's cave
3	Penetrate	Advancing the catheter with damping feedback
4	Inflation	Tentatively injecting the balloon to anticipate a pear shape
5	Compression	Focusing on the ganglion

lower half, with the head serving as a reference for balloon positioning. Finally, delicately pulling the catheter with your other hand can be employed to apply additional pressure on the ganglion (Fig. 12.6) [13]. This PBC procedure was condensed into a concise five-step algorithm, as illustrated in Table 12.1.

12.2.7.1 Volume

As a capsule-like structure of Meckel's cavity with inherent elasticity, the pressure–volume relationship exhibits nonlinearity beyond a certain threshold, leading to subsequent pressure reduction despite ongoing volume expansion. The effective injection volume varies among patients due to interindividual differences in size and elasticity. Typically, a volume range of 0.3–0.7 mL can ensure complete coverage of the cavity; however, it is advisable to discontinue the injection once fluoroscopy indicates cessation of pear growth.

12.2.7.2 Time

Reconsidering the impact of prolonged compression on heightened numbness, the time parameter should not be disregarded. Based on our empirical findings, a compressive duration of 1½ min was determined to be sufficient in achieving fluoroscopic evidence of a solid-bottom-pear shape. To prevent pressure loss, it is recommended to manually hold the syringe instead of relying on a three-way valve, thereby enabling supplementary injection in accordance with pressure feedback and fluoroscopic images.

12.3 Conclusion

The ultimate objective of PBC is to compress the Gasserian ganglion rather than occupy Meckel's cave. A comprehensive understanding of the local anatomy in relation to fluoroscopic projection is crucial prior to commencing the process. Typically, this process involves five essential steps: precise cannula engagement with the foramen ovale at an optimal angle, accurate puncturing of Meckel's cave, catheter penetration with effective damping feedback, tentative inflation of the balloon to anticipate a desired pear shape, and focused compression targeting the bottom (Table 12.1). By applying precise pressure to the semilunar ganglion in the correct direction and for an appropriate duration, long-term effectiveness can be achieved without significant residual numbness.

References

1. Mingxing L, Jun Z. Mechanism underlying cranial nerve rhizopathy. Med Hypotheses. 2020;142:109801.
2. Giorgio C, Giulia DS, Andrea T. Trigeminal neuralgia. N Engl J Med. 2020;383(8):754–62.
3. Brown JA, Hoeflinger B, Long PB, et al. Axon and ganglion cell injury in rabbits after percutaneous trigeminal balloon compression. Neurosurgery. 1996;38(5):993.
4. Mullan S, Lichtor T. Percutaneous microcompression of the trigeminal ganglion for trigeminal neuralgia. J Neurosurg. 1983;59(6):1007–12.
5. Jun Z. Targeting the foramen ovale is the point of percutaneous balloon compression? Comment on: robot-assisted percutaneous balloon compression for trigeminal neuralgia-preliminary experiences. BMC Neurol. 2024;24(1):79.
6. Zhou YI, Ning-NiNG D, Xue-Lai L, et al. A Comparative review of the outcome following MVD and PBC in patients with trigeminal neuralgia. J Neurol Surg A Cent Eur Neurosurg. 2023;84(5):470–6.
7. Goto Tetsuya O, Bae S, Mamoru T, et al. Recent advances in basic research on the trigeminal ganglion. J Physiol Sci. 2016;66(5):381–6.
8. Qiu X, Haitao H, Ma YI, et al. Relationship between compression time and long-term hypoesthesia in primary trigeminal neuralgia treated with percutaneous balloon compression. Neurosurg Rev. 2023;46(1):212.
9. Imran N, Amanda L, Girish V, et al. Comparing percutaneous treatments of trigeminal neuralgia: 19 years of experience in a single centre. Stereotact Funct Neurosurg. 2016;94(2):75–85.
10. Jun Z. The key to a successful PBC in treatment of trigeminal neuralgia. Acta Neurochir Suppl. 2023;135:161–5.
11. Shaozhen H, Zhengnan H, Haolin W, et al. The value of a headless pear shape in percutaneous balloon compression for trigeminal neuralgia. Oper Neurosurg (Hagerstown). 2023;25(4):372–8.
12. Yingying D, Yue W, Yuhai W, et al. A retrospective study to examine the association of different pear-shaped balloons with efficacy and postoperative complications in percutaneous balloon compression for trigeminal neuralgia. Neurosurg Rev. 2023;46(1):60.
13. Haolin W, Shaozhen H, Nan HZ, et al. Riveting technique in percutaneous balloon compression for trigeminal neuralgia remedy. Clin Neurol Neurosurg. 2024;240:108245.

Gamma Knife Application in the Treatment of Trigeminal Neuralgia

13

Jin Woo Chang

Trigeminal neuralgia (TN) is defined by the International Headache Society as "recurrent unilateral brief electric shock-like pains, abrupt in onset and termination, limited to the distribution of one or more divisions of the trigeminal nerve and triggered by innocuous stimuli." Treatments for TN are divided into the following three categories: pharmacological treatments; surgical treatments, including microvascular decompression (MVD) and percutaneous procedures, such as radiofrequency rhizotomy (RFR), balloon microcompression, and glycerol injection; and stereotactic radiosurgery. Gamma knife radiosurgery (GKRS) can be used for drug-resistant TN patients who are poor surgical candidates due to medical comorbidities or age or for those who refuse invasive therapy, especially in the absence of other primary indications, such as neurovascular conflict. In this chapter, we aim to explore the history of gamma knife radiosurgery (GKRS) for TN, the rationale of treatment, relevant literature, and the specific methods and outcomes of GKRS.

J. W. Chang (✉)
Center for Innovative Functional Neurosurgery, Brain Research Institute, Department of Neurosurgery, Yonsei University College of Medicine, Seoul, South Korea
e-mail: jchang@yuhs.ac

13.1 Historical Perspective of Gamma Knife in Trigeminal Neuralgia

The Swedish neurosurgeon Lars Leksell began treating TN patients in 1951 using a prototype guiding device linked to a dental X-ray machine. Lindquist reported on the progress of TN patients who had undergone GKRS in 1991, and several studies have documented the safety and efficacy of GKRS, including long-term results, for TN. Other techniques of radiosurgery, such as cyber knife surgery and linear accelerator, were introduced in the 2000s and have shown effectiveness, compared to other surgical treatments. Several modifications have been made to the treatment regimens for GKRS over the past few decades. The development of high-quality magnetic resonance imaging (MRI) enabled a better imaging of the trigeminal nerve and root entry zone and renewed interest in radiosurgery for TN.

13.2 Rationale of Radiosurgery for Trigeminal Neuralgia

The pathogenesis of TN is not fully understood, and its exact pathophysiology remains controversial. However, in general, it is described by a mixed peripheral and central mechanism.

S.-T. Li et al. (eds.), *Microvascular Decompression Surgery*,
https://doi.org/10.1007/978-981-96-0767-9_13

Neurovascular conflict is the most accepted theory, as it is related to TN in a vast majority of cases. Chronic nerve compression results in demyelination of trigeminal sensory fibers within the proximal nerve root, with progressive axonal degeneration. Demyelination can lead to ephaptic transmission, and the reentry mechanism causes an amplification of sensory inputs. Meanwhile, nerve injury leads to a release of mediators that sensitize peripheral nerve terminations, resulting in neurochemical and phenotypic changes and increased excitability of trigeminal neurons and trigeminal nuclei (central sensitization). Ultrastructural and biochemical changes in axons and myelin are seen in the root, the Gasserian ganglion, or both. The rationale for achieving pain relief after GKRS is related to focal axonal degeneration of the trigeminal nerve associated with nociceptive sensibility, destruction of ionic channels, and electrophysiological blocking initially after nerve irradiation. Additionally, a delayed radiation effect with axonal degeneration has been proposed, as some patients experience a late response after GKRS.

13.3 Pain Relief, Complications and Repeated GKRS

Table 13.1 lists studies with more than 100 patients who underwent GKRS for TN. GKRS showed high rates of pain relief, ranging from 70–98% in large studies of over 100 patients. Pain control was achieved in 69–85% of cases at 1 year, 59% at 2 years, and 38–52% at 5 years. Regarding long-term results, rates of pain control maintenance were 32–59.7% at 7 years and 30–45.3% at 10 years. Although follow-up periods vary among the studies, making direct comparison difficult, the average pain free duration was 7–58 months. The mean recurrence rate was 26.9%, with a range of 3.3–45.1%.

Complications due to GKRS are uncommon, with hypesthesia being the most common adverse event. The incidence of hypesthesia is reported to be up to 2.7–55.0%, with a mean occurrence rate of 22.55%. Similar to the latency period for GKRS to be effective, there may also be a latency period between the procedure and the development of complications. The mean time to hypesthesia occurrence ranged from 6 to

Table 13.1 Review of studies with more than 100 cases of gamma knife radiosurgery for trigeminal neuralgia

Study (year)	Number of patients	Mean or median follow-up period (months)	Pain relief (%)	Complications (%)	Recurrence (%)
Young et al. [1]	110	19.8	95.5	2.7	3.3
Maesawa et al. [2]	220	22	78.6	10.2	13.6
Pollock et al. [3]	117	26	75	37	16
Petit et al. [4]	112	30	77	7.3	29
Sheehan et al. [5]	136	19	70	19	24
Urgosik et al. [6]	107	60	96	20	25
Longhi et al. [7]	170	37.4	90	8.75	18
Fountas et al. [8]	106	34.3	89.6	16	32.1
Kondziolka et al. [9]	503	24	89	10.5	42.9
Hayashi et al. [10]	130	38	98	24	18.0
Marshall et al. [11]	448	20.9	86	44	40
Young et al. [12]	315	68.9	85.6	32.9	14.3
Lucas et al. [13]	446	21.2	84.5	42	45.1
Régis et al. [14]	497	43.8	91.75	21.1	34.4
Taich et al.	263	24	79	NA	39.8
Martínez Moreno et al. [15]	117	66	91	32.5	19
Zhao et al. [16]	247	49.7	87.9	31.9	3.6
Gagliardi et al. [17]	166	64.7	78	24	31.2
Lee et al. [18]	108	17	80	55	22

36 months. Other complications include dysesthesia, deafferentation pain, dysgeusia, dry eye syndrome, keratitis, hearing impairment, and masticator weakness. Rarely, significant injury to adjacent vasculature due to high doses have been reported. Terms used in each article related to complications had a lack of precision; hence, there may be differences in the rate of complications.

Due to the low incidence of complications associated with GKRS, rather than other procedures, repeat GKRS may be considered for pain recurrence. Repeat GKRS appears to have a similar efficacy to initial GKRS for TN, with rates of complete and partial pain relief ranging from 78% to 85%. There is a report that prior GKRS is associated with bothersome facial numbness after GKRS. The main complications after repeat GKRS are new facial sensory symptoms caused by partial trigeminal nerve injury, seen in 11–69% of patients. Therefore, to reduce complications due to repeat GKRS, decreasing the dose of the second GKRS would be helpful, as would moving the target to not overlap with the previous target, so that a previously treated nerve is not exposed to a high dose of radiation.

13.4 GKRS Policy: Dose and Target

When GKRS was first used for TN, Leksell targeted the Gasserian ganglion. After that, Lindquist, et al. reported the results of GKRS targeting the Gasserian ganglion in 1991 and then stated the results of treatment of the trigeminal REZ, where peripheral myelination with Schwann cells transits to central myelination with oligodendrocytes. Rand, et al. reported the results of the GKRS targeting the retrogasserian area, anterior to REZ, in 1993. Since then, both the REZ and retrogasserian area have been used to treat TN with GKRS (Fig. 13.1).

There is still controversy regarding which target is better. The major difference between the targets is the dose received by the REZ and the brainstem. However, the effect and complications related to the target and the dose are not established. Several studies have compared the complications and effects between anterior and posterior targets. They reported that an anterior target has lower complications than a posterior target, showing similar or better pain relief. However, since there is a difference between

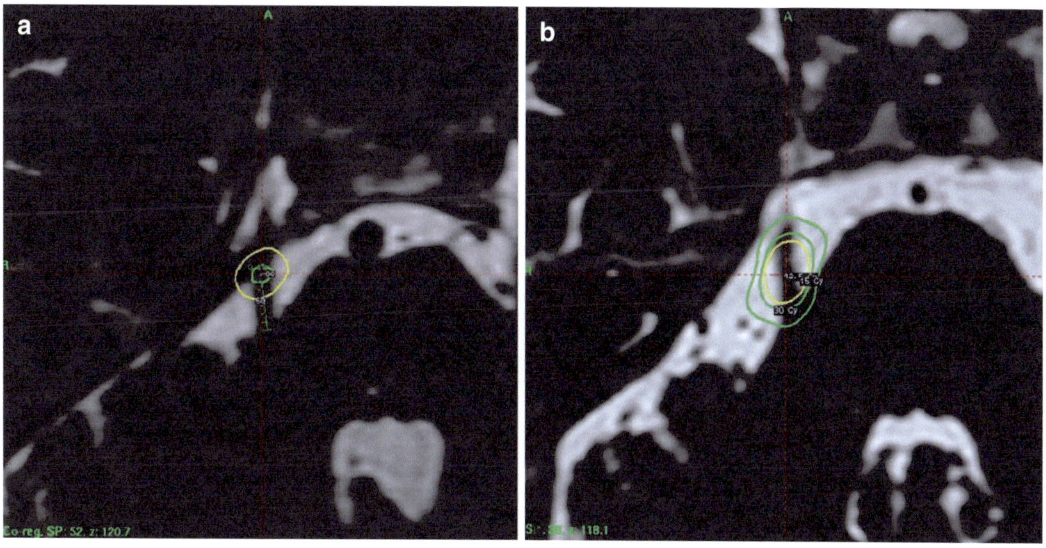

Fig. 13.1 Targets used in gamma knife radiosurgery for trigeminal neuralgia. Retrogasserian area (**a**) and trigeminal root entry zone (**b**)

doses among studies and targets and the appropriate dose has not yet been established for the target, it is difficult to directly determine which target is better. Determination of the treatment dose may vary according to the target. However, studies have shown that a dose of 70 Gy failed to control pain in 100% and that radiation below 70 Gy had little effect on the structure of the trigeminal nerve. A radiation dose of more than 80 Gy causes partial degeneration with loss of axons and demyelination, which is the mechanism of pain relief in GKRS. Therefore, GKRS with 80 Gy or higher is usually performed. In addition, many studies have shown that higher doses lead to greater pain control. However, a high dose of more than 90 Gy is related to a higher complication rate with similar pain control effects; hence, they are not usually used. Recently, a dose between 80 and 90 Gy is generally used, with modification depending the circumstances.

13.5 Conclusion

GKRS has been used for TN for a long time with low complication rates and high success rates. Over time, technical refinements have improved its safety and efficacy. GKRS is being increasingly used as a primary intervention for TN for patients who cannot undergo surgery due to medical comorbidities and age or for those who refuse invasive therapy. To further increase safety and efficiency, discussions are underway on the treatment policy to be applied. In the future, advances in imaging modalities and in GKRS technique, as well as accumulation of long-term results and experience will yield better results of GRKS for TN.

References

1. Young RF, Vermulen S, Posewitz A. Gamma knife radiosurgery for the treatment of trigeminal neuralgia. Stereotact Funct Neurosurg. 1998;70(Suppl 1):192–9.
2. Maesawa S, Salame C, Flickinger JC, Pirris S, Kondziolka D, Lunsford LD. Clinical outcomes after stereotactic radiosurgery for idiopathic trigeminal neuralgia. J Neurosurg. 2001;94:14–20.
3. Pollock BE, Phuong LK, Gorman DA, Foote RL, Stafford SL. Stereotactic radiosurgery for idiopathic trigeminal neuralgia. J Neurosurg. 2002;97:347–53.
4. Petit JH, Herman JM, Nagda S, DiBiase SJ, Chin LS. Radiosurgical treatment of trigeminal neuralgia: evaluating quality of life and treatment outcomes. Int J Radiat Oncol Biol Phys. 2003;56:1147–53.
5. Sheehan J, Pan HC, Stroila M, Steiner L. Gamma knife surgery for trigeminal neuralgia: outcomes and prognostic factors. J Neurosurg. 2005;102:434–41.
6. Urgosik D, Liscak R, Novotny J Jr, Vymazal J, Vladyka V. Treatment of essential trigeminal neuralgia with gamma knife surgery. J Neurosurg. 2005;102:29–33.
7. Longhi M, Rizzo P, Nicolato A, Foroni R, Reggio M, Gerosa M. Gamma knife radiosurgery for trigeminal neuralgia: results and potentially predictive parameters—part I: idiopathic trigeminal neuralgia. Neurosurgery. 2007;61:1254–61.
8. Fountas KN, Smith JR, Lee GP, Jenkins PD, Cantrell RR, Sheils WC. Gamma knife stereotactic radiosurgical treatment of idiopathic trigeminal neuralgia: long-term outcome and complications. Neurosurg Focus. 2007;23:E8.
9. Kondziolka D, Zorro O, Lobato-Polo J, Kano H, Flannery TJ, Flickinger JC, et al. Gamma knife stereotactic radiosurgery for idiopathic trigeminal neuralgia. J Neurosurg. 2010;112:758–65.
10. Hayashi M, Chernov M, Tamura N, Taira T, Izawa M, Yomo S, et al. Stereotactic radiosurgery of essential trigeminal neuralgia using Leksell gamma knife model C with automatic positioning system: technical nuances and evaluation of outcome in 130 patients with at least 2 years follow-up after treatment. Neurosurg Rev. 2011;34:497.
11. Marshall K, Chan MD, McCoy TP, Aubuchon AC, Bourland JD, McMullen KP, et al. Predictive variables for the successful treatment of trigeminal neuralgia with gamma knife radiosurgery. Neurosurgery. 2012;70:566–73.
12. Young B, Shivazad A, Kryscio RJ, St Clair W, Bush HM. Long-term outcome of high-dose γ knife surgery in treatment of trigeminal neuralgia. J Neurosurg. 2013;119:1166–75.
13. Lucas JT Jr, Nida AM, Isom S, Marshall K, Bourland JD, Laxton AW, et al. Predictive nomogram for the durability of pain relief from gamma knife radiation surgery in the treatment of trigeminal neuralgia. Int J Radiat Oncol Biol Phys. 2014;89:120–6.49.
14. Régis J, Tuleasca C, Resseguier N, Carron R, Donnet A, Gaudart J, et al. Long-term safety and efficacy of gamma knife surgery in classical trigeminal neuralgia: a 497-patient historical cohort study. J Neurosurg. 2016;124:1079–87.
15. Martínez Moreno NE, Gutiérrez-Sárraga J, Rey-Portolés G, Jiménez-Huete A, Martínez ÁR. Long-term outcomes in the treatment of classical trigeminal neuralgia by gamma knife radiosurgery: a retrospective study in patients with minimum 2-year follow up. Neurosurgery. 2016;79:879–88.

16. Zhao H, Shen Y, Yao D, Xiong N, Abdelmaksoud A, Wang H. Outcomes of two-isocenter gamma knife radiosurgery for patients with typical trigeminal neuralgia: pain response and quality of life. World Neurosurg. 2018;109:e531–8.
17. Gagliardi F, Spina A, Bailo M, Boari N, Cavalli A, Franzin A, et al. Effectiveness of gamma knife radiosurgery in improving psychophysical performance and patient's quality of life in idiopathic trigeminal neuralgia. World Neurosurg. 2018;110:e776–85.
18. Lee CC, Chen CJ, Chong ST, Hung SC, Yang HC, Lin CJ, et al. Early stereotactic radiosurgery for medically refractory trigeminal neuralgia. World Neurosurg. 2018;112:e569–75.

Intermediate Nerve Neuralgia

14

V. S. Dementevsky, E. A. Lekchnov, D. A. Rzaev, and K. V. Slavin

14.1 History

The intermediate nerve (nervus inermedius, Wrisberg's nerve) was first documented in 1777 by the German anatomy professor Heinrich August Wrisberg. Although Eustachius discovered NI as early as 1563, he did not define it as a separate structure [1, 2]. Later, in 1881, an Italian physician Giuseppe Sapolini identified the NI as the 13th cranial nerve, and accurately sketched its anatomy in 1883 [2]. In 1989, based on embryological and anatomical data, NI was shown to be a separate cranial nerve [3]. NIN or geniculate neuralgia is a very rare disease with only 174 cases published between 1932 and 2018 [4]. NIN was mentioned for the first time by John Nottingham in 1857 as "tic douloureux of the ear" with subsequent description by multiple other authors [2]. In 1907, Ramsey Hunt systematized NIN data, described its anatomical and physiological features, and proposed the term geniculate neuralgia [2, 5].

14.2 The Nervus Intermedius Anatomy

Studies show that NI microanatomy can be extremely variable. Detailed knowledge of NI anatomy and physiology as well as its relationship with the surrounding anatomical structures of the cerebello-pontine angle (AICA and the VII–VIII complex) is very relevant to NIN treatment [6]. NI is quite thin and short with the average diameter of 0.62 mm and average length—14 mm from the brain stem to the internal auditory canal (IAC) [1]. Rhoton divided NI into proximal, intermediate, and distal segments [7]. NI is frequently tightly fused with only the upper medial part of the VIII nerve in the proximal segment near the brainstem, but sometimes it runs with the VIII nerve all the way up to IAC [8]. In the intermediate segment, NI separates from nerve VIII, runs apart between nerves VIII and VII, and can be identified on 3 T MRI. According to some data, NI often can be present in this segment as a single root [1, 2] or, according to other data, as a set of 4 roots [6]; less often, the number of NI roots in this segment may be 5 or 6 [1, 2]. In 57% of cases, NI roots are seen in the proxim-

V. S. Dementevsky
Federal State Budgetary Institution "Federal Scientific and Clinical Center for Reanimatology and Rehabilitology", Solnechnogorsk, Russia
e-mail: vdementevskiy@fnkcrr.ru

E. A. Lekchnov (✉) · D. A. Rzaev
Federal State Budgetary Institution "Federal Neurosurgical Center", Novosibirsk, Russia
e-mail: e_lekhnov@neuronsk.ru; d_rzaev@neuronsk.ru

K. V. Slavin
Department of Neurosur gery, University of Illinois at Chicago, Chicago, IL, USA

Neurology Section, Jesse Brown Veterans Administration Medical Center, Chicago, IL, USA
e-mail: kslavin@uic.edu

S.-T. Li et al. (eds.), *Microvascular Decompression Surgery*,
https://doi.org/10.1007/978-981-96-0767-9_14

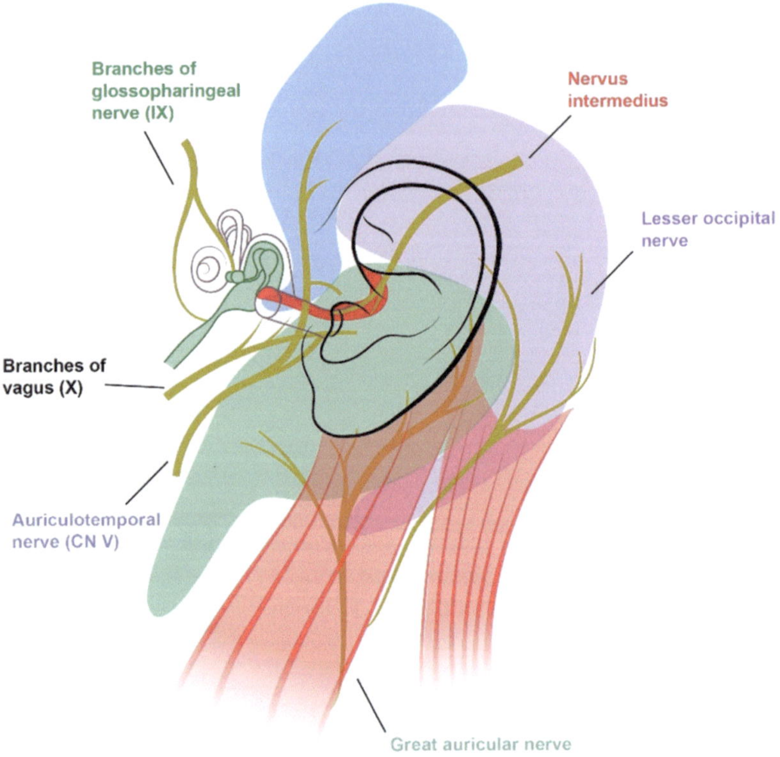

Fig. 14.1 Innervation of pinna, retroauricular region and internal auditory canal

ity of the premeatal segment of the VIII nerve and, less often, next to the brainstem and distal premeatal and intrameatal segments of the VIII nerve [6]. It should be noted that NI is not visualized as a separate structure due to tight fusion with the VII–VIII complex in about 20–22% of cases [2]. In its distal segment inside IAC, NI joins the facial nerve and cannot be clearly defined [1, 8]. In 90% of cases, NI joins the VII nerve within IAC, and in 10%—in the premeatal segment of the VII nerve [6].

Numerous cadaver studies and intraoperative findings in patients show that NI gives rise to a number of fine anastomoses to the facial and vestibulocochlear nerves [2]. Further, in the facial nerve canal, where NI, greater petrosal nerve, and facial nerve join, a geniculate ganglion (GG) is formed [9]. GG sends fibers to the tongue through the facial nerve, chorda tympani, and lingual nerve; through the large superficial petrosal nerve, Vidian nerve, and pterygopalatine nerves—to the palate and related areas, and through the facial nerve and posterior auricular nerve—to the inner surface of the pinna [9]. NI contains parasympathetic secretory fibers to the glands (lacrimal, sublingual, submandibular, salivary glands, glands of the nasal mucosa, and palate), taste fibers to the anterior two-thirds of the tongue and hard palate, as well as sensory fibers from the posterior-upper part of the external auditory canal [6, 10, 11]. It is worth noting that pinna, internal auditory canal, and retroauricular region have complex innervation through greater and lesser occipital, trigeminal (auriculotemporal branches), glossopharyngeal (tympanic branch), and vagus (auricular branch) nerves [12–14] (Fig. 14.1), and this creates significant difficulty in NIN diagnosis.

14.3 Intermediate Nerve Neuralgia Mechanism

There is plenty of evidence that NI involvement plays a key role in NIN development [11]. However, the NIN etiology is complex and is not fully understood [9, 15]. Various NIN origin theories have been proposed, including neurovascular conflict (NVC) with NI, which is most accepted and confirmed by numerous observations [6, 15]. Local demyelination and chronic inflammation lead to NI irritation and increase level of pain perception [11, 15]. High resolution MR imaging and MR angiography are capable of detecting NI NVC [11]. Microvascular decompression (MVD) of the NI in such cases can relieve pain immediately after surgery [6]. NIN and the other cranial nerves hyperactivity syndromes have much in common in etiological and pathophysiological aspects [16–18]. Previously, different pathological discharge mechanisms due to injury or inflammation in mechanoreceptive conduction system in cranial neuralgias including NIN were discussed [9].

14.4 Nervus Intermedius Neuralgia

NIN is a rare disease for which there is no generally accepted management protocol. Clinically, NIN manifests by short attacks of electric shock-like pain paroxysms in the depth of the ear with radiation to the retroauricular and temporal regions [19]. The pain is severe and rivaled only by that of trigeminal neuralgia (TN), glossopharyngeal neuralgia (GPN), and cluster headache. The description of pain is that of an ice pick repeatedly jabbed into the ear. Uncontrolled pain of this severity has been associated with suicide and should therefore be treated with a sense of urgency. These pain paroxysms may be accompanied by lacrimation, salivation, and changes in taste. The pain can have a gradual or paroxysmal onset, be dull, persistent, or sharp, stabbing, and ultimately significantly reduces the patient's quality of life [20]. Attacks are commonly triggered by daily activities involving contact with or light touch of the external acoustic meatus, auricle and/or periauricular region. Patients have also noted that NIN attacks may be triggered by lying on the affected side. NIN patients prefer to avoid any contact with trigger areas. Between attacks, patients are relatively pain free. A dull ache remaining after the intense pain subsides may be suggestive of persistent NI compression by a structural lesion. This disease is rarely seen in persons younger than 30 years. Patients with NIN often have severe comorbidities, such as depression, anxiety, and sleep disturbances that accompany painful episodes.

There are two most commonly used classification systems proposed by the International Headache Society (IHS) and International Association for the Study of Pain (IASP) [21].

According to the International Headache Classification, there are three NIN subtypes that are similar to TN subtypes: Classical, Secondary, and Idiopathic. Idiopathic NIN denotes a condition of pain without any identifiable cause. In Secondary NIN, the involvement of NI is attributed to neurological diseases like multiple sclerosis or tumors of the cerebellopontine angle. In the latter case, neurological deficits arising from damage to other nerves in close proximity tend to dominate the clinical presentation, leading to tinnitus, hearing loss, vertigo, nausea, hoarseness, and dysphagia. Classical NIN develops without apparent cause other than neurovascular compression demonstrated on MRI or during surgery. Main difference between NIN and NI neuropathy is a type of pain. In NI neuropathy, the pain is within NI distribution, and is described by the patient as dull, deep in the ear, and continuous or near-continuous. Brief paroxysms may be superimposed, but they are not the predominant pain type. This combination distinguishes painful NI neuropathy from NIN. Intermedius neuropathy can be associated with Herpes Zoster infection and other disorders, or be idiopathic with unknown etiology. Neuropathy caused by herpes zoster infection is commonly associated with facial paresis and other symptoms and/or clinical signs of the infection or its aftermath [21].

14.5 Diagnosis and Different Diagnosis

Every patient presenting with ear pain should be evaluated by otolaryngologists to exclude underlying ear pathology. The pain may also be referred

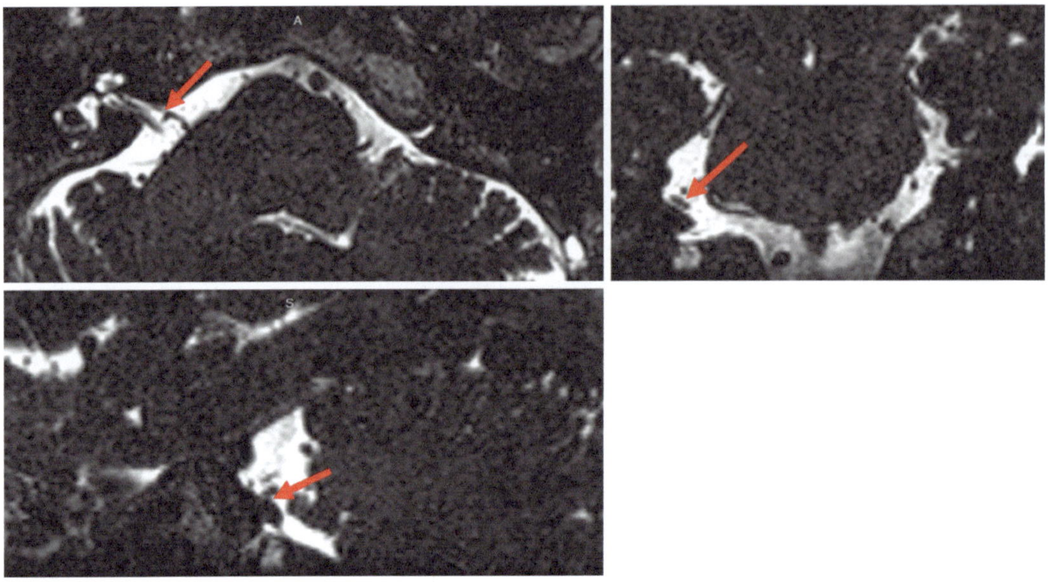

Fig. 14.2 Clinical example of a patient with NIN. 3 T-MRI revealed NVC between VII–VIII complex and AICA (red arrow)

to the ear from surrounding structures, such as teeth, throat, parotid gland, neck vessels, or upper cervical roots and occipital nerves. Neuralgic ear pain can be associated with injury of six different nerves that innervate ear region, often with overlapping dermatomes. Trauma or local structural irritation, such as infection, neoplasms, inflammation, and compression, of these nerves could contribute to pain within innervation zones [22]. Clinical and instrumental evaluation of all patients with a new diagnosis of NIN should include high-resolution magnetic resonance imaging (MRI) or magnetic resonance angiography of brain with gadolinium contrast to rule out posterior fossa or brainstem lesions and demyelinating disease [23]. In contrast to computed tomography or MRI at 1.5 T, high-resolution MRI at 3 T visualize NI in 70% patients [6] (Fig. 14.2). At the same time, 3 T MRI cannot delineate individual NI rootlets [6]. MRI combined with computer-assisted reconstruction allows visualization of vessels and nerves with a specificity of 83–96% and a sensitivity of 83–100% [24]. It is necessary to confirm neurovascular conflict as the most likely cause of classical NIN with MRI with special thin-slices sequences for visualization of cranial nerve (3D-FIESTA or CISS).

Additional CT or MRI scan of the sinuses should be considered in case of any question of occult or coexisting sinus disease. Screening laboratory tests consisting of a complete blood count, erythrocyte sedimentation rate, and automated blood chemistry should be performed. A complete blood count is required for baseline comparisons before starting treatment with carbamazepine as a conservative treatment option.

14.6 Therapy

Drug therapy of NIN is prescribed prior to surgical consideration. Medications can relieve symptoms in many patients, especially in early stages of the disease [15, 25], and include carbamazepine, gabapentin, pregabalin and baclofen. Carbamazepine and oxcarbazepine are considered a first-line treatment for NIN. Rapid response to these drugs helps to confirm the clinical diagnosis. In 70% of cases, carbamazepine use allows to suppress chronic neuropathic pain [25].

Carbamazepine should be initiated slowly with a starting dose of 100 to 200 mg at bedtime for 2 nights and increased in 200 mg increments over 2 days. Effective dose is 1200 mg or more per day, if no side effects occur. The patient should be cautioned about side effects, including dizziness, sedation, confusion, and rash. Careful monitoring of laboratory parameters is mandatory. When pain relief is obtained, the patient should be kept at that dosage of carbamazepine for at least 6 months before the medication tapering is considered [26]. If carbamazepine does not adequately control patient's pain or has intolerable side effects, gabapentin may be considered as the second-line therapy. The initial dose is 300 mg at bedtime for 1–2 days. The drug is then increased in 300 mg increments given in equally divided doses over 2 days, as side effects allow, until pain relief is obtained or a total dose of 2400 mg per day is reached. The dosage greater than 3600 mg per day is rarely required. Pregabalin represents a reasonable alternative to gabapentin and is better tolerated by some patients. Pregabalin is started at 50 mg three times per day and may be titrated upward to 100 mg three times per day if side effects allow [26]. In cases when pain persists despite medical therapy, surgical intervention is considered [25].

14.7 Surgery

Despite existence of various surgical approaches in NIN, currently there is no generally accepted treatment algorithm. In addition, due to NIN extreme rarity, the majority of studies contain small sample groups and study designs differ from each other, generally making them difficult to compare. Current surgical approaches are summarized in Table 14.1 and include NI transection, NI MVD, GG excision, and V, IX, X cranial nerves rhizotomy. Among them, the most commonly used surgical approaches today are NI transection and NI MVD (VII–VIII complex) [27, 28]. Despite a low level of evidence, accumulated surgical experience suggests overall effectiveness of these procedures in NIN patients with drug-resistant pain syndrome [29]. As seen in our summary (Table 14.1), NI rhizotomy was performed in 116 (%) and MVD in 59 (%) patients, with both procedures being done for the same purpose [27, 30–34]. Pain improved in 146 cases (90.1%) (all surgical techniques), it persisted after surgery in 6 cases (3.7%), there was a recurrence of the pain syndrome in 14 cases (8.6%) (Table 14.1).

14.7.1 NI MVD

It is believed that the main cause of NIN is a vascular conflict in NI root entry zone (REZ) similar to neurovascular conflict affecting other cranial nerves [12, 35]. Due to their anatomical proximity, AICA, PICA or the vertebral arteries can cause compression of the VII/VIII complex, including NI [27, 29, 35]. Among published cases, AICA compression was observed in 75%, PICA and vertebral arteries—in 25% of cases [14, 27, 29, 35]. MVD alone has been demonstrated to be effective and providing excellent results [15, 23]. Arterial transposition leads to nerve decompression and immediate pain syndrome regression [14]. In the presence of NVC, there is no need to perform NI transection and other cranial nerves exploration [11, 23], but this issue is still open for debate [23]. Postoperative NI MVD complications include transient neurological deficits (partial hearing loss and/or facial nerve palsy), which may be explained by VII/VIII complex traction [15, 23].

14.7.2 NI Transection

A more complicated situation arises when there is no clear NI NVC on imaging, but typical NIN symptoms exist. Moreover, it is not always possible to intraoperatively identify the offending vessel adjacent to VII/VIII complex. In these cases, NI transection is a possible surgical alternative (Table 14.1). Surgery success largely depends on microanatomy knowledge of NI and surrounding anatomical structures (Fig. 14.3).

During this procedure, the surgeon may face a number of difficulties and risk postoperative neurological complications. For example, to visualize NI, it is necessary to dissect NI from the VII-VIII complex with possible facial and/or vestibulocochlear nerves injury leading to postoper-

Table 14.1 Surgical techniques in NIN treatment, presence of concomitant cranial nerve neuralgia, and treatment results

							V CN		IX CN		X CN		Outcomes				
No	Author, year	Patients	Transection NI	MVD NI	GG excision	Concomitant neuralgias	Rhizotomy	MVD	Rhizotomy	MVD	Rhizotomy	MVD	Clinical improvement	Pain relieved	Pain persisted	Pain recurrence	Follow up
1	Tatit 2022 [30]	1	1	1										1			12 months
2	Zheng 2021 [12]	23		23										22		1	6 months
3	Witters 2021 [23]	1		1										1			7 days clinicaly
4	Zenonos 2020 [25]	1	1							1		1					5 years
5	Onoda 2020 [14]	1		1										1			12 months
6	George 2020 [31]	1	1	1						1		1		1			18 months (L), 10 months (R)
7	Clifton 2019 [32]	12	11	7										10		2	Not indicated
8	Peris-Celda 2018 [27]	11	9	2		7	1	4	2	3	2[a]		4	8[b]		5	37 months
9	Holste 2018 [33]	15	14	5		10		8	2	2	2	2		13[c]		6	6.4 years
10	Fernandes 2017 [35]	8		8										7	1		35 months
11	Tubbs 2013 [20]	1	1							1				1			16 months
12	Saers 2011 [24]	1		1										1			12 months
13	Younes 2010 [15]	1		1										1			12 months
14	Özer 2009 [36]	1		1										1			4 years
15	Sakas 2007 [11]	1		1										1			6 months

16	Pulec 2002 [13]	64	64		64	[e]	16						1	63			Not indicated
17	Rupa 1991 [34]	18	14[d]	5	10	[e]		3	14	5	11	5		13	5		3.3 years
18	Bellotti 1978 [37]	1		1		1	1							1			12 months
	Total	162	116	59	74	18	18	15	18	13	15	9	5	146	6	14	

[a]Part root rhizotomy
[b]Pain completely relieved in the early postoperative period
[c]Pain completely relieved during the first 2 weeks
[d]Also tympanic nerve section (4 patients) and chorda tympani section has been made (1 patient); *L* left side, *R* right side
[e]Exact number is not indicated

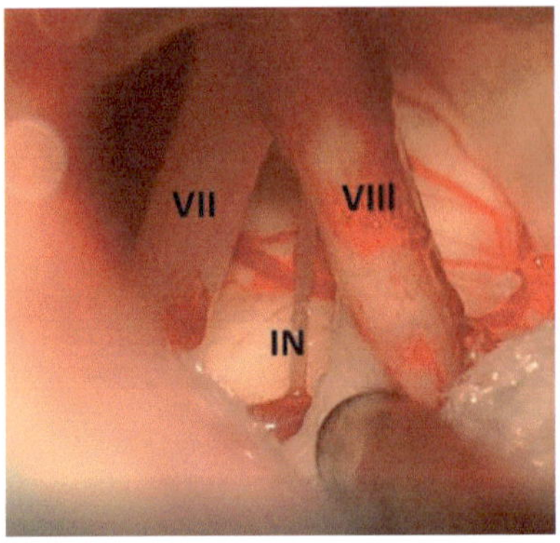

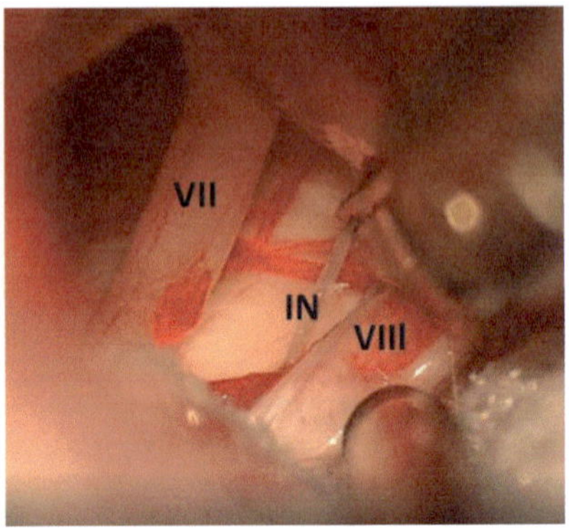

Fig. 14.3 Intraoperatively NI was dissected from the VII/VIII complex (left picture) and transected (right picture)

ative facial weakness, hearing loss, or vertigo [12, 15, 23, 35]. In addition, patients after NI transection may have so-called minor complications such as taste and lacrimation disorder or transient weakness of the m. levator labialis on the side of the approach [12], buttaste or lacrimation changes tend to be insignificant [25]. To minimize the risk of postoperative neurological deficits of during dissection of VII–VIII complex, special care should be exercised and neurophysiological monitoring must be used. NI transection was used almost twice as often as the NI MVD in patients with NIN (Table 14.1).

14.7.3 Other Surgical Techniques

In addition to the above-described techniques for NIN and concomitant neuralgias, other surgical approaches have been proposed in the past, including MVD or rhizotomy of the V, IX, X cranial nerves, GG excision [5, 34], that may be combined with NI transection. Anatomical and microscopic studies revealed that GG collects sensory and autonomic fibers entering through the chorda tympani and greater petrosal nerve with subsequent transmission of pain impulses through NI [5, 34]. GG excision procedure showed good postoperative results with pain relief after unsuccessful NI transection [5, 34]. The GG excision technique consists in resection of the internal knee of the facial nerve (but not more than 20%) and partial excision of the large petrosal nerve in order to reduce risk of developing postoperative facial nerve deficit [5]. In addition to GG excision and NI transection, exploration and rhizotomy of the V, IX, X cranial nerves, as well as entire surgical algorithms, have been proposed. The combination of GG excision with transection of NI, chorda tympani, tympanic nerve branch of IX nerve, and upper roots of X nerve shows best results and helps to eliminate the most severe pain [34]. It is worth noting that such approaches (exploratory craniotomies and MVDs, rhizotomy of V, IX, X cranial nerves, GG removal, etc.) were applied in the past when high-quality preoperative neuroimaging was not available [11], as a result, such patients without clear preoperative diagnosis had to be reoperated, since the pain syndrome in some of them persisted [34]. These surgical procedures are quite complex and present mainly a historical interest; current surgical approaches (NI MVD and NI transection) may be supplemented by MVD of V, IX, X cranial nerves if needed [27, 33].

14.7.4 NIN Treatment Algorithm

From a practical point of view, a number of key issues that could influence treatment efficacy and help patients to get rid of excruciating pain need to be highlighted in NIN surgery. First of all, a comprehensive clinical and neuroimaging examination aimed to exclude concomitant neuralgias mimicking NIN or other primary pathology is required. This will help in avoiding diagnostic mistakes and unnecessary procedures, such as diagnostic cranial nerve exploration. More detailed imaging analysis makes it possible to define a need in specific interventions, such as NI MVD or NI transection and/or additional procedures such as MVD of other cranial nerves (e.g., in case of concurrent TN or GPN). The second question concerns surgical strategies and tactics. With clear NI NVC, MVD of the VII–VIII complex is justified. However, in absence of NI NVC (both with neuroimaging and intraoperative findings), but with clear clinical signs of NIN (when other possible causes of pain have been excluded), NI transection should be performed. Such approaches alone (MVD or NI transection) are acceptable only in case of NIN without concomitant disorders. In case of concomitant neuralgia, it is necessary to perform MVD of a clinically relevant nerve. From our point of view, a "prophylactic" exploration of other cranial nerves without any signs of neuralgia is inappropriate since proximity of a vessel to a cranial nerve may occur in asymptomatic people without any symptoms of neuralgia [16, 17].

14.8 Neurophysiological Monitoring

As mentioned earlier, NI and its rootlets can usually be identified intraoperatively due to their anatomical features [12]. Since NI can be present in multiple branches mixed within VII–VIII nerve complex, an incomplete NI transection may result in pain persistence [12]. Therefore, proper use of intraoperative neurophysiological monitoring (IONM) may help in NI identification, functional assessment of other cranial nerves (i.e., VII and VIII), and avoidance of neurological deficit after the surgery. Previous histological studies of human cadavers showed that NI contains 86.45% myelinated and 13.55% unmyelinated fibers. Up to 0.5% large (>12 μm in diameter) motor fibers, comparable in size to those in the facial nerve, are found among NI myelinated fibers [38]. NI may be responsible for the perioral muscles activation, in particular for the elevation of the corner of the mouth [39] due to selective innervation of individual muscle bundles in that region [32, 33, 39]. Thus, NI can be detected using during the surgery with recording from lower perinasal and perioral musculature. During NI stimulation, muscular responses have statistically significant greater latency (8.5 ms–11.1 ms) and lower amplitude (10.8–11.1 mV) compared to the facial nerve (5.6 ± 1.5 ms and 740 ± 123.7 μV) [8, 38]. Moreover, NI stimulation threshold is higher (0.4 ± 0.1 V) compared to the threshold of the facial nerve (0.08 ± 0.01 V) [8]. Time-amplitude parameters of the stimulation responses differ for NI and facial nerve [38, 39], and this difference can be used for intraoperative NI detection, especially in those cases where intraoperative visualization is challenging [8]. For example, short-latency, low-threshold, and high-amplitude responses are characteristic for the facial nerve, while long-latency, high-threshold, and low-amplitude responses belong to NI [8]. These neurophysiological differences (between the NI and facial nerve) are of great importance when there are no anatomical landmarks due to altered CPA anatomy (e.g., in vestibular schwannomas) [8] or absence of NI direct visualization [8].

14.9 Conclusion

NIN is a very rare disease that may be challenging to diagnose. Special attention should be paid to modern additional diagnostic methods, such as 3 T MRI and MR angiography, in order to determine the existence of NVC and the exact location of NI. Use of IONM during NI surgery is mandatory, as it facilitates identification of NI and its neighbors. Appropriately chosen and performed surgery translates into highly effective treatment outcome while minimizing the risk of postoperative complications such as facial palsy or hearing loss. Proper strategy and attention to surgical nuances will generally improve operative results and preserve patients' quality of life.

References

1. Elakkad SE, Yetto JM, Landon MD, Cathey MR. Stuck in the middle: nervus intermedius-related neuropathologic imaging spectrum. Neurograph. 2019;9:330–43.
2. Alfieri A, Strauss C, Prell J, Peschke E. History of the nervus intermedius of Wrisberg. Ann Anat. 2010;192:139–44.

3. Lobko PI, Khil'kevich SI. The intermediate nerve and its place in the system of cranial nerves. Arkh Anat Gistol Embriol. 1989;97:37–46.
4. Baldauf J, Rosenstengel C, Schroeder HWS. Nerve compression syndromes in the posterior cranial fossa. Dtsch Arztebl Int. 2019;116:54–60.
5. Pulec JL. Geniculate neuralgia: diagnosis and surgical management. Laryngoscope. 1976;86:955–64.
6. Meybodi AT, Liang AS, Mokhtari P, Moreira LB, Zhao X, Lawton MT, Preul MC. Nervus intermedius: microsurgical and anatomic relationships to the cerebellopontine angle neurovascular complex. Surg Neurol Int. 2023;14:37.
7. Rhoton AL, Kobayashi S, Hollinshead WH. Nervus intermedius. J Neurosurg. 1968;29:609–18.
8. Ashram YA, Jackler RK, Pitts LH, Yingling CD. Intraoperative electrophysiologic identification of the nervus intermedius. Otol Neurotol. 2005;26:274–9.
9. Boudreau JC, Oravec J, White TD, Madigan C, Chu SP. Geniculate neuralgia and facial nerve sensory systems. Arch Otolaryngol. 1977;103:473–81.
10. Irving RM, Viani L, Hardy DG, Baguley DM, Moffat DA. Nervus intermedius function after vestibular schwannoma removal: clinical features and pathophysiological mechanisms. Laryngoscope. 1995;105:809–13.
11. Sakas DE, Panourias IG, Stranjalis G, Stefanatou MP, Maratheftis N, Bontozoglou N. Paroxysmal otalgia due to compression of the intermediate nerve: a distinct syndrome of neurovascular conflict confirmed by neuroimaging: case report. J Neurosurg. 2007;107:1228–30.
12. Zheng R, Zhao C, Zhao Z, Li X. Case report: direct visualization of the nervus intermedius during the microvascular decompression procedure: should we take it seriously? Front Neurol. 2021;12:666427.
13. Pulec JL. Geniculate neuralgia: long-term results of surgical treatment. Ear Nose Throat J. 2002;81:30–3.
14. Onoda K, Kawaguchi A, Takaya Y, Saito Y, Ishikawa H, Uno T, Miyamoto M, Oyama K, Matsuno A. A case of nervus intermedius neuralgia. World Neurosurg. 2020;137:89–92.
15. Younes WM, Capelle H-H, Krauss JK. Microvascular decompression of the anterior inferior cerebellar artery for intermediate nerve neuralgia. Stereotact Funct Neurosurg. 2010;88:193–5.
16. Jannetta P. Observations on the etiology of trigeminal neuralgia, Hemifacial spasm, acoustic nerve dysfunction and glossopharyngeal neuralgia. Definitive microsurgical treatment and results in 117 patients. Minim Invasive Neurosurg. 1977;20:145–54.
17. De Simone R, Ranieri A, Bilo L, Fiorillo C, Bonavita V. Cranial neuralgias: from physiopathology to pharmacological treatment. Neurol Sci. 2008;29(Suppl 1):S69–78.
18. Love S, Coakham HB. Trigeminal neuralgia: pathology and pathogenesis. Brain. 2001;124:2347–60.
19. DeLange JM, Garza I, Robertson CE. Clinical reasoning: a 50-year-old woman with deep stabbing ear pain. Neurology. 2014;83:e152–7.
20. Tubbs RS, Steck DT, Mortazavi MM, Cohen-Gadol AA. The nervus intermedius: a review of its anatomy, function, pathology, and role in neurosurgery. World Neurosurg. 2013;79:763–7.
21. Headache Classification Committee of the International Headache Society (IHS). The International Classification of Headache Disorders, 3rd edition. Cephalalgia. 2018;38:1–211.
22. Fernandez-Vial D, Sangalli L, Perez C. A rare case of idiopathic painful nervus intermedius neuropathy in a 13-year-old female: a case report and discussion in the context of the literature. Children. 2022;9:1234.
23. Witters L, Lukes A, Menovsky T. Paroxysmal otalgia treated with microvascular decompression of the intermediate nerve: illustrative case. J Neurosurg Case Lessons. 2021;1:CASE2155.
24. Saers SJF, Han KS, de Ru JA. Microvascular decompression may be an effective treatment for nervus intermedius neuralgia. J Laryngol Otol. 2011;125:520–2.
25. Zenonos G, McDowell MM, Abou-Al-Shaar H, Alkhalili K, Gardner PA. A case report of pediatric geniculate neuralgia treated with sectioning of the nervus intermedius and microvascular decompression of cranial nerves IX and X. Pediatr Neurosurg. 2020;55:439–43.
26. Atlas of uncommon pain syndromes. 2014. https://doi.org/10.1016/C2011-0-69791-1.
27. Peris-Celda M, Oushy S, Perry A, Graffeo CS, Carlstrom LP, Zimmerman RS, Meyer FB, Pollock BE, Link MJ. Nervus intermedius and the surgical management of geniculate neuralgia. J Neurosurg. 2018;131:343–51.
28. Inoue T, Shima A, Hirai H, Suzuki F, Matsuda M. Nervus intermedius neuralgia treated with microvascular decompression: a case report and review of the literature. NMC Case Rep J. 2017;4:75–8.
29. Tang IP, Freeman SR, Kontorinis G, Tang MY, Rutherford SA, King AT, Lloyd SKW. Geniculate neuralgia: a systematic review. J Laryngol Otol. 2014;128:394–9.
30. Tatit RT, Raffa PEAZ, Seba MCC, Franceschini PR, De Aguiar PHP. Geniculate neuralgia: a case report and systematic review. Neurosurg Open. 2022:3(4). https://doi.org/10.1227/neuopn.0000000000000022.
31. George DD, Ridder TS. Geniculate neuralgia in an adolescent treated via sectioning of the nervus intermedius and microvascular decompression. J Neurosurg Pediatr. 2020;26:189–92.
32. Clifton WE, Grewal S, Lundy L, Cheshire WP, Tubbs RS, Wharen RE. Clinical implications of nervus intermedius variants in patients with geniculate neuralgia: let anatomy be the guide. Clin Anat. 2020;33:1056–61.
33. Holste KG, Hardaway FA, Raslan AM, Burchiel KJ. Pain-free and pain-controlled survival after sectioning the nervus intermedius in nervus intermedius neuralgia: a single-institution review. J Neurosurg. 2019;131:352–9.

34. Goulin Lippi Fernandes E, van Doormaal T, de Ru S, Miller K, Han KS. Microvascular decompression of the VII/VIII cranial nerve complex for the treatment of intermediate nerve neuralgia: a retrospective case series. Oper Neurosurg (Hagerstown). 2018;15:378–85.
35. Özer FD, Duransoy YK, Çamlar M. Atypic geniculate neuralgia: atypic anatomic correlation of cranial nerve roots and AICA. Acta Neurochir. 2009;151:1003–4.
36. Rupa V, Saunders RL, Weider DJ. Geniculate neuralgia: the surgical management of primary otalgia. J Neurosurg. 1991;75:505–11.
37. Bellotti C, Medina M, Oliveri G, Ettorre F, Barrale S, Sturiale C, Melcarne A. Neuralgia of the intermediate nerve combined with trigeminal neuralgia: case report. Acta Neurochir. 1988;91:142–3.
38. Alfieri A, Strauss C. Microvascular decompression may be an effective treatment for nervus intermedius neuralgia. J Laryngol Otol. 2011;125:765; author reply 765.
39. Alfieri A, Rampp S, Strauss C, Fleischhammer J, Rachinger J, Scheller C, Prell J. The relationship between nervus intermedius anatomy, ultrastructure, electrophysiology, and clinical function. Usefulness in cerebellopontine microsurgery. Acta Neurochir. 2014;156:403–8.

15 Glossopharyngeal Neuralgia

Raviteja Bethamcharla, Geoffrey Reeves, and Raymond F. Sekula

15.1 Introduction

Glossopharyngeal neuralgia (GPN), is a painful cranial nerve disorder with an estimated annual incidence of 0.2–0.7 per 100,000 [1, 2]. Although rare, GPN is a most debilitating condition due to lancinating and severe paroxysms of pain in the sensory afferents of the pharyngeal and auricular branches of the glossopharyngeal and vagus nerves (CN IX and X) [3–5]. The term vagoglossopharyngeal neuralgia has been used to describe paroxysmal pain attacks, primarily involving the palantine tonsil and posterior area of tongue, accompanied by "vagal" symptoms (e.g., syncope, bradycardia, and asystole).

GPN is infrequently misdiagnosed as trigeminal neuralgia (TN) involving the mandibular division of the trigeminal nerve. GPN may be differentiated from TN with a swallowing test, since swallowing is a common trigger of GPN, or by pain referred to the deep ear, which is partially innervated by cranial nerves IX and X. Signs and symptoms of glossopharyngeal neuralgia along with vascular compression of the centrally myelinated portions of cranial nerves IX and X, respectively, is classified as classical GPN (cGPN). Microvascular decompression (MVD) of an offending vessel is a potentially curative surgical treatment for cGPN.

15.2 Clinical Considerations and Diagnosis

Similar to TN, diagnosis of GPN is a clinical diagnosis dependent upon pain location and characteristics. During initial examination with suspicion of glossopharyngeal neuralgia, it is important to confirm that the patient's description of the pain meets certain criteria. The pain type, duration, trigger zones, and location should be taken into consideration. According to the latest guidelines established by the International Headache Society, GPN is a relapsing-remitting disorder characterized by severe, unilateral, electric shock-like pain lasting a maximum of 2 min in the distribution of the glossopharyngeal nerve as well as the auricular and pharyngeal branches of the vagus nerve [5]. The pain localizes to sensory areas of the aforementioned nerves (i.e., the posterior portion of the tongue, tonsillar fossa, pharynx, beneath the angle of the mandible, and ear). Pain associated with GPN is usually triggered by otherwise innocuous actions such as swallowing,

R. Bethamcharla
Department of Neurological Surgery, Columbia University, New York, NY, USA

G. Reeves
College of Physicians and Surgeons, Columbia University, New York, NY, USA

R. F. Sekula (✉)
Department of Neurosurgery, Columbia University Irving Medical Center, New York, NY, USA
e-mail: rfs2155@cumc.columbia.edu

S.-T. Li et al. (eds.), *Microvascular Decompression Surgery*,
https://doi.org/10.1007/978-981-96-0767-9_15

coughing, talking, yawning, or hearing loud sounds [3]. In severe cases of GPN, patients may avoid eating or drinking in an effort to avoid triggering the paroxysmal attacks. Prolonged lack of consumption of food and water can lead to weight loss and dehydration that may become life-threatening.

Physical examination of the patient with GPN confirms an absence of sensory deficits in the glossopharyngeal and vagal nerve distributions, but mild sensory deficits have been noted by quantitative sensory testing in trigeminal neuralgia patients [6]. If major sensory changes such as reduced/missing gag reflex are found during examination, glossopharyngeal neuropathy should be considered a more likely diagnosis. The frequency of GPN attacks is variable, and exacerbations in the form of paroxysmal pain attacks and periods of remission are unpredictable. Approximately 10% of patients with GPN develop pain-induced vagal symptoms of bradycardia, syncope, and, very rarely, asystole, a condition sometimes referred to as vagoglossopharyngeal neuralgia. The IHS does not, however, currently classify glossopharyngeal neuralgia with vagal symptoms as a separate entity.

Once the clinical characteristics of GPN have been established, GPN is then classified as classical, secondary, or idiopathic. Classical GPN (cGPN) requires the demonstration of neurovascular compression (NVC) of the glossopharyngeal nerve root either by high-resolution MRI [7] or during surgery [5]. Cases of GPN associated with neurovascular compression (NVC) were first reported by Laha and Jannetta in 1977 [8]. Similar to our understanding of classical and idiopathic TN (i.e., TN secondary to NVC with or without morphological changes), degree of NVC is likely an important finding in these patients. A study conducted by Sindou et al. measured the lengths and volumes of central myelin in trigeminal, facial, glossopharyngeal, and vagus nerves respectively, and the authors found that the incidence of hyperactive cranial neuralgias (i.e., trigeminal neuralgia, hemifacial spasm (HFS), and glossopharyngeal neuralgia) corresponded to the average lengths and volumes of the central myelin along the cisternal segment of the respective cranial nerves [9]. The vagal and glossopharyngeal nerves have the shortest length and volume of central myelin, which corresponds to the incidence of GPN being the least among the cranial neuralgias (i.e., incidence of GPN < HFS < TN). This study lends support to the idea that vascular compression along the centrally myelinated portions of the glossopharyngeal and vagus nerves causes cGPN. High resolution MR imaging techniques, and interpretation at our institution to delineate proximal vascular compression of cranial nerves IX and X to diagnose cGPN is discussed later in this chapter. Secondary GPN refers to paroxysmal pain syndrome caused by an underlying etiology other than NVC including inflammation, infarction, tumor (i.e., most likely malignant carcinoma), type I Chiari malformation, tonsillectomy, and vertebral artery dissection. GPN from these etiologies often presents with continuous pain of longer duration compared to GPN secondary to NVC [5]. When there is no evidence of either NVC or other etiology GPN is classified as idiopathic.

Differential diagnoses of GPN includes other neuralgias (i.e., TN, superior laryngeal neuralgia), painful glossopharyngeal neuropathy, and non-neuropathic pains (i.e., pharyngeal tumors, tonsillitis, pharyngitis, parapharyngeal abscess, post-tonsillectomy pain, retropharyngeal tendinitis, and Eagle's syndrome). Painful glossopharyngeal neuropathy is characterized by continuous or near-continuous burning pain often equated to pins and needles in the distribution of the glossopharyngeal nerve (i.e., posterior tongue, tonsillar fossa, pharynx, or beneath the angle of the mandible) [3]. Patients may have brief paroxysms, but are not the predominant type of pain, and sensory deficits are often present on the ipsilateral posterior tongue and/or tonsillar fossa (i.e., the gag reflex may be weak or missing). Glossopharyngeal neuropathy may be secondary to tumors at the CPA or iatrogenic injury, respectively. Exclusion of non-neuropathic pains is essential to confirm GPN. A laryngoscopy is necessary to exclude a pharyngeal tumor or parapharyngeal abscess that may be causing the pain.

15.3 Management

Carbamazepine and oxcarbazepine are considered first-line medications similar to the management of trigeminal neuralgia [1, 10, 11]. Other medications that may be considered in patients with poor tolerability or lack of effect are phenytoin, gabapentin, topiramate, lamotrigine, and baclofen. However, patients with GPN may become refractory to medical management or develop serious adverse effects with first-line drugs, and neurosurgical intervention should be considered as an early option. In patients with NVC confirmed by high-resolution MRI, MVD should be considered the first-line treatment. GPN responsive to MVD is most commonly caused by arterial compression along the centrally myelinated portion of the ninth and tenth cranial nerves, respectively [12]. Ablative procedures including stereotactic radiosurgery (SRS), peripheral glycerol rhizotomy [13, 14], CT-guided percutaneous tractotomy-nucleotomy [15], and percutaneous thermorhizotomy [13, 16] may be considered in the rare patient unwilling or unfit to undergo MVD. Some centers may still utilize endocranial sectioning of the glossopharyngeal nerve along with a small rostral portion of the vagus nerve [16], but experienced centers typically avoid rhizotomy [7, 17].

15.4 Anatomy

The glossopharyngeal nerve consists of a cisternal, jugular foramen, and extracranial segment, respectively [18]. The cisternal segment originates from the rostral portion of the post-olivary sulcus of the medulla as one or more rootlets and traverses the subarachnoid space. The point of origination of the cisternal segment is referred to as the root entry point (REP). The REP is ventral and caudal to the choroid plexus protruding from the Foramen of Luschka and immediately inferior to the root exit point of the facial nerve [18, 19]. Cranial nerve IX central myelination comprises 4.8–13.3% of the length of its cisternal segment (i.e., the proximal region beginning at the REP) [9]. The most distal extent of central myelination along the glossopharngyeal nerve is 1.51 ± 0.39 millimeters on average from the brainstem [9, 20, 21]. The glossopharyngeal nerve continues anterolaterally as the jugular foramen segment along the medial aspect of the intrajugular ridge. At the jugular foramen, cranial nerve IX enters a dural meatus becomes the extracranial segment. The extracranial segment exits the dural meatus and crosses the internal carotid artery laterally beneath the styloid process and eventually forms the superior and inferior ganglia [18, 19].

The vagus nerve arises as approximately eight to ten rootlets immediately inferior to the glossopharyngeal nerve and superior to the accessory nerve rootlets, posterior to the rostral third of the inferior olive, and ventral to the choroid plexus. The rootlets enter the vagal meatus, a dural meatus separated from the superiorly situated glossopharyngeal meatus, by a dural septum. Cranial nerve X traverses the jugular foramen and enlarges to form a superior ganglion. The nerve continues to proceed inferiorly to communicate with cranial nerve XI. The cranial fibers of the accessory nerve emerge from the postolivary sulcus of the medulla inferior to the vagus nerve and join the vagus nerve rootlets entering the jugular foramen at the vagal meatus. The cervical fibers of cranial nerve XI originate in the upper cervical spinal cord and form a common trunk posterior to the dentate ligament. The cervical trunk traverses the foramen magnum and courses superiorily towards the jugular foramen. The hypoglossal nerve rootlets originate in the ventrolateral medullary sulcus (i.e., between the rostral two-thirds of the inferior olive and medullary pyramid). Cranial nerve XII rootlets continue anterolaterally through the subarachnoid space prior to entering the hypoglossal canal [18, 19].

The most common offending arteries in order of decreasing frequency are the posterior inferior cerebellar artery (PICA) (Fig. 15.1), vertebral artery, or anterior inferior cerebellar artery (AICA) [22, 23]. CN X upper rootlets have also been associated with GPN secondary to NVC [19]. Analogous to trigeminal neuralgia, focal demyelination of proximal centrally derived

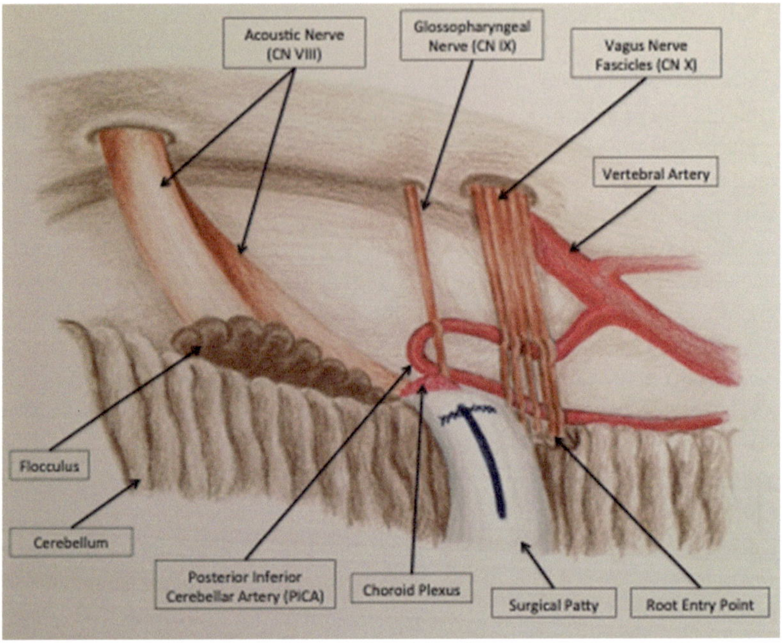

Fig. 15.1 This illustration depicts the relationship between the glossopharyngeal nerve (CN IX), vagus nerve (CN X), and the posterior inferior cerebellar artery (PICA). GPN secondary to neurovascular compression can be caused by compression of CN IX or the upper rootlets of CN X

myelin has been implicated in the etiopathogenesis of GPN with much objective data [24].

15.5 Imaging

After the exclusion of structural lesions, patients with GPN are evaluated with a dedicated MRI protocol optimized to delineate the lower cranial nerves and adjacent vessels. The protocol includes heavily T2 weighted, thin-section multiplanar steady state free precession (SSFP) sequences, which result in excellent resolution between cerebrospinal fluid (CSF) and the adjacent cranial nerves [25]. Additionally, the protocol consists of whole brain sagittal T1, axial FLAIR, and DWI sequences. Thin-section SSFP images of the brainstem are obtained in all three planes (i.e., axial, coronal, sagittal). Sagittal T1-weighted imaging parameters are as follows: TR/TE, 600/default to minimum; slice thickness, 5 mm; gap, 1 mm; FOV, 22 cm; and matrix, 256 × 192. Axial imaging parameters are as follows: TR/TE, 2200/150; slice thickness, 5 mm; gap, 1 mm; FOV, 22 cm; and matrix, 256 × 192. SSFP sequences in axial, coronal, and sagittal acquisitions are obtained with the following parameters: TR/TE, default to minimum; flip angle, 65°; slice thickness, 1 mm; matrix, 384 × 256; number of excitations, 2; and FOV, 18–20 cm.

This protocol is used to evaluate patients with suspected vascular compression causing GPN as well as trigeminal neuralgia and hemifacial spasm at our institution [30, 31]. The evaluation of vascular compression in cranial nerve disorders utilizing SSFP imaging has been well described in syndromes other than GPN [26–29]. Since SSFP sequences are a volumetric acquisition, multiplanar reformats in oblique planes are also possible. At our institution, MRIs protocoled to delineate the cranial nerves are performed on a 3 T MR scanner (Discovery MR, GE) since the shorter scan times result in less motion degradation versus a 1.5 T MR examination. Additionally, we employ the slice zero filling interpolation processing, which reconstructs twice as many slices by overlapping half of the slice thickness for the reconstructions [25]. The SSFP sequences are reviewed in all three planes to identify NVC of the glossopharyngeal nerve and to determine if the offending vessel is an artery or a vein. Compressive arteries, almost always the posterior inferior cerebellar artery, can be traced back to a parent vessel (i.e., vertebral artery). This is often best visualized on the coronal SSFP sequences. Veins, however, cannot be followed back to a parent artery. Other centers routinely include MR angiography, which is unhelpful as inclusion and exclusion of MR angiography have led to similar reported sensitivities (>95%) for detecting neurovascular compression, respectively [30].

If NVC of the IX and/or X cranial nerves is found on MRI, a diagnosis of cGPN can be made. There is a growing body of evidence in the trigeminal neuralgia literature that symptoms are associated with more severe NVC [30–32]. As an analogous cranial nerve disorder, the degree of NVC visualized on MR examination may be of significance in GPN. Therefore, at our institution, two different grades of NVC severity are considered when evaluating CN IX imaging. "Contact" is defined as a vessel touching the nerve with no CSF visualized separating the two. "Deformation" is defined as deviation or distortion of the nerve away from its normal course by an offending vessel. Further studies are required to accurately assess the clinical significance of contact versus deformation in the setting of cGPN. Additionally, because dedicated MRI protocols have a high sensitivity for the detection of NVC in trigeminal neuralgia, it is assumed that sensitivity for detection of NVC in GPN is correspondingly high [30]. Vascular contact with the glossopharyngeal nerve (i.e., of the peripherally myelinated portion of the nerve) likely occurs in asymptomatic individuals, therefore, clinical correlation with radiologic findings is essential.

15.6 Surgical Technique

At our institution, MVD for GPN is performed using techniques described in prior studies [33, 34], with modifications to avoid fixed cerebellar retraction [35]. In fact, this senior author has avoided fixed retractors for MVD of all cranial nerves since approximately 2005. Strict management of fluids is initiated in the preoperative holding area. The administration of intravenous fluids is limited to only the amount necessary to maintain a normotensive state prior to dural opening, which is usually less than 500 mL [35]. Additionally, a modification of the physiological dose of mannitol (0.25 g/kg) and an 8-mg dose of dexamethasone are given 30 min prior to the start of the procedure. The patient is turned in the lateral decubitus position, all pressure points are padded, and rigid fixation of the head is avoided. A 4-cm incision is planned just posterior to the digastric groove. The incision is made with a 15-blade knife down to the subcutaneous fat and a 15-mm Weitlaner retractor is inserted. The fascia and muscles are then opened down to the bone. Next, a cerebellar retractor is placed in the opening, and a burr-hole craniostomy is made at the asterion. The craniostomy is subsequently widened to 1.5 × 2.0 cm using a 5-mm coarse diamond drill bit (Midas; Stryker). A caudal and lateral suboccipital craniectomy is achieved, and any breached mastoid air cells are waxed. Next the dura is opened in a T-shaped fashion and reflected back with suture. A cotton patty is placed over the cerebellum to gently release CSF from the cerebellomedullary cistern, and the use of a self-retaining retractor is avoided. The lower cranial nerves are identified, and the arachnoid is sharply dissected. No tributaries of the superior petrosal vein complex are sacrificed. In our experience, the sacrifice of veins should be avoided to minimize complications. After the glossopharyngeal and vagus nerves come into view, the arachnoid about the nerves is also sharply dissected. The surgeon then identifies compressive vessels along the first few millimeters of CN IX and rostral rootlets of CN X near the brainstem and decompresses the nerves by decompressing the artery away from the nerves. The vessel may be permanently separated from the nerves by interposition or transposition. The craniectomy defect is then closed with a suitable material, such as titanium mesh or calcium phosphate cement [36, 37].

15.7 Postoperative Course

Patients are observed on a regular inpatient neurological surgery floor unit following microvascular decompression surgery, maintaining close attention to any alteration of vital signs or neurological examination. In patients with classical glossopharyngeal neuralgia, immediate pain relief following surgery is anticipated. Most patients are ambulatory and eating well on the first postoperative day and discharged from the hospital. Patients may have moderate headaches and nausea that typically subsides over a couple of days, such that the overall average length of stay is short. As soon as postoperative fatigue and intermittent headaches resolve, usually over the course of 4 weeks, patients may resume full levels of activity. At the time of discharge, patients should be advised to look out for delayed complications such as cerebrospinal fluid leak or wound infection. Preoperatively prescribed anticonvulsants are generally tapered over 10 to 14 days to minimize any potential drug withdrawal effects.

15.8 Outcomes

Jannetta first reported MVD of the vagus and glossopharyngeal nerves to treat GPN [8]. In Jannetta's series of 41 GPN patients who underwent MVD, immediate and long-term pain relief was noted in 79% and 76% of patients, respectively. With further improvements in preoperative imaging workup [7] and surgical technique [35], MVD has proven an even more effective surgical treatment with low morbidity for GPN [7, 16, 38–40]. In a 2015 literature review of 211 patients undergoing MVD for GPN, 97% were immediately pain-free and 93% of patients at a mean follow-up of 8.9 years were pain-free without medication or with occasional pain not requiring medication. Of these patients, 2% had permanent hoarseness and dysphagia, respectively. Another 1% of patients had permanent facial paresis. There were no mortalities after MVD for GPN.

References

1. Rushton JG, Stevens JC, Miller RH. Glossopharyngeal (vagoglossopharyngeal) neuralgia: a study of 217 cases. Arch Neurol. 1981;38(4):201–5.
2. Katusic S, Williams DB, Beard CM, Bergstralh E, Kurland LT. Incidence and clinical features of glossopharyngeal neuralgia, Rochester, Minnesota, 1945-1984. Neuroepidemiology. 1991;10(5–6):266–75.
3. Sicard R, Robineau M. Algie vélo-pharyngée essentielle. Traitement chirurgical. Rev Neurol. 1920;36:256–7.
4. Weisenburg TH. Cerebello-pontile tumor diagnosed for six years as tic douloureux: the symptoms of irritation of the ninth and twelfth cranial nerves. JAMA J Am Med Assoc. 1910;54(20):1600–4.
5. Society IH. International Classification of Headache Disorders-3. https://ichd-3.org/13-painful-cranial-neuropathies-and-other-facial-pains/13-2-glossopharyngeal-neuralgia/. Accessed 10 Dec 2023.
6. Younis S, Maarbjerg S, Reimer M, et al. Quantitative sensory testing in classical trigeminal neuralgia-a blinded study in patients with and without concomitant persistent pain. Pain. 2016;157(7):1407–14.
7. Jani RH, Hughes MA, Ligus ZE, Nikas A, Sekula RF. MRI findings and outcomes in patients undergoing microvascular decompression for glossopharyngeal neuralgia. J Neuroimaging. 2018;28(5):477–82.
8. Laha RK, Jannetta PJ. Glossopharyngeal neuralgia. J Neurosurg. 1977;47(3):316–20.
9. Guclu B, Sindou M, Meyronet D, Streichenberger N, Simon E, Mertens P. Cranial nerve vascular compression syndromes of the trigeminal, facial and vago-glossopharyngeal nerves: comparative anatomical study of the central myelin portion and transitional zone; correlations with incidences of corresponding hyperactive dysfunctional syndromes. Acta Neurochir. 2011;153(12):2365–75.
10. Blumenfeld A, Nikolskaya G. Glossopharyngeal neuralgia. Curr Pain Headache Rep. 2013;17(7):343.
11. Fromm GH. Clinical pharmacology of drugs used to treat head and face pain. Neurol Clin. 1990;8(1):143–51.
12. Jannetta PJ. Microsurgery of cranial nerve cross-compression. Clin Neurosurg. 1979;26:607–15.
13. Yomo S, Arkha Y, Donnet A, Regis J. Gamma knife surgery for glossopharyngeal neuralgia. J Neurosurg. 2009;110(3):559–63.
14. Williams BJ, Schlesinger D, Sheehan J. Glossopharyngeal neuralgia treated with gamma knife radiosurgery. World Neurosurg. 2010;73(4):413–7.
15. Kanpolat Y, Savas A, Batay F, Sinav A. Computed tomography-guided trigeminal tractotomy-nucleotomy in the management of vagoglossopharyngeal and geniculate neuralgias. Neurosurgery. 1998;43(3):484–9; discussion 490.
16. Rey-Dios R, Cohen-Gadol AA. Current neurosurgical management of glossopharyngeal neuralgia and technical nuances for microvascular decompression surgery. Neurosurg Focus. 2013;34(3):E8.
17. Zheng X, Wei XY, Zhu J, Yuan Y, Ying TT, Li ST. Microvascular decompression alone without rhizotomy is an effective way of treating glossopharyngeal neuralgia: clinical analysis of 46 cases. Stereotact Funct Neurosurg. 2020;98(2):129–35.

18. Ozveren MF, Ture U. The microsurgical anatomy of the glossopharyngeal nerve with respect to the jugular foramen lesions. Neurosurg Focus. 2004;17(2):E3.
19. Rhoton AL Jr. The cerebellopontine angle and posterior fossa cranial nerves by the retrosigmoid approach. Neurosurgery. 2000;47(3 Suppl):S93–129.
20. Lang J. Anatomy, length and blood vessel relations of "central" and "peripheral" paths of intracisternal cranial nerves. Zentralbl Neurochir. 1982;43(3):217–58.
21. Tarlov IM. Structure of the nerve root: ii. Differentiation of sensory from motor roots; observations on identification of function in roots of mixed cranial nerves. Arch Neurol Psychiatry. 1937;37(6):1338–55.
22. Resnick DK, Jannetta PJ, Bissonnette D, Jho HD, Lanzino G. Microvascular decompression for glossopharyngeal neuralgia. Neurosurgery. 1995;36(1):64–8; discussion 68–69.
23. Sampson JH, Grossi PM, Asaoka K, Fukushima T. Microvascular decompression for glossopharyngeal neuralgia: long-term effectiveness and complication avoidance. Neurosurgery. 2004;54(4):884–9; discussion 889–890.
24. Bethamcharla R, Reddy H, Teich AF, Sekula RF Jr. Histopathology of the trigeminal ganglion and nerve: a historical review. J Neurosci Res. 2023;101(8):1203–4.
25. Hughes MA, Frederickson AM, Branstetter BF, Zhu X, Sekula RF Jr. MRI of the trigeminal nerve in patients with trigeminal neuralgia secondary to vascular compression. AJR Am J Roentgenol. 2016;206(3):595–600.
26. Jo KW, Kong DS, Hong KS, Lee JA, Park K. Long-term prognostic factors for microvascular decompression for trigeminal neuralgia. J Clin Neurosci. 2013;20(3):440–5.
27. Garcia M, Naraghi R, Zumbrunn T, Rosch J, Hastreiter P, Dorfler A. High-resolution 3D-constructive interference in steady-state MR imaging and 3D time-of-flight MR angiography in neurovascular compression: a comparison between 3T and 1.5T. AJNR Am J Neuroradiol. 2012;33(7):1251–6.
28. Zeng Q, Zhou Q, Liu Z, Li C, Ni S, Xue F. Preoperative detection of the neurovascular relationship in trigeminal neuralgia using three-dimensional fast imaging employing steady-state acquisition (FIESTA) and magnetic resonance angiography (MRA). J Clin Neurosci. 2013;20(1):107–11.
29. Borges A, Casselman J. Imaging the trigeminal nerve. Eur J Radiol. 2010;74(2):323–40.
30. Jani RH, Hughes MA, Gold MS, Branstetter BF, Ligus ZE, Sekula RF Jr. Trigeminal nerve compression without trigeminal neuralgia: intraoperative vs imaging evidence. Neurosurgery. 2019;84(1):60–5.
31. Maarbjerg S, Wolfram F, Gozalov A, Olesen J, Bendtsen L. Significance of neurovascular contact in classical trigeminal neuralgia. Brain. 2015;138(Pt 2):311–9.
32. Leal PR, Hermier M, Souza MA, Cristino-Filho G, Froment JC, Sindou M. Visualization of vascular compression of the trigeminal nerve with high-resolution 3T MRI: a prospective study comparing preoperative imaging analysis to surgical findings in 40 consecutive patients who underwent microvascular decompression for trigeminal neuralgia. Neurosurgery. 2011;69(1):15–25; discussion 26.
33. Jannetta PJ. Trigeminal neuralgia. 1st ed. Oxford: Oxford University Press; 2010. p. 18.
34. McLaughlin MR, Jannetta PJ, Clyde BL, Subach BR, Comey CH, Resnick DK. Microvascular decompression of cranial nerves: lessons learned after 4400 operations. J Neurosurg. 1999;90(1):1–8.
35. Thirumala P, Frederickson AM, Balzer J, et al. Reduction in high-frequency hearing loss following technical modifications to microvascular decompression for hemifacial spasm. J Neurosurg. 2015;123(4):1059–64.
36. Frederickson AM, Sekula RF Jr. The utility of calcium phosphate cement in cranioplasty following retromastoid craniectomy for cranial neuralgias. Br J Neurosurg. 2013;27(6):808–11.
37. Foster KA, Shin SS, Prabhu B, Fredrickson A, Sekula RF Jr. Calcium phosphate cement cranioplasty decreases the rate of cerebrospinal fluid leak and wound infection compared with titanium mesh cranioplasty: retrospective study of 672 patients. World Neurosurg. 2016;95:414–8.
38. Kondo A. Follow-up results of using microvascular decompression for treatment of glossopharyngeal neuralgia. J Neurosurg. 1998;88(2):221–5.
39. Ferroli P, Fioravanti A, Schiariti M, et al. Microvascular decompression for glossopharyngeal neuralgia: a long-term retrospectic review of the Milan-Bologna experience in 31 consecutive cases. Acta Neurochir. 2009;151(10):1245–50.
40. Xia L, Li YS, Liu MX, et al. Microvascular decompression for glossopharyngeal neuralgia: a retrospective analysis of 228 cases. Acta Neurochir. 2018;160(1):117–23.

16 Internal Neurolysis for Trigeminal Neuralgia Without Vascular Conflict

Kim Burchiel

16.1 Trigeminal Neuralgia Without Vascular Conflict

Trigeminal neuralgia is a craniofacial pain condition characterized by severe paroxysm pain, often described as lancinating or electrical, lasting seconds to minutes in the trigeminal distribution. Dandy first proposed that neurovascular compression of the trigeminal nerve was a potential cause of trigeminal neuralgia [1]. Compression of the trigeminal nerve at the root entry zone by a blood vessel is clearly the most common "anatomical" association in patients with trigeminal neuralgia. Vascular compression may lead to hyperexcitability of injured or demyelinated axons [2], which may result in ectopic high-frequency discharges large enough to trigger spreading depolarization in ganglionic nociceptive neurons [3]. Jannetta established microvascular decompression (MVD), i.e., separating the conflicting vessel from the injured nerve, as one of the most important surgical treatments of trigeminal neuralgia [4].

Neurovascular compression (NVC) is also not a monolithic condition. Sindou has produced a grading scale for NVC: Grade I is mere vascular contact, grade II is vascular indentation into the nerve, and grade III is anatomic deviation of the nerve based on vascular conflict [5]. It also appears that around 17% of an age-matched population has some form of NVC [6]. Given that trigeminal neuralgia has a prevalence of 0.01–0.02% of the population, this means that roughly 99.96% of NVC is *asymptomatic*. Maarbjerg has shown that in patients with trigeminal neuralgia, NVC was prevalent both on the symptomatic and asymptomatic side (89% vs. 78%, $p = 0.017$), while severe NVC (nerve displacement or atrophy) was highly prevalent on the symptomatic compared to the asymptomatic side (53% vs. 13%, $p < 0.001$) [7]. From this work, it appears that with trigeminal neuralgia can be the result of severe NVC, but possibly not the cause in all cases with *any* degree of NVC. In cases of less severe NVC it is possible, even likely, that MVD may also not address the etiology of with trigeminal neuralgia.

It has become increasing clear that trigeminal neuralgia is not a homogenous disorder. There is no question that vascular compression of the nerve is an important etiology with trigeminal neuralgia. However, the evidence suggests that the "theoretical support for a vascular compressive etiology of with trigeminal neuralgia is weak, albeit the surgical outcome data are relatively convincing" [8]. Multiple sclerosis, and rarely vascular malformations and tumors, can also be associated with trigeminal neuralgia. Numerous studies have now demonstrated genetic polymorphisms that seem to predispose

K. Burchiel (✉)
Oregon Health and Science University, Portland, OR, USA
e-mail: burchiek@ohsu.edu

S.-T. Li et al. (eds.), *Microvascular Decompression Surgery*,
https://doi.org/10.1007/978-981-96-0767-9_16

to the development of trigeminal neuralgia [9, 10]. Trigeminal neuralgia occurs and recurs in the absence of neurovascular conflict [12]. Trigeminal neuralgia patients without NVC are younger at onset of symptoms than patients with NVC, and they are predominantly female [11]. It seems that neurovascular conflict is neither a *necessary* nor a *sufficient* condition for the development of trigeminal neuralgia.

16.2 Treatment Options of Trigeminal Neuralgia Without Vascular Compression

The advent of high-resolution brainstem, nerve, and vascular structure imaging has made it possible to ascertain with a very high level of certainty (96% sensitivity, 90% specificity) whether neurovascular compression is present prior to any invasive procedure [12]. In the absence of NVC on imaging, microvascular decompression is not a viable option. Given the considerable evidence that classic trigeminal neuralgia (TN1) can and does occur in the absence of NVC, it is reasonable to ask what the strategy for these patients might be if the condition becomes medically intractable [13].

Partial sensory rhizotomy is one type of posterior fossa exploration ablative procedure. This procedure entails division of the lateral one-half to two-thirds of the sensory root, 2–5 mm from the pons. It was reported by Dandy as a way to preserve some facial sensation and mastication strength with partial transection of the trigeminal nerve in the treatment of trigeminal neuralgia [1]. However, the ablative nature of the procedure can result in permanent sensory deficits in up to 83% of cases with a pain recurrence rate greater than 40%. Moreover, 4.9% of these patients may experience anesthesia dolorosa [14].

By avoiding transecting the nerves, internal neurolysis emerged as another option to alleviate the irritation of the trigeminal nerve in case neurovascular conflict was not identified. The procedure involves "combing" or brushing the nerve by longitudinally splitting portions of the trigeminal nerve bundles between the pons and the porus trigeminus. The mechanism by which internal neurolysis produces pain relief is unclear. Internal neurolysis is a destructive procedure in comparison with MVD. Possible mechanism for its effectiveness is the reduction of triggering of lancinating pain, much like RFL, partial sensory rhizotomy, and other ablative procedures. Internal neurolysis traumatizes the nerve and potentially reduces its abnormal signal to the brainstem.

Internal neurolysis disrupts the nerve across its entirety, rather than only the lateral third or half. By disrupting a larger cross-section of nerve fibers that could be contributing to the triggered, lancinating pain, internal neurolysis increases the chance of pain relief. Furthermore, internal neurolysis leaves the nerve by and large in continuity. This may mitigate the severity of numbness which is relevant, since patients who underwent partial sensory rhizotomy reported lower patient satisfaction in comparison to those who underwent microvascular decompression due to persistence of facial numbness [15].

In patients without neurovascular conflict, other percutaneous ablative therapies targeting gasserian ganglion include radiofrequency gangliolysis, chemoablation using retrogasserian glycerol, physical pressure using balloon microcompression, and radiation-induced degeneration produced by stereotactic radiosurgery. All these options are appropriate second-line therapy in patients who cannot tolerate posterior fossa exploration or who have failed microvascular decompression.

16.3 Surgical Techniques for Internal Neurolysis

Internal neurolysis is performed under general endotracheal anesthesia, using a minimum of inhalational anesthetic to facilitate monitoring of Brainstem Auditory Evoked Responses (BAERs) and no paralytic agents to allow monitoring of facial electromyogram. A bipolar facial electromyogram is recorded ipsilaterally from the orbicularis oris and orbicularis oculi. BAERs are recorded bilaterally.

The patient is placed supine, with the head placed in the Mayfield head holder. The head is rotated away from the side of surgery, and the neck is slightly flexed and elevated. After sterile preparation of the skin, a curved retroauricular incision is made from approximately the top of the pinna to the mastoid notch and the skin edges are retracted using "fish hooks."

A small craniectomy is then created by drilling, starting inferior and posterior to the asterion. Once dura is exposed, the craniectomy is then enlarged with Kerrison rongeurs to the point that the edges of the anterior transverse sinus, transverse-sigmoid junction, and the superior aspect of the sigmoid sinus are minimally exposed. Any bleeding points are controlled with small pieces of Gelfoam (Pfizer, New York, NY, USA) soaked in thrombin. The final size of the craniectomy should be 2.5 to 3 cm in diameter. Open mastoid air cells must be fully waxed.

The dura is then opened in a curvilinear fashion paralleling the transverse-sigmoid junction, and the dura anterior to the incision is tacked up using three or four sutures. A cottonoid patty is then inserted through the incision and over the cerebellum to facilitate cerebrospinal fluid (CSF) drainage. A flexible retractor is used to hold a small rounded brain retractor blade, and this is inserted to exert gentle pressure on the cerebellum and to augment CSF drainage. At this point the operating microscope is brought into position.

Under magnification and direct vision, the retractor blade is then inserted over the cerebellum pointing directly at the interval between the tentorium and the petrous ridge. Care should be taken not to inadvertently injure any branches of the petrosal vein from retraction. Most commonly, the petrous vein branches (2–3) converge to a common entry into the superior petrosal sinus. The entirety of the petrous vein is typically coagulated by bipolar cautery, then divided away from the tentorium. The retractor is then inserted deeper over the cerebellum to expose the trigeminal nerve and its entry into the brainstem.

The trigeminal nerve and root entry zone are carefully examined for conflict by an artery or vein. When no neurovascular compression is confirmed, internal neurolysis is then performed. The trigeminal nerve itself is then longitudinally divided along its fibers, using a straight blunt-tip bayonet probe, into 5–10 bundles between the pons and the porus trigeminus (Fig. 16.1). We include both the portio minor and portio major in the neurolysis, as the portio minor has been shown to carry unmyelinated fibers implicated in pathological facial pain, and neural anastomoses exist between these components of the trigeminal nerve. Internal neurolysis may trigger trigeminocardiac reflex, leading to sudden lowering of heart rate, mean arterial blood pressure (MABP), cardiac arrhythmia, or even brief asystole. Thus, anesthesiologist should be notified prior to starting to split the trigeminal nerve fibers. In cases where bradycardia is induced, glycopyrrolate is used to correct the bradycardia, and the heart rate is carefully monitored.

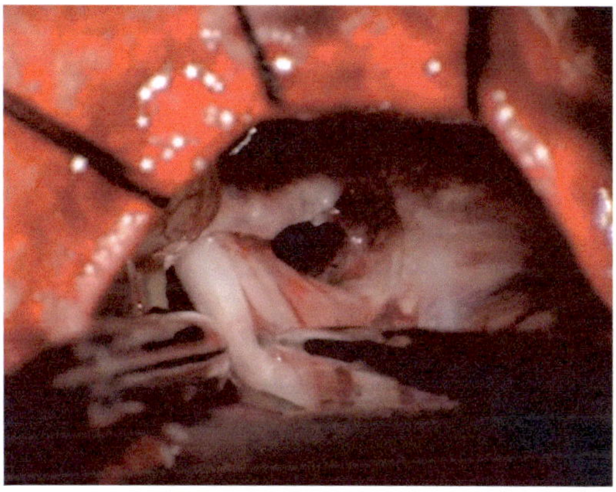

Fig. 16.1 The trigeminal nerve, including portio major and minor, is longitudinally divided along its fibers into 5–10 bundles between the pons and the porus trigeminus

During the procedure careful attention is paid to the ipsilateral BAERs. A latency change of less than 10% in waves IV and V is not unusual and is almost immediately reversible at the conclusion of the procedure. If the BAER latency is delayed beyond 10%, or if amplitude changes in the BAERs are observed, the retractor is removed, and typically the procedure can proceed without additional retraction.

Once the internal neurolysis is accomplished, hemostasis is ensured, and all retractors are removed. The dura is dosed and sealed with fibrin glue. All exposed air cells are waxed again. The small skull defect is repaired with hydroxyapatite cement. The muscle and skin are dosed in layers.

16.4 Outcomes and Efficacy

Internal neurolysis is a safe and efficacious treatment for trigeminal neuralgia when there is no neurovascular conflict found on imaging or at surgery. This procedure resulted in immediate relief of all pain in 85% of patients and significant pain relief in 96% of patients [16, 17]. The success rate is durable, with an estimated 72% - 82% of patients maintaining significant pain relief without medications at 5 years [16, 18, 19]. Systematic review of internal neurolysis showed 85% to 94.6% of patients were pain-free immediately after the procedure [20]. These immediate results nearly equivalent to those for MVD since the largest MVD series reported that 82% of patients were pain-free immediately after MVD, with partial relief in 98% [21].

Previous treatment for trigeminal neuralgia is a poor prognostic factor for successful treatment. Patients with a previous procedure were more likely to have experienced pain recurrence compared with patients who had not undergone a previous procedure [22]. A median time to treatment failure of 8.7 months was seen in those treated with MVD, GKS, or RFL. In comparison, a median time to failure of 24.4 months was seen in those without previous treatment [16].

Short-term pain-free results appear to be similar among partial sensory rhizotomy, RFL, and internal neurolysis. Internal neurolysis covers all distributions of the trigeminal nerve, unlike partial sensory rhizotomy and RFL. Reported long-term pain RFL outcome has varied widely across literature [23–25]. Our practice generally counsel patients that 50% of patients develop pain recurrence 5 years after RFL. A long-term follow-up study of partial sensory rhizotomy reports a success rate of 60% at 5 years [15]. In patients without neurovascular conflict, internal neurolysis appears to provide more durable pain relief compared to RFL and partial sensory rhizotomy.

Hypesthesia is an expected complication of internal neurolysis due to the manipulation of the trigeminal nerve and should be carefully evaluated. Almost all patients develop some facial numbness after internal neurolysis in the immediate postoperative [16, 18]. The success of internal neurolysis at relieving pain is predicated on producing some degree of sensory loss. Numbness or hypesthesia is generally limited in severity and well tolerated by patients. The degree of reported numbness generally diminishes at long-term follow-up. Given the ablative nature of internal neurolysis to the trigeminal nerve, other important complications to consider and discuss with the patients include corneal hypesthesia, loss of corneal reflex, keratitis, and corneal ulcer. Patients with preoperative facial numbness are also at risk of developing anesthesia dolorosa, although this complication appears to be uncommon, and on par with partial sensory rhizotomy [14, 20].

16.5 Conclusion

Internal neurolysis is more durable than RFL, and more efficacious than GKS. Thus, it may be a better option in a younger patient population. Because of its durability, internal neurolysis may be the most appropriate initial treatment for younger patients with trigeminal neuralgia without neurovascular conflict, with RFL held in reserve for recurrences.

References

1. Dandy WE. An operation for the cure of tic douloureux partial section of the sensory root at the pons. Arch Surg. 1929;18:687–734.
2. Burchiel KJ, Baumann TK. Pathophysiology of trigeminal neuralgia: new evidence from a trigeminal ganglion intraoperative microneurographic recording. Case report. J Neurosurg. 2004;101:872–3.
3. Devor M, Amir R, Rappaport ZH. Pathophysiology of trigeminal neuralgia: the ignition hypothesis. Clin J Pain. 2002;18:4–13.
4. Jannetta PJ. Arterial compression of the trigeminal nerve at the pons in patients with trigeminal neuralgia. J Neurosurg. 1967;26(Suppl):159–62.

5. Sindou M, Howeidy T, Acevedo G. Anatomical observations during microvascular decompression for idiopathic trigeminal neuralgia (with correlations between topography of pain and site of the neurovascular conflict). Prospective study in a series of 579 patients. Acta Neurochir. 2002;144:1–12; discussion 12–13.
6. Miller JP, Acar F, Hamilton BE, et al. Radiographic evaluation of trigeminal neurovascular compression in patients with and without trigeminal neuralgia. J Neurosurg. 2009;110:627–32.
7. Maarbjerg S, Gozalov A, Olesen J, et al. Trigeminal neuralgia—a prospective systematic study of clinical characteristics in 158 patients. Headache. 2014;54:1574–82.
8. Thomas KL, Vilensky JA. The anatomy of vascular compression in trigeminal neuralgia. Clin Anat. 2014;27:89–93.
9. Mannerak MA, Lashkarivand A, Eide PK. Trigeminal neuralgia and genetics: a systematic review. Mol Pain. 2021;17:17448069211016139.
10. Siqueira SR, Alves B, Malpartida HM, et al. Abnormal expression of voltage-gated sodium channels Nav1.7, Nav1.3 and Nav1.8 in trigeminal neuralgia. Neuroscience. 2009;164:573–7.
11. Ko AL, Lee A, Raslan AM, et al. Trigeminal neuralgia without neurovascular compression presents earlier than trigeminal neuralgia with neurovascular compression. J Neurosurg. 2015;123:1519–27.
12. Lee A, Mccartney S, Burbidge C, et al. Trigeminal neuralgia occurs and recurs in the absence of neurovascular compression. J Neurosurg. 2014;120:1048–54.
13. Burchiel KJ. A new classification for facial pain. Neurosurgery. 2003;53:1164–6; discussion 1166–1167.
14. Bederson JB, Wilson CB. Evaluation of microvascular decompression and partial sensory rhizotomy in 252 cases of trigeminal neuralgia. J Neurosurg. 1989;71:359–67.
15. Zakrzewska JM, Lopez BC, Kim SE, et al. Patient reports of satisfaction after microvascular decompression and partial sensory rhizotomy for trigeminal neuralgia. Neurosurgery. 2005;56:1304–11; discussion 1311–1302.
16. Ko AL, Ozpinar A, Lee A, et al. Long-term efficacy and safety of internal neurolysis for trigeminal neuralgia without neurovascular compression. J Neurosurg. 2015;122:1048–57.
17. Xu R, Materi J, Raj D, et al. Internal neurolysis versus intraoperative glycerin rhizotomy for trigeminal neuralgia. J Neurosurg. 2023;138:270–5.
18. Jie H, Xuanchen Z, Deheng L, et al. The long-term outcome of nerve combing for trigeminal neuralgia. Acta Neurochir. 2013;155:1703–8; discussion 1707.
19. Ma Z, Li M. "Nerve combing" for trigeminal neuralgia without vascular compression: report of 10 cases. Clin J Pain. 2009;25:44–7.
20. Sabourin V, Lavergne P, Mazza J, et al. Internal neurolysis for the treatment of trigeminal neuralgia: a systematic review. World Neurosurg. 2022;158:e829–42.
21. Barker FG 2nd, Jannetta PJ, Bissonette DJ, et al. The long-term outcome of microvascular decompression for trigeminal neuralgia. N Engl J Med. 1996;334:1077–83.
22. Sabourin V, Mazza J, Garzon T, et al. Internal neurolysis with and without microvascular decompression for trigeminal neuralgia: case series. World Neurosurg. 2020;143:e70–7.
23. Fraioli B, Esposito V, Guidetti B, et al. Treatment of trigeminal neuralgia by thermocoagulation, glycerolization, and percutaneous compression of the gasserian ganglion and/or retrogasserian rootlets: long-term results and therapeutic protocol. Neurosurgery. 1989;24:239–45.
24. Noorani I, Lodge A, Vajramani G, et al. Comparing percutaneous treatments of trigeminal neuralgia: 19 years of experience in a single centre. Stereotact Funct Neurosurg. 2016;94:75–85.
25. Onofrio BM. Radiofrequency percutaneous Gasserian ganglion lesions. Results in 140 patients with trigeminal pain. J Neurosurg. 1975;42:132–9.

17 Surgical Anatomy of the Triangular Plexus and Trigeminal Root. Implications for RF-Thermo-Rhizotomy

Marc Sindou and Andrei Brinzeu

17.1 Introduction

Surgical indications for the several types of trigeminal neuralgias (TNs) depend on their respective mechanisms, reflected in their definitions and classification [1, 2]. Thus not all TNs are eligible for microvascular decompression (MVD), the current "gold standard" for Classical TNs.

It is recognized that these **Classical TNs**, by definition hypothesized on imaging to be due to a neurovascular conflict (NVC), have MVD as the first option for treatment. This is especially true when the NVC has a high grade of compression. When the suspected vascular agent corresponds to a simple contact on the trigeminal root (Grade I), i.e., not responsible of displacement of the root (Grade II), nor does it create an engrooving into it (Grade III), an alternative surgical procedure to MVD might be considered.

Of course, **Idiopathic TNs** (i.e., without any identifiable etiology) do not justify open surgery for MVD. For those, percutaneous lesioning or stereotactic radiosurgical procedures are indicated.

Secondary TNs should be treated by having recourse to their respective specific therapies. However, when the neuralgic component of the pain remains refractory, recourse to an open or percutaneous lesioning procedure may be considered.

Among the various percutaneous lesioning procedures (glycerol injection introduced by Hakanson; balloon compression by Mullan or thermocoagulation by Sweet), the Radio-Frequency Thermo-Rhizotomy procedure (RF-Th-Rh) has a well-established place with specific indications [3].

RF-Th-Rh was pioneered by Kirschner under the term "Electrocoagulation of the Gasserian Ganglion" in 1933 [4]. The method was refined in the 1960s by Sweet [5] with the name of "Controlled thermocoagulation of trigeminal ganglion and rootlets for differential destruction of pain fibers." Sweet's technique was based on the three following principles.

1. **Location should be retrogasserian** on the trigeminal pathways (on the portion of the trigeminal pathways situated between the ganglion and the brainstem immediately after the ganglion i.e. the triangular plexus or begining of the trigeminal root),
2. **To limit the lesioning effect** to the sole territory affected with the neuralgic pain, **target must take into account the somatotopic organization of the TGN**. The somatotopic

M. Sindou (✉)
Department of Neurosurgery, University of Lyon, Lyon, France

A. Brinzeu
Neuroscience Research Center, Department of Neurosciences, University of Medicine "Victor Babes", Timisoara, Romania

S.-T. Li et al. (eds.), *Microvascular Decompression Surgery*,
https://doi.org/10.1007/978-981-96-0767-9_17

distribution of the ophthalmic (V1), the maxillary (V2), and the mandibular (V3) divisions is at the level of not only the ganglion but also the retrogasserian portion of the root, clearly in the triangular plexus, and—although to a lesser degree—in the cisternal and the TREZ (Trigeminal Root Entry Zone) portions of the sensory root. Such somatotopy permits targeting the thermal lesion to obtain an *analgesia/hypoesthesia limited to the trigger zone(s)* and covering the trigeminal division(s) involved, whilst sparing the rootlets not related to the clinical manifestations.

3. **In an attempt to make the procedure as selective as possible**, i.e., reduce the harmful consequences of the sensory fibers lesioning, Sweet used an **electrode doted of a thermocouple** to control the temperature delivered at the tip of the electrode. He qualified his method:" Controlled thermocoagulation of trigeminal ganglion and rootlets for differential destruction of pain fibers" [5]. The attempt to have a differential effect of the temperature on the fine unmyelinated fibers (considered as the pain, i.e., nociceptive, fibers) was based on acute experiments showing the earlier and preferential disappearance of the potentials corresponding to the slow-conducting (fine, unmyelinated) fibers [6, 7]. Actually, chronic physiological experiments and histological studies after thermo-lesioning in animals showed that all types of fibers (the large myelinated ones as well as the fine unmyelinated ones) were similarly attained [8, 9]. Nevertheless, *the thermal control allows to limit the intensity of the sensory deficit*, and therefore decreases the risk of producing an anesthesia dolorosa phenomenon.

17.2 Surgical Anatomy of the TGN

The trigeminal nerve (TGN), the fifth cranial nerve, has three components, for the sensory innervation of the face: the ophthalmic (V1), the maxillary (V2), and the mandibular (V3) divisions. The ophthalmic nerve enters the cranial cavity from the orbit via the superior orbital fissure and runs between the two layers of the dural lateral wall of the cavernous sinus. The maxillary nerve penetrates the skull base via the foramen rotundum. The mandibular nerve becomes endocranial through the foramen ovale, accompanied by the motor nerve responsible for the masticatory function. Then the TGN extends from the trigeminal cave (TC), which is located in the middle fossa, to enter the cerebellopontine cistern in the posterior fossa through the porus trigeminus. Finally, the TGN penetrates into the ventral surface of the pons, with a large sensory and a smaller motor component.

The TGN presents gross anatomical, microanatomical, electrophysiological, and histological particularities dominated by its somatotopic organization, not only at level of the ganglion and the triangular plexus part of the retrogasserian portion of the root but also—although to a lesser degree—in its cisternal and TREZ (Trigeminal Root Entry Zone) portions. This somatotopic organization permits targeting the lesioning of the RF-thermorhizotomy (RF-Th-Rh) procedure so as to obtain a selective analgesia/hypoesthesia corresponding to the trigger zone(s) and covering the trigeminal division(s) involved, whilst sparing the rootlets not related to the clinical manifestations.

17.2.1 Descriptive Anatomy

17.2.1.1 The Trigeminal Nerve in the Trigeminal Cave

The trigeminal cave of Meckel (TC) is the anatomical space, containing CSF, where the trigeminal ganglion of Gasser (TGgl) and the retrogasserian portion of the sensory rootlets are located. There, the TGgl is crossed inferiorly by the motor nerve. The TC is formed by an expansion of the dura and the arachnoid of the posterior fossa that developed an anterior evagination laterally to the parasellar lodge, the latter being the so-called cavernous sinus.

The TC contains cerebrospinal fluid which corresponds to the trigeminal cistern; this cistern is identifiable on high-resolution T2-MRI. The TC harbors the trigeminal ganglion—in its anterior part—and the triangular plexus of the trigeminal sensory root—in its posterior part. There, the trigeminal motor root runs inferiorly to the triangular plexus and the TGgl to exit with the V3 mandibular sensory nerve through the foramen ovale to innervate the masticatory muscles (Fig. 17.1).

The trigeminal ganglion has a semi-lunar shape with a convex anterior edge where the three peripheral nerves enter, and a concave posterior margin from which the sensory root emerges. Between their emergence from the TGgl and the upper petrous ridge, rootlets form a triangle, named the triangular plexus (TP) because of its anastomoses (Fig. 17.2). At the TP level, the sensory fibers have a somatotopic organization—similarly to the one of the ganglion level—before merging into the posterior root. Fibers of V3 are inferior-lateral, fibers of V1 are superior-medial, fibers of V2 course in between. Noteworthy, inside the trigeminal cave, the trigeminal ganglion, as well as the triangular plexus, are identifiable and dissectible [10, 11].

17.2.1.2 The Trigeminal Root in the Cerebellopontine Angle

The trigeminal root crosses the upper part of the cerebellopontine angle (CPA) over 2 cm length on average, to penetrate into the ventrolateral aspect of brainstem. The exit of root from the trigeminal cave is through the trigeminal porus, which is circumscribed by the upper petrous ridge, inferiorly, and the peripheral border of the tentorium, which contains the superior petrosal sinus, superiorly.

On crossing over the petrous ridge, the root is somewhat flat in the horizontal plane. In the CPA cistern it becomes cylindrical, approximately 5 mm in diameter in healthy nerves, then elliptical before attaining the pons.

At entry into brainstem, at the so-called trigeminal root entry zone (TREZ), the sensory root divides into two components: (1) the pars major—the more voluminous—inferolaterally located and (2) the pars intermediaris formed by tiny rootlets, located in between the pars major and the emergence of the motor root, superomedially located, and named pars minor (Fig. 17.3).

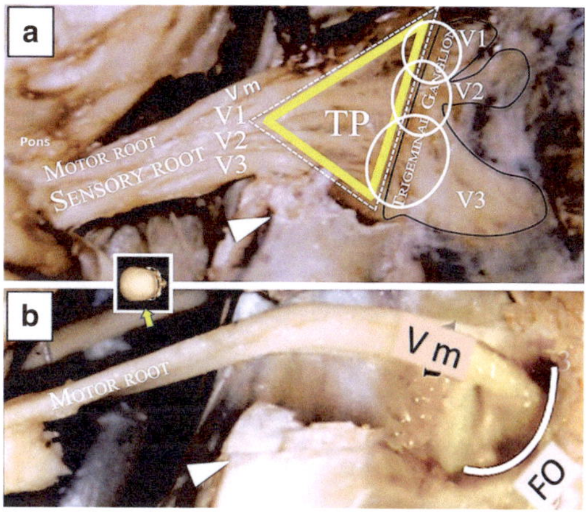

Fig. 17.1 General view of the trigeminal nerve (TGN). Laboratory dissection of the (right) TGN; superior/lateral view after resection of the dural roof of the trigeminal cave. **Upper view (a)**, from periphery to cerebello-pontine cistern: (1) The **ophthalmic nerve (V1)** entering the parasellar lodge through the *superior orbital fissure;* the **maxillary nerve (V2)** through the *foramen rotundum;* the **mandibular nerve (V3)** through the *foramen ovale*. (2) The **Trigeminal Ganglion of Gasser (Ggl)** has a semilunar shape and is trifoliated *(as delineated by the three ovalar circles)*. It presents a convex anterior margin which receives the fibers of the peripheral branches and a concave posterior margin from which the axons of the sensory rootlets arise to reach the brain stem through the trigeminal root. The trigeminal Ggl has a clearcut somatotopia with V1 medial and V3 lateral. (3) The **Triangular plexus (TP)** (*yellow triangle*) is the initial part of the retrogasserian portion of the trigeminal root, from the posterior margin of the trigeminal ganglion (anteriorly) to the crossing of the root over the petrous ridge (posteriorly). The triangular plexus is characterized by (tiny) anastomoses between the sensory rootlets. In spite of these anastomoses the triangular plexus has still a clearcut somatotopia, with V1 medially, V3 laterally, and V2 in between. (4) The **Cisternal portion of the sensory root** (with all its constituting rootlets) crosses the cerebello-pontine angle cistern, from the porus of the trigeminal cave of Meckel (*arrow head*) to the trigeminal root entry zone ot the TGN in the pons (*Pons*). **Lower view (b)**, **The Motor Root and Nerve (Vm)**, after resection of the sensory root and trigeminal ganglion. The motor root emerges from the pons at the superomedial border of the sensory trigeminal root, to course medially along the cisternal portion of the sensory root; then its travels below the triangular plexus (TP) and the ganglion (Ggl) to reach the foramen ovale together with the mandibular nerve (V3). See exit of Vm through the foramen ovale (*FO*)

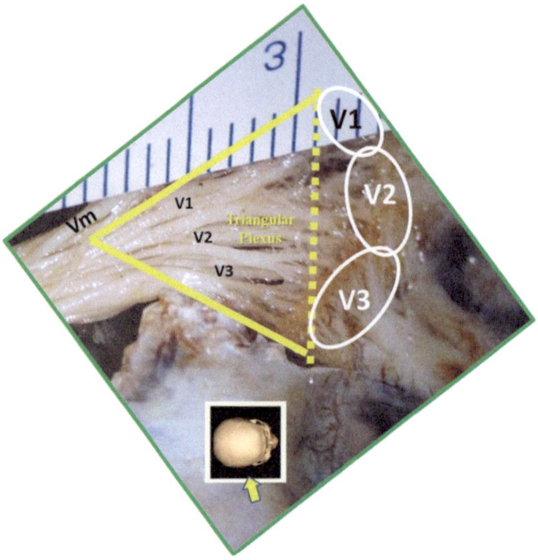

Fig. 17.2 The Triangular Plexus. The triangular plexus (yellow triangle) extends from the posterior margin of the (trifoliated) trigeminal ganglion with its three components from V1, V2 and V3 origins (anteriorly) to the crossing of the root over the upper petrous ridge (posteriorly). The triangular plexus is characterized by (tiny) anastomoses between the sensory rootlets. In spite of these anastomoses the triangular plexus keeps there a clearcut somatotopy, with V1 supero-medially, V3 infero-laterally, and V2 in between

To our knowledge, TREZ has not received any official taxonomic definition. However, for most authors TREZ corresponds essentially to that portion of the root which is of central myelin nature. In our view, TREZ should include the transitional zone, the central myelin portion of the root, and the adjacent region of brainstem where root fibers have subpial paths on their way from or to their respective nuclei [12].

These structures are likely to be considered as a whole harboring anatomical-physiological higher sensitiveness and excitability, likely explaining the respective incidences of the cranial nerve hyperactive syndromes according to the length and volume of this portion in the CPA cistern [12, 13].

To be recalled, in the cerebellopontine cistern the trigeminal root has several important anatomical relationships: rostrally, the superior cerebellar artery and the (tiny) trochlear cranial nerve coursing along the tentorium incisura and caudally, the cochleo-vestibular-facial nerve complex together with the anterior inferior cerebellar artery and its tributary: the labyrinthine artery. In

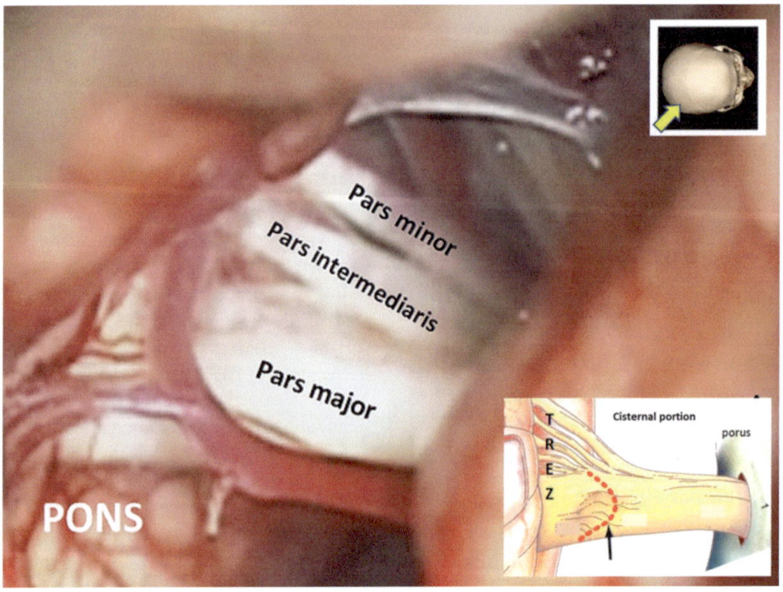

Fig. 17.3 The Trigeminal Root Entry Zone (TREZ) via a posterior view of the juxta-pontine portion of the root, on right side. Microsurgical operative view of TREZ in the right cerebellopontine angle, with its different components: Pars minor (= motor root), Pars intermediaris, and Pars major (sensory), at pons. Schematic drawing of the TREZ; the arrow indicates the transitional zone between central myelin portion and schwannian peripheral myelin portion of the sensory root (dotted curve)

its cisternal portion the trigeminal root is vascularized by small branches of the superior cerebellar artery. Posteriorly, the root is in close relationship with the superior petrosal vein and its affluents, often stuck to the root.

17.2.2 Functional Anatomy

The primary function of the trigeminal nerve is sensory input from the face and head cavities. The T-cells (which are rather pseudo-unipolar sensory neurons), contained in the trigeminal ganglion, send their axonal extensions toward the sensory nuclei in brainstem; their peripheral (= dendritic) extensions form the fibers of the three nerves of the TGN. Thus, the tactile and thermo-algesic fibers of the three divisions originate in the primary neurons situated in the trigeminal ganglion. From it the centrifugal fibers run to the pons.

Inside the brainstem two sensory nuclei receive the fibers from the trigeminal ganglion: in the pons, the principal trigeminal nucleus receiving the large tactile fibers, and in the medulla oblongata and upper cervical spinal cord, the spinal nucleus of the trigeminal tract which receives the small fibers related to nociception and temperature sensation [14].

A somatotopic organization of the sensory fibers has been recognized not only in the trigeminal ganglion but also in the trigeminal root, particularly in its retrogasserian portion, named the triangular plexus. There, the fibers from V3 (mandibular afferent fibers) are situated in a lateral position, with the V1 (ophthalmic) afferent fibers in a medial position, and the V2 (maxillary) afferent fibers taking an intermediate position (Fig. 17.4). These fibers then traverse the major sensory root of the trigeminal nerve to reach the pons. This cisternal portion of the nerve has an elliptical cross-section with the fibers having still relatively somatotopic and not-yet-functional organization with the V1 fibers situated superomedially, the V3 fibers inferolaterally, and the V2 fibers somewhat intermediate to these (Fig. 17.4).

This view of a somatotopic organization of the retro-gasserian trigeminal root is corroborated by data from anatomical and surgical studies. Microsurgical dissection studies in cadavers [11, 15, 16] showed that the three trigeminal topographical divisions are well-delineated in the root at least immediately posteriorly to the trigeminal ganglion, i.e., in the so-called triangular plexus. Also, during percutaneous RF-thermo-rhizotomy, it was observed that direct stimulation of the root at triangular plexus level—for strict placement of the electrode in the sensory rootlets corresponding to the trigger zone—elicits sensory responses under the form of paresthesias somatotopically distributed [5, 17–20]. Furthermore, subsequent thermo-lesioning, when performed inferolaterally in the triangular plexus or in the neighboring cisternal portion of the root, produces hypoesthesia mainly in the V3 and more or less in the V2 territories, and when performed more superomedially, preferentially in the V2/V1 territories. This somatotopic organization is also in accordance with the neurophysiological studies by Sindou et al., who—for guiding the targeting of thermo-rhizotomies—performed direct stimulation of the sensory root with EMG-recordings together with video recordings of the face [21, 22]. According to the placement of the probe in the trigeminal root (as described above), stimulation provoked not only paresthesias in the expected V1, V2, or V3 territories but also twitches in the orbicularis oculi, levator labii, or orbicularis oris muscles, respectively. These clinically observable phenomena were considered trigemino-facial reflexes, and were subsequently used for intraoperative neurophysiological guidance because of their localizing value [10, 23].

On penetrating the pons, the root undergoes a functional rearrangement with three distinct components: the pars minor (superomedial), with a motor function, the pars major (inferolateral), sensory and mostly thermo-algesic, and in between, the pars intermediaris considered as specially harboring the corneal sensory fibers (Fig. 17.4).

At the juxta-pontine level, the sensory fibers tend to locate according to their destiny and therefore function (Fig. 17.4). The thermo-algesic fibers regroup in the pars major to then follow the descending tract down to the spinal trigeminal nucleus at the spinal cord–medullary junction. Also classically, the epicritic and proprioceptive

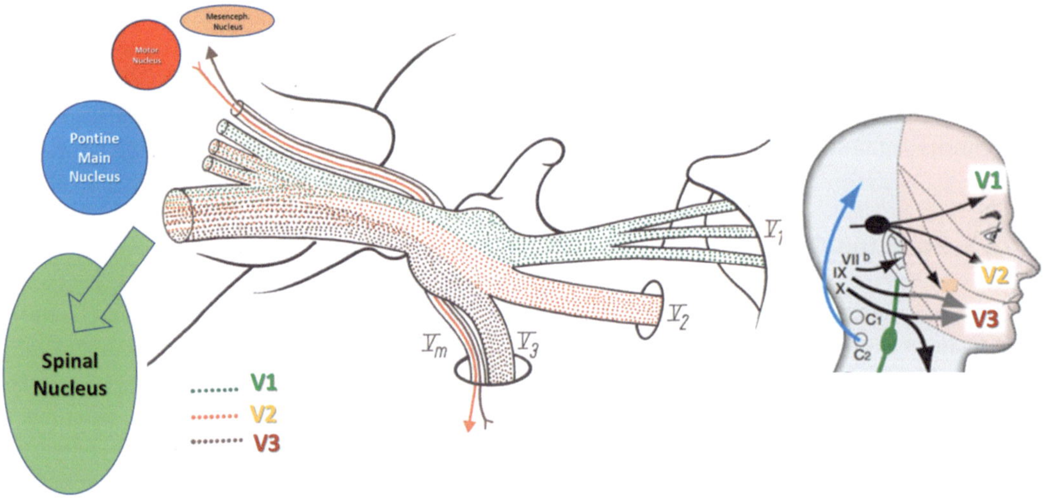

Fig. 17.4 Somatotopy of the trigeminal fibers (Schematic lateral view, on right side). At the triangular plexus and the initial retrogasserian portion of the **sensory root**, the axonal fibers issued from the ganglionic bipolar T-shaped cells have a clearcut somatotopic organization. In the root the fibers from the mandibular nerve cells (V_3) predominate infero-laterally, those originating from the ophtalmic nerve (V_1) supero-medially, and those from the maxillary nerve (V_2) in between. This arrangement is clearer in the retrogasserian than in the juxta-pontine portion of the root, where the fibers are redistributed according to their destination in the brainstem, by means of anastomoses between the three contingents from the three branches. The epicritic and proprioceptive fibers are more supero-medially situated, to reach the main pontine nucleus; these fibers can be individualized and termed as the pars intermediaris. The small myelinated and the unmyelinated fibers, mostly thermal and nociceptive, mainly placed with an inferolateral predominance and forming the pars major, go through the descending spinal tract to the spinal nucleus. Both are located as far as the third segment of the spinal cord. The spinal nucleus comprises the interpolaris and the caudalis subnuclei. A rostro-caudal somatotopic organization of the subnucleus caudalis has been described, corresponding to an "onion-rings" pattern (Drake and McKenzie [24]; McKenzie [25]), the lips and lower nose territory being highest in the subnucleus, the most lateral regions of the face being more caudal in the subnucleus. Noteworthy, the superomedial "third" of the pars major and the pars intermediaris contain the sensory corneal fibers. This repartition explains the analgesic effect—without complete tactile anesthesia and without corneal anesthesia—obtained after partial section of the pars major in the selective juxtapontine rhizotomy procedure. Of paramount importance, the spinal nucleus is a region of convergent projections from the entire cephalic extremity. The nociceptive fibers from the VIIth, IXth, and Xth cranial nerves, and also the fibers from the upper cervical spinal nerves, join the descending spinal tract and the caudalis part of the spinal nucleus. To be noted, the caudalis part of the nucleus is in continuity with the gray of the dorsal horn of the spinal cord, and is hypothesized playing some role in the pain control. Then the fibers arising from the spinal nucleus project to a large number of encephalic structures, especially the reticular formation and the thalamus (similarly to the ascending spinoreticular tracts). The **motor root** emerges from the pons in a superomedial position to the sensory root constituting the pars minor of the Vth cranial nerve, then crosses the trigeminal cave below the gasserian ganglion, to become satellite of the mandibular nerve at exit through the foramen ovale. The proprioceptive and myotatic fibers of the Vth—most from the masticatory muscles after having travelled retrogradely in the pars minor, form the mesencephalic tract in brainstem to terminate into the mesencephalic nucleus. The cells of this nucleus send fibers onto the (pontine) motor nucleus, thus playing a role in relaying information for the regulation of the Vth motor nerve

fibers would preferentially transit in the pars intermediaris to reach the pontine principal nucleus.

Despite such functional rearrangement, clinical and surgical observations show—at this level of the root—a still relative somatotopic organization of the fibers. After partial juxta-pontine rhizotomy, by definition performed just at the entry of the nerve in brainstem, it was observed that a section of only the inferolateral portion of the pars major allows preservation of the sensory function in V1 and more or less V2 [26, 27].

Regarding the cornea innervation, the corneal reflex, which is the substratum of a protective autonomic and somatic function including blinking and lacrimation, obeys to nociceptive mechanisms. Electrophysiological and histological studies have shown that cornea is innervated by A delta and C fibers. Classically it is considered that corneal fibers run into the pars intermediaris. Differently, Terrier et al. on their surgical experience assume that all corneal fibers run along the dorsomedial third of the pars major [27, 28]. Whatever, limiting the rhizotomy to the inferolateral two-thirds of the pars major would likely be the way to avoid corneal ulcer caused by sensory impairment.

Actually, the exact transition point between the two types of organization, somatotopic vs. functional, is still uncertain, and remains to be further studied. Whatever, good knowledge of the morphological and functional anatomy of the TGN has important surgical implications.

17.3 The RF-Thermo-Rhizotomy Procedure

The somatotopic organization permits targeting the thermo-lesioning so as to obtain a selective analgesia/hypoesthesia corresponding to the trigger zone(s) and covering the trigeminal division(s) involved, whilst sparing the rootlets not related to the clinical manifestations.

17.3.1 Technique

The patient is installed supine in a comfortable position, with equipment for safe anesthesiologic conditions and head positioned for intraoperative X-ray control, as well as easy surgical maneuvers. The trocar is introduced through the cheek up to the Foramen Ovale following the Hartel percutaneous approach (Fig. 17.5). Then the trocar is pushed under X-ray fluoroscopic control to the upper ridge of the petrous bone. Because it is painful, this phase needs brief intravenous boluses of anesthetics (historically: Methohexital/Brevital, followed by: Propanidide/Epontol, and now: Propofol/Diprivan). After passing through the Foramen Ovale under fluoroscopic guidance, the trocar enters the trigeminal cave in relation with the trigeminal system.

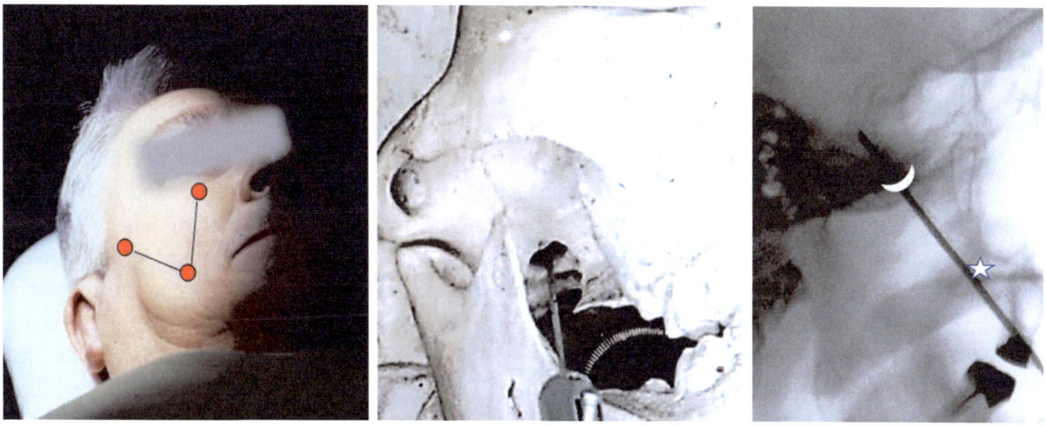

Fig. 17.5 The transjugal-transoval Hartel route for percutaneous access to trigeminal cave and nerve. *Left*: Cutaneous landmarks: 30 ± 5 mm lateral to the labial commissure (60 mm from the middle of the intercommisssural line). The foramen ovale is targeted by aiming: on lateral view, a point at 35 mm anterior to the anterior wall of the external auditory meatus (= tragus) on the orbito-meatal line along the inferior border of the zygoma; in frontal view, the medial border of the pupilla. Depth is guided by X-ray. For targetting V1, the cutaneous entry point can be 5 mm more laterally and inferiorly, for targetting V3, 5 mm more medially and superiorly. *Center*: Exocranial view of the needle trajectory, successively transjugal and through the pterygomaxillary fossa, up to the foramen ovale. Note that trajectory passes close to the lateral pterygoid process, which can be—if hypertrophied—an obstacle to access the foramen. *Right*: Hartel route performed under fluoroscopy (lateral view). The tip of the needle should target the intersection between the clivus and the upper petrous ridge. Note that trajectory passes in front of the inferior/posterior angle of the maxillary sinus (star) and through the axis of the foramen ovale (semilunar shape)

The anatomical region crossed by the trocar—and corresponding to the trans-jugal, trans-pterygomaxillary, trans-oval route of Hartel—may be considered an inverted, three-sided, pyramidal volume, with its apex at a cheek cutaneous point, 3 cm lateral to the labial commissure. Its triangular base, located at skull base, is delineated by the three following landmarks. The superolateral one is a cutaneous point on the orbito-meatal line along the inferior border of the zygoma, 3 cm anterior to the tragus. The superomesial one corresponds to the pupilla. The deep-seated one is the Foramen Ovale itself. An anatomical detailed description has been given in already published articles [29].

Wrong trajectories might lead to vital complications, especially if puncturing the internal carotid artery. Even with a correct trajectory, the needle may encounter the parotid duct, the maxillary artery, the auditory tube, with the following respective consequences: hemo-sialorrhea, hematoma of the cheek and the pterygomaxillary region, serous otitis, all generally without durable severity.

Knowledge of surgical anatomy and imaging are of paramount help to understand the potential risks of the percutaneous Hartel approach. At skull base the following structures can be endangered: the internal jugular vein located 27 mm postero-laterally to the trocar trajectory, the internal carotid artery at its entry into the petrous carotid canal (25 mm posterior to the needle axis), again the internal carotid artery at Foramen Lacerum if trajectory would be deviated of 10° medially from its correct pathway, and also the membranous portion of the auditory tube if trajectory would be deviated of a 9° angle in the anteromedial direction. The inferior orbital fissure can be encountered firstly with its contents, then if pushed more deeply upward the superior orbital fissure with the paraclinoidal portion of the internal carotid artery, might be attained if needle would be placed 17° too anteriorly from its correct trajectory.

Importantly, before any decision to use the percutaneous route, it is necessary to ensure by imaging of the skull base (CT scan and/or MRI) that there are no arterial structures at risk in the path of the trocar such as intracavernous aneurysm, mega-dolicho-carotid and/or megadolicho-vertebrobasilar arteries, or persistent trigeminal artery (that may be found in 0.5% of the cases).

Accessing and puncturing the foramen ovale may be difficult in some patients, especially those with *a hypertrophic pterygoid process* or those harboring *platybasia*. In such circumstances trajectory guided by neuro-navigation systems, or better by performing catheterization of the foramen under CT-control, can be helpful.

After locating the extremity of the trocar under lateral radio-fluoroscopy at the cross-section of the upper ridge of the petrous apex and the clival plane (Fig. 17.6), the electrode is inserted into the trocar-needle. There, the uninsulated extremity of the active electrode is supposed to be placed at the level of the triangular plexus, the optimal target for performing the thermo-lesion [20].

At this level the fibers of the V3 (mandibular) division are located in an inferolateral position, those of the V2 (maxillary) division in an intermediate position, and those of the V1 (ophthalmic) division superomedially. A reference needle electrode (anode) is inserted subcutaneously in the middle of the hairline at the forehead or at level of one shoulder.

After positioning the electrode in the estimated appropriate location on the radiological basis, stimulation for physiological localization is performed in an awake patient using an electrical current, at a frequency of 5 Hz in our technique [22] (Fig. 17.7). The final placement is adjusted until the evoked paresthesias correspond with the territory of pain, *particularly its trigger-zone*. Stimulation is delivered using a train lasting 3 to 5 s. When the intensity threshold to obtain paresthesias is greater than 0.4 V on first attempt(s), further trials with different trajectories of the electrode are made until the proper threshold (a lower one, +/− 0.3 V) is found. When stimulation provokes masticatory responses with a threshold below 0.3 V, relocation of the electrode away from the trigeminal motor fibers is attempted.

Noteworthy, at 5 Hz, electrical stimulation additionally produces muscle twitches in the

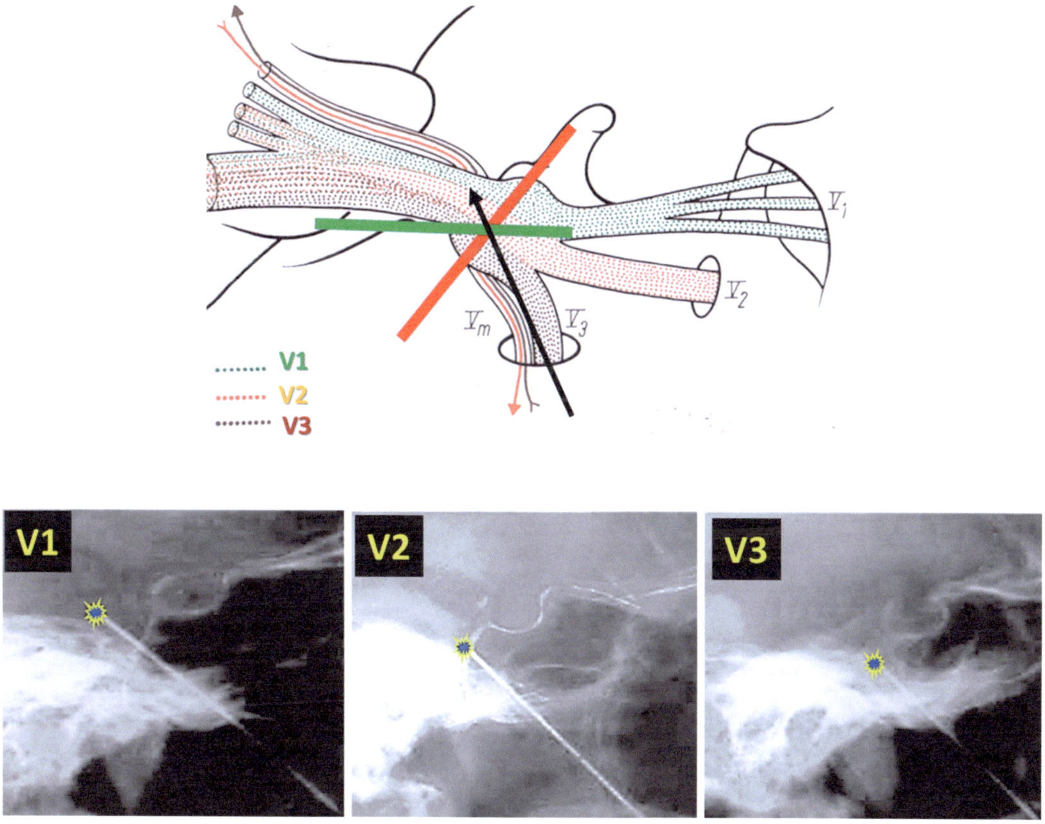

Fig. 17.6 Fluoroscopic control of the electrode location. *Upper*: Schematic representation of the landmarks of the trigeminal fibers at the gasserian ganglion, the triangular plexus and the root. The red line corresponds to the dorsum sellae and the clivus, and the green line to the upper petrous ridge. The black arrow represents the trajectory of the trocard and electrode inside the trigeminal system. *Lower*: Lateral X-ray projections of the tip of the electrode in the V_3, V_2, V_1 trigeminal components at the triangular plexus level

facial nerve territory, clinically well-visible in approximately one-half of the patients. These evoked muscular twitches, that we named facial Evoked Motor Responses (EMRs), and that we attributed to *trigeminal-facial reflexes*, can be evidenced by video-recordings and electromyographic recordings [21]. Their localizing value was demonstrated by correlating the territory of the EMR with the location of the evoked paresthesias and the topography of the postoperative hypoesthesia. It was established that EMRs in the Orbicularis oculi indicate situation of the electrode in the V1 fibers, in Levator labii in the V2 fibers, and in Orbicularis oris in the V3 fibers (Fig. 17.8). These clinically observable EMRs were hypothesized to be owing to trigemino-facial reflexes The EMRs noted in the upper territory resemble the classic blink-reflex. Those observed in the lower territories, (reported for the first time) were hypothesized—according to our electrophysiological studies—to be trigemino-facial reflexes generated in brainstem, similar to the well-known aforementioned blink reflex. On these bases, we integrated the concept of "Neurophysiological navigation" guidance inside the protocol learned from Professor Sweet at MGH in Boston [23]. Importantly, observation of muscle twitches in the Orbicularis oculi under stimulation at low intensity indicates that the uninsulated extremity of the electrode is (too) close to the ophthalmic fibers; consequently, electrode must be relocated appropriately, so that to avoid harmful corneal anesthesia [23].

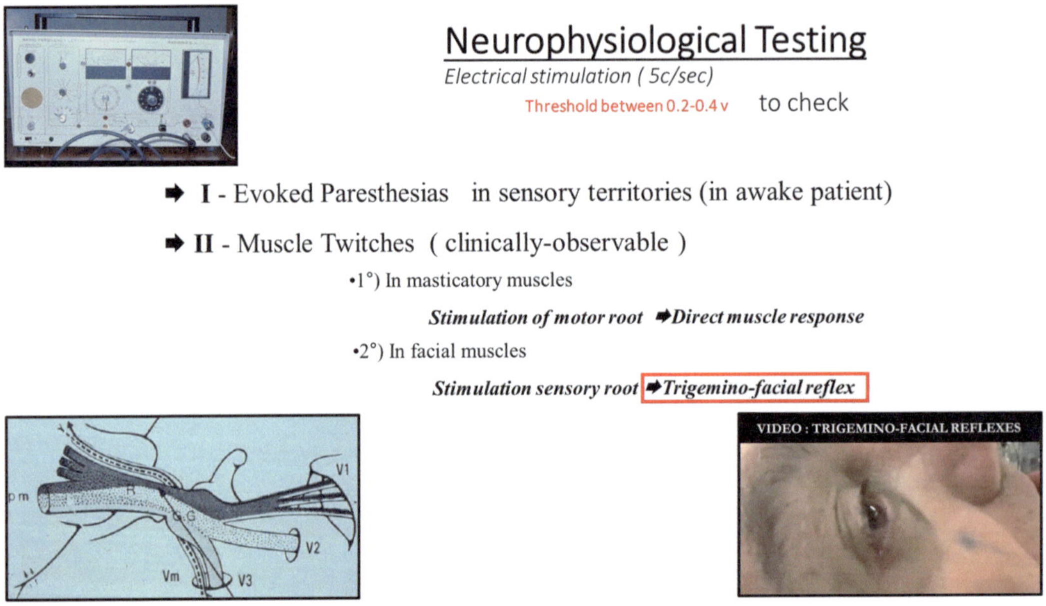

Fig. 17.7 Neurophysiological control of the electrode location. When root stimulation provokes intense **masticatory responses** under a threshold of 0.3 V, relocation of the electrode away from the trigeminal motor fibers is attempted. Stimulation to **evoke paresthesias** for physiological localization is performed in an awake patient, using an electrical current at a frequency of 50 Hz (according to the initial description by Sweet) or 5 Hz (according to our personal modification). The placement of the electrode is adjusted until the evoked paresthesias correspond with the area of the pain. If intensity threshold to elicit paresthesias is greater than 0.4 V, modification of the location of the electrode is searched until proper threshold (approximately 0.2 V) is found. Electrical stimulation of the root produces muscle twitches in the facial nerve territory, well-observable at 5 Hz, especially in the orbicularis oculi (= blink-reflex). They could be clearly observed in the lower facial territories in approximately one-half of the patients. We named these evoked twitches: **facial evoked motor responses (EMRs)** [21, 23]. EMRs were demonstrated using video recordings and electromyographic recordings. These responses were interpreted as trigemino-facial reflexes at brainstem level. By correlating these EMRs with the location of the evoked paresthesias and also with the territories of postoperative hypoesthesia, it could be established that the EMRs in the orbicularis oculi indicate electrode location in V_1, EMRs in the levator labii in V_2, and EMRs in the orbicularis oris location in V_3 [21]

Then, to check the accurate location of the electrode before definitive lesioning, a minimal thermal lesion is added as a test. This thermal test is performed at the painful threshold of approximately 45–50 °C, and lasts—approximately of a duration of 3 to 5 s- until the patient complains of a burning sensation., This thermal test, if not prolonged and surpassing 50 °C, produces only a very transient hypoesthesia. Good correlation of the site of the induced burning pain and the observed (transient) hypoesthesia with the territory of the neuralgia and the trigger zone are considered an additional indication of accurate electrode placement. Otherwise, attempts to reposition the electrode should be made. Appearance of a cutaneous redness/vasodilatation in a trigeminal division would signify location of the uninsulated tip of the electrode (too) close to the ganglion (Fig. 17.9).

After it's the final neurophysiological control, the location of the electrode is radiographically verified on lateral cranial X-ray. Then the therapeutic thermal lesioning is performed under (one or more frequently several) brief intravenous anesthesia(s) light enough to permit concomitant testing of the corneal reflex (+++).

NB: In our practice, we currently use a straight electrode, of 0.6 mm in diameter, with an uninsulated tip over 6 mm. Lesioning is usually made at a temperature of 55° to

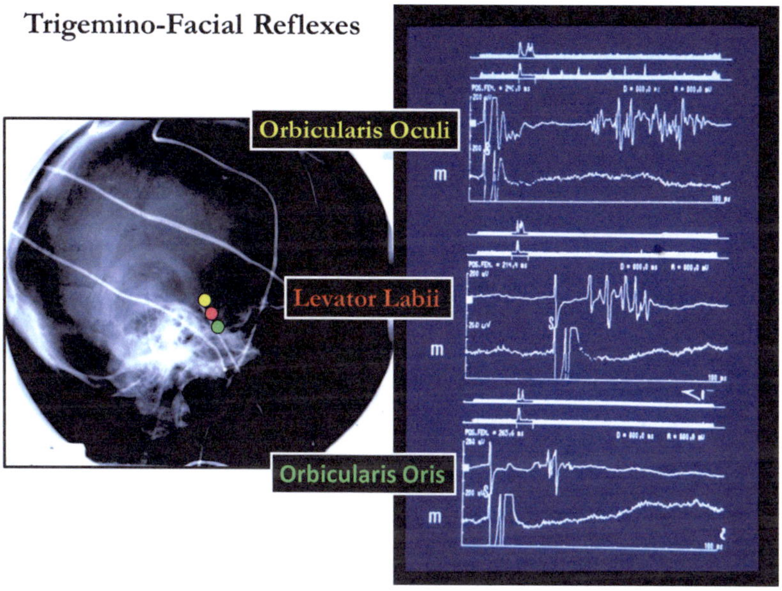

Fig. 17.8 EMG-recordings of Evoked Motor Responses (EMRs): localizing value. EMRs are predominantly in orbicularis oris for stimulation of the fibers corresponding to the V_3 division of the root (green), in levator labii for stimulation of the V_2 fibers (red) and in orbicularis oculi for stimulation of the V_1 fibers (i.e., direct blink-reflex) (yellow) [21]. Study of correlation with the territory of the hypoesthesia obtained by the thermolesion allowed to attribute to these EMR that are clinically observable a practical, localizing value for surgical guidance [23]. Observation of these EMRs revealed useful in surgical practice due to their high localizing value, especially in drowsy and confused patients not cooperating [23]

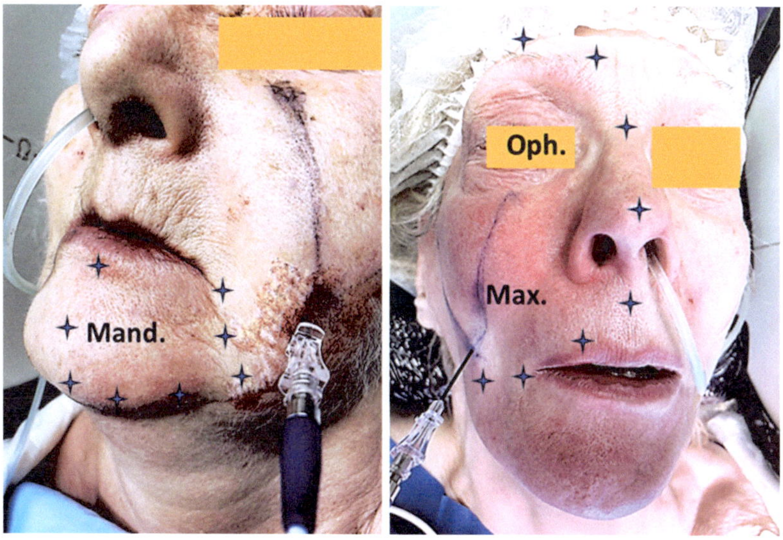

Fig. 17.9 The meaning of vasodilatation under thermal stimulation test in the trigeminal territory. Figure shows two examples of redness localized in trigeminal territories under elevation (# 55 °C) of the thermal lesioning process, on the left in the V3 division, on the right in the V2 and V1 divisions. In our experience, such an event-considered an axon reflex-revealed to be of a high localizing value. However, its occurence means that the uninsulated tip of the electrode is located toward the peripheral side of the trigeminal system, at least in the vicinity of the trigeminal ganglion. Its observation should incite to push the electrode (slightly) deeper, so that it rather be retrogasserian

75 °C. Temperature of heating is gradually increased by 5 °C increments, depending on the sensory loss produced after each lesion; a temperature of 75 °C is not exceeded during the procedure. Usually when the electrode tip is inside the trigeminal system, there is no need to exceed 70 °C. Paresthesias and EMRs elicited by an electrical stimulation of less than 0.5 V testify that the electrode tip is inside or in close contact with the trigeminal system.

The one or several thermo-lesion(s) are made until a marked hypoesthesia covers the entire area of pain. If the corneal reflex disappears during the heating, thermal lesioning is immediately stopped.

For us, the criterion for effectiveness of thermo-lesion is the obtention of analgesia to pinprick without complete loss of tactile sensation to for instance a pencil, and without alteration of the corneal reflex tested with a cotonoid. The analgesia/hypoesthesia should be centered on the trigger zone and cover the whole neuralgic territory.

A wise precaution is to prescribe, as soon as surgery is completed, eye drops of artificial tears, and if necessary to indicate a close ophthalmologic surveillance, which would be the more so important as the thermolesion has produced corneal hypoesthesia.

17.3.2 Therapeutic Effects

A retrospective analysis of an initial personal series of 583 patients [20] showed that the best location of the electrode to perform the thermo-lesion was at the triangular plexus level, not only for achieving an optimal effect on pain (Fig. 17.10) but also for minimizing the side effects and complications (Fig. 17.10). At this target, an effect qualified as "excellent"—that is, corresponding to the suppression of the neuralgia, with a strong analgesia at pin-prink testing and without complete loss of the tactile sensation, and covering the painful territory without trespassing the involved trigeminal divisions—was obtained in 70% of the patients. A result qualified of "good" (additionally 17% of the cases) was same, but not totally well-centered and/or not so well limited to the painful territory. At this triangular plexus target, the side effects and the complications were much less than at the neighboring locations of the electrode, as shown in the figure. Patients with dysesthesias amounted at 7% with 3% with a distressing anesthesia dolorosa; keratitis occurred in 5% of the patients of whom one case evolved to corneal ulcer with blindness (i.e., in 0.17% of the series).

In our total series of 3250 cases who had a thermo-rhizotomy procedure over a 40-year period of full-time activity [30], initial pain relief was achieved in 97% of the patients; overall, recurrent rate amounted at 7% with a survey of up to 28 years for the earliest patient operated on (17 years on average). This relatively low rate of recurrences can be put in relation to the fact that our aim was to create a noticeable hypoesthesia to nociception with only some degree of tactile hypoesthesia, in spite of a more or less (announced) bothering numbness, so as to minimize recurrence occurrence.

A review that we carried out on ten literature series, totaling 7483 patients and followed from 3 to 26 years depending on the series (9 years on average), showed an average rate with immediate pain relief of 94% of the cases (from 81 to 99% depending on the series) and an average rate with long-term efficacy of 60.4% (from 20 to 93% depending on the series) [30]. The side effects and neurological complications were reported at very different frequencies among the various publications reviewed: bothering facial hypoesthesia at 5–98% depending on the series and masticatory deficit at 4–24%, for the side effects and keratitis (1–8%) and dysesthesias/anesthesia dolorosa (0.8–7% for the later), for the complications. The reported mortality was 0.1%, by carotid artery injury.

A more recent review, in 2019, which collected seven literature studies including 4533 patients with an average FU from 3 to 9.3 years according to series, reports pain-free and recurrence rates ranging from 26 to 82% and 16 to 74%, respectively [31, 32]. In this review, mortality was zero;

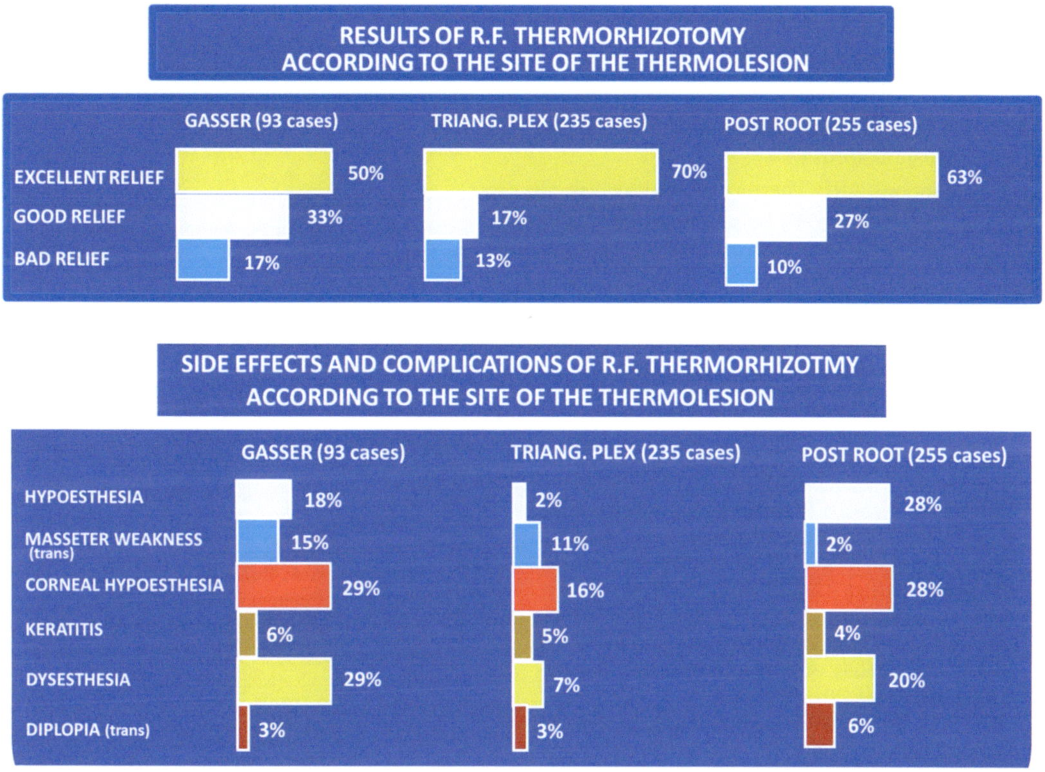

Fig. 17.10 Effects of RF-Thermohizotomy according to the location of the thermolesion. **Results on pain according to the site of the thermolesion**. Pain relief was better achieved when the uninsulated tip of the electrode was located in the triangular plexus rather than in the gasserian ganglion or in the root in the cerebello-pontine angle [20]. **Side-effects and complications according to the site of the thermolesion**. Location of the thermolesion in the triangular plexus was safer than in root in the cerebello-pontine angle or in the ganglion [20]

patients with sequelae of hearing loss were 6, cranial nerve palsy 36, corneal hypoesthesia 300, keratitis 55, masticatory weakness 280, facial hypoesthesia 853, anesthesia dolorosa 29.

Disparity of the rates of the long-term relief and recurrences among authors can be—logically -linked to the degree of the hypoesthesia left by the thermo-lesion. The important dilemma with this method is to decide between strong hypoesthesia with low probability of (early) recurrence, but bothersome numbness, and, mild hypoesthesia with less side effects, but high rate of pain return. Decision should be discussed with the patient, and clearly written down in the signed informed consent.

Nonetheless, the method—which has almost no contraindication even in elderly patients—is very operator-dependent and requires specific training.

17.4 Conclusions

The purpose of the percutaneous lesioning techniques is to suppress the conduction of the trigeminal fibers that carry the neuralgic pain to the brainstem. RF-Thermo-rhizotomy is one of those. Thanks to modern interventional neuradiology techniques allowing for a safe navigation through the FO by Hartel's classical trajectory, to anaesthesilogic techniques means of modulating the patient's conscience level and the successively developed surgical and neurophysiologic refinements, a certain selectivity can be obtained.

RF-Thermo-rhizotomy, like the other lesioning techniques including the stereotactic radiosurgery modality, is effective on pain transmission, but generates side effects, of which numbness is the dominant component, and corneal anesthesia with keratitis a subsequent risk. The lesser the postoperative hypesthesia, the higher the risk of recurrence. The stronger the hypoesthesia, the more risk of bothering paresthesias and secondary anesthesia dolorosa.

Percutaneous RF-Thermo-rhizotomy is a demanding technique. To be selective, i.e., accurate and long-term effective without harmful side effects, it necessitates detailed knowledge on its surgical anatomical substratum.

References

1. Cruccu G, Finnerup NB, Jensen TS, Scholz J, Sindou M, Svensson P, Treede RD, Zakrzewska JM, Nurmikko T. Trigeminal neuralgia: new classification and diagnostic grading for practice and research. Neurology. 2016;87(2):220–8.
2. IHS C. Headache classification Committee of the International Headache Society (IHS) the international classification of headache disorders, 3rd edition. Cephalalgia. 2018;38(1):1–211.
3. Sindou M, Brinzeu A. Trigeminal neuralgias: a neurosurgical illustrated guide. Cham: Springer; 2023.
4. Kirschner M. The puncturing technique and the electrocoagulation of the ganglion Gasseri: transferred. Operations (DiePunktiostechnik und die Elektrocoagulation des ganglion Gasseri: übergez Operationen) German. Arch Klin Chir. 1933;176:620.
5. Sweet WH, Wepsic JG. Controlled thermocoagulation of trigeminal ganglion and rootlets for differential destruction of pain fibers. 1. Trigeminal neuralgia. J Neurosurg. 1974;40(2):143–56.
6. Frigyesi TL, Siegfried J, Broggi G. The selective vulnerability of evoked potentials in the trigeminal sensory root of graded thermocoagulation. Exp Neurol. 1975;49(1 Pt 1):11–21.
7. Letcher FS, Goldring S. The effect of radiofrequency current and heat on peripheral nerve action potential in the cat. J Neurosurg. 1968;29(1):42–7.
8. Kanpolat Y, Onol B. Experimental percutaneous approach to the trigeminal ganglion in dogs with histopathological evaluation of radiofrequency lesions. Acta Neurochir Suppl (Wien). 1980;30:363–6.
9. Smith HP, McWhorter JM, Challa VR. Radiofrequency neurolysis in a clinical model. Neuropathological correlation. J Neurosurg. 1981;55(2):246–53.
10. Bernard F, Mercier P, Sindou M. Morphological and functional anatomy of the trigeminal triangular plexus as an anatomical entity: a systematic review. Surg Radiol Anat. 2019;41(6):625–37.
11. Emmons WF, Rhoton AL Jr. Functional subdivision of the trigeminal sensory root. Surg Forum. 1968;19:440–1.
12. Guclu B, Sindou M, Meyronet D, Streichenberger N, Simon E, Mertens P. Cranial nerve vascular compression syndromes of the trigeminal, facial and Vago-glossopharyngeal nerves: comparative anatomical study of the central myelin portion and transitional zone; correlations with incidences of corresponding hyperactive dysfunctional syndromes. Acta Neurochir. 2011;153(12):2365–75.
13. De Ridder D, Møller A, Verlooy J, Cornelissen M, De Ridder L. Is the root entry/exit zone important in microvascular compression syndromes? Neurosurgery. 2002;51(2):427–33; discussion 433-424.
14. Haskel RBL, Berry MM, Standing SM. Nervous system. In: Gray's anatomy. 38th ed. London: Churchill Livingstone; 1995. p. 1158–60.
15. Gudmundsson K, Rhoton AL Jr, Rushton JG. Detailed anatomy of the intracranial portion of the trigeminal nerve. J Neurosurg. 1971;35(5):592–600.
16. Joo W, Yoshioka F, Funaki T, Mizokami K, Rhoton AL Jr. Microsurgical anatomy of the trigeminal nerve. Clin Anat. 2014;27(1):61–88.
17. Kanpolat Y, Savas A, Bekar A, Berk C. Percutaneous controlled radiofrequency trigeminal rhizotomy for the treatment of idiopathic trigeminal neuralgia: 25-year experience with 1,600 patients. Neurosurgery. 2001;48(3):524–32; discussion 532-524.
18. Karol EA, Sanz OP, Rey RD. Sensory and motor trigeminal evoked potentials to localize the position of trigeminal electrodes. Acta Neurochir. 1991;108(3–4):110–5.
19. Peris-Celda M, Graziano F, Russo V, Mericle RA, Ulm AJ. Foramen ovale puncture, lesioning accuracy, and avoiding complications: microsurgical anatomy study with clinical implications. J Neurosurg. 2013;119(5):1176–93.
20. Sindou M, Keravel Y. Trigeminal neuralgia. Percutaneous thermocoagulation of the trigeminal nerve (author's transl). Neurochirurgie. 1979;25(3):166–72.
21. Sindou M, Fobe JL, Berthier E, Vial C. Facial motor responses evoked by direct electrical stimulation of the trigeminal root. Localizing value for radiofrequency thermorhizotomy. Acta Neurochir. 1994;128(1–4):57–67.
22. Tatli M, Sindou M. Anatomoradiological landmarks for accuracy of radiofrequency thermorhizotomy in the treatment of trigeminal neuralgia. Neurosurgery. 2008;63(1 Suppl 1):ONS129–37; discussion ONS137-128.
23. Sindou MP. Neurophysiological navigation in the trigeminal nerve: use of masticatory responses and facial motor responses evoked by electrical stimulation of the trigeminal rootlets for RF-thermorhizotomy guidance. Stereotact Funct Neurosurg. 1999;73(1–4):117–21.
24. Drake CG, Mckenzie KG. Mesencephalic tractotomy for pain: experience with six cases. J Neurosurg. 1953;10(5):457–62. https://doi.org/10.3171/jns.1953.10.5.0457. PMID: 13097205.
25. Mckenzie KG. Trigeminal tractotomy. Clin Neurosurg. 1954;2:50–69; discussion, 69–70. PMID: 13270405.

26. Dandy W. Section of the sensory root of the trigeminal nerve at the pons; preliminary report of the operative procedure. Bull Jhons Hokins Hospital; 1925.
27. Terrier LM, Amelot A, François P, Destrieux C, Zemmoura I, Velut S. Therapeutic failure in trigeminal neuralgia: from a clarification of trigeminal nerve somatotopy to a targeted partial sensory rhizotomy. World Neurosurg. 2018;117:e138–45.
28. Terrier L-M, Zemmoura I, Amelot A, Destrieux C, François P, Velut S. New insights into the trigeminal nerve somatotopy: lessons from partial sensory rhizotomy. Morphologie. 2017;101(335):195.
29. Alvernia JE, Sindou MP, Dang ND, Maley JH, Mertens P. Percutaneous approach to the foramen ovale: an anatomical study of the extracranial trajectory with the incorrect trajectories to be avoided. Acta Neurochir. 2010;152(6):1043–53.
30. Tatli M, Satici O, Kanpolat Y, Sindou M. Various surgical modalities for trigeminal neuralgia: literature study of respective long-term outcomes. Acta Neurochir. 2008;150(3):243–55.
31. Bendtsen L, Zakrzewska JM, Abbott J, Braschinsky M, Di Stefano G, Donnet A, Eide PK, Leal PRL, Maarbjerg S, May A, Nurmikko T, Obermann M, Jensen TS, Cruccu G. European academy of neurology guideline on trigeminal neuralgia. Eur J Neurol. 2019;26(6):831–49.
32. Maarbjerg S, Di Stefano G, Bendtsen L, Cruccu G. Trigeminal neuralgia—diagnosis and treatment. Cephalalgia. 2017;37(7):648–57.

18 Surgical Treatment of Masseter Spasm

Hua Zhao and Shi-Ting Li

18.1 Introduction

Hemimasticatory spasm (HMS) was originally named as Romberg spasm 1987 by Gowers WR [1]. It is a relatively rare type of unilateral trigeminal nerve (TN) motor branch dysfunction, whose pathogenesis is currently unclear [2]. It causes unilateral paroxysmal contractions in the jaw-closing muscles that prevent voluntary closing of the mouth, which may persist during sleep, and is accompanied by muscle pain, with compensatory hypertrophy changes also often seen in the muscles affected by spasms (Fig. 18.1). The medial pterygoid, masseter, and temporalis muscles are affected by this condition [3, 4].

HMS is usually precipitated by talking, laughing, etc. Due to the lack of sensory processing, it is different from hemifacial spasm (HFS). One of the proposed mechanisms is the involvement of trigeminal motor fibers in the form of focal demyelination and ectopic pulse generation. Others have also proposed that HMS should be considered a peripheral entrapment neuropathy [5]. Cruccu et al. reported two cases of HMS and indicated that HMS is induced by ectopic activity secondary to focal demyelination of trigeminal motor nerve fibers [6]. In addition, some researchers speculate that HMS may originate from damage to the trigeminal motor root or motor nucleus, similar to the nonautonomous movement of HFS, although the location and cause of ectopic excitation are different. Some authors reported that some cases of HMS were related to pontine infarction [7]. Xu [8] pointed that Parry-Romberg syndrome (PRS) could result in HMS. The above research results indicate that the etiology of HMS is diverse; therefore, specific treatment strategies should be considered and implemented accordingly.

At present, there are various treatment methods for HMS [9]. Local injection of botulinum toxin (BT) A is considered a favorable treatment for symptom relief. In a previously reported case, although the symptoms of BT were significantly improved, patients needed to receive regular injections of BT to primarily alleviate the symptoms. The improvement of the patient's symptoms may also be due to the self-limiting nature of the disease, rather than the influence of BT [10, 11]. In addition, some authors have attempted treating HMS with carbamazepine and phenytoin with some success. Contrary to the failure of botulinum toxin and drug therapy, some authors reported that the introduction of microvascular decompression (MVD) in these HMS patients has shown good results. The first successful cure of HMS via MVD by Kyu-Hyon Chon supported the similarity between HMS and HFS in mechanism, which was further demonstrated in six cases of HMS with MVD treatment from

H. Zhao · S.-T. Li (✉)
Department of Neurosurgery, XinHua Hospital, Shanghai JiaoTong University School of Medicine, Shanghai, China

S.-T. Li et al. (eds.), *Microvascular Decompression Surgery*,
https://doi.org/10.1007/978-981-96-0767-9_18

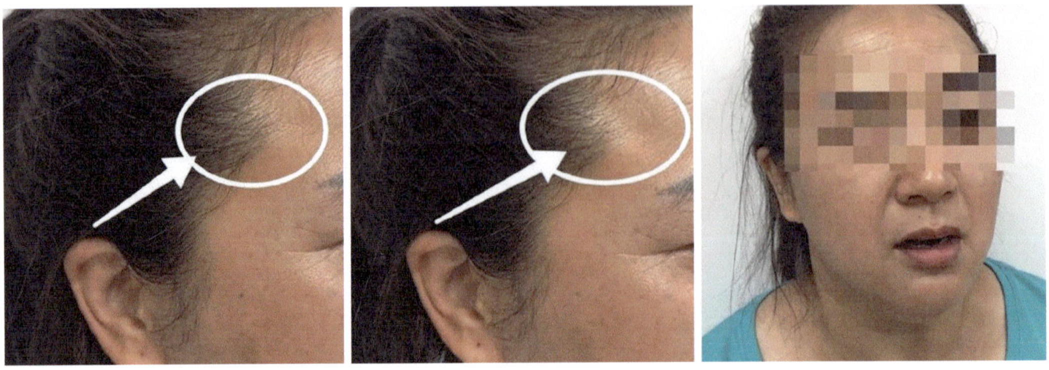

Fig. 18.1 Intermittent local protrusion in the right temporal region, Intermittent period with normal mandibular movement

Table 18.1 Summary of the patients with HMS treated by MVD

Authors	Age	Gender	Involved muscles	Treatment	Offending vessels	Outcomes
Chon et al. [12]	54	M	Right temporalis/masseter	MVD	SCA	Relief
Wang et al. [13]	50	F	Left masseter	MVD	AICA in 2 patients SCA in 2 patients Both AICA and SCA in 2 patients	Not relief
	42	F	Right temporalis/masseter	MVD		Relief
	38	M	Right masseter	MVD		Relief
	48	F	Right masseter	MVD		Relief
	57	F	Left temporalis/masseter	MVD		Delayed relief
	53	F	Right temporalis/masseter	MVD		Relief
Dou et al. [14]	56	F	Left masseter	MVD	SCA	Relief
Sun et al. [15]	22	M	Left masseter	MVD	SCA	Relief
Chen et al. [16]	44	M	Right temporalis/masseter	MVD	SCA	Relief
	36	M	Left temporalis/masseter	MVD	Pontine artery and lateral pontine vein	Delayed relief
	62	M	Right temporalis/masseter	MVD	SCA	Relief
	48	F	Left temporalis/masseter	MVD	SCA	Relief
	57	F	Right temporalis/masseter	MVD	SCA	Relief
	30	F	Right temporalis/masseter	MVD	SCA	Relief

Yong-Nan Wang et al. (Table 18.1). As shown in Table 18.1, not all patients can be cured through MVD surgery. At our center, we use MVD combined with highly selective trigeminal rhizotomy (HSTR) to treat this disease. After long-term follow-up (>2 years), all patients have been completely cured.

18.2 Clinical Characteristics

1. Unilateral, involuntary, and paroxysmal contractions of the muscles of mastication. Each episode lasted from a few seconds to several minutes.

2. Voluntary closing of the mouth, which may persist during sleep, and is accompanied by muscle pain.
3. Spasms were painful and triggered by activities like chewing, talking, clenching of teeth, or voluntary tapping of the involved muscles.

18.3 Neurophysiological Examination

Electromyography (EMG) has extremely important value in the diagnosis and differential diagnosis of masticatory muscle spasms in clinical practice, with characteristic changes in the quiescent and episodic phases. The affected muscles are mainly the masseter and temporal muscles, with some involving the medial pterygoid muscles and very few involving the lateral pterygoid muscles [17].

Using a Nikolai multichannel electromyography device and a concentric circular needle electrode, the spontaneous potential, motor unit potential phase, amplitude, and recruitment form of bilateral masseter, temporal muscle, and lateral pterygoid muscle were examined.

Blink reflex examination: Place the stimulation electrode on one side of the orbital notch and record the electrode on both sides of the orbicularis oculi muscle. Record R1 recorded on the same side of stimulation and R2 recorded on both sides.

The electromyography shows explosive discharges during the onset of muscle spasms, and a large number of motor unit potentials are visible during the resting period. The EMG shows a group discharge potential that occurs synchronously with spasms, and the affected muscles are innervated by the motor branches of the trigeminal nerve. No obvious abnormalities were observed in the blink reflex (Fig. 18.2).

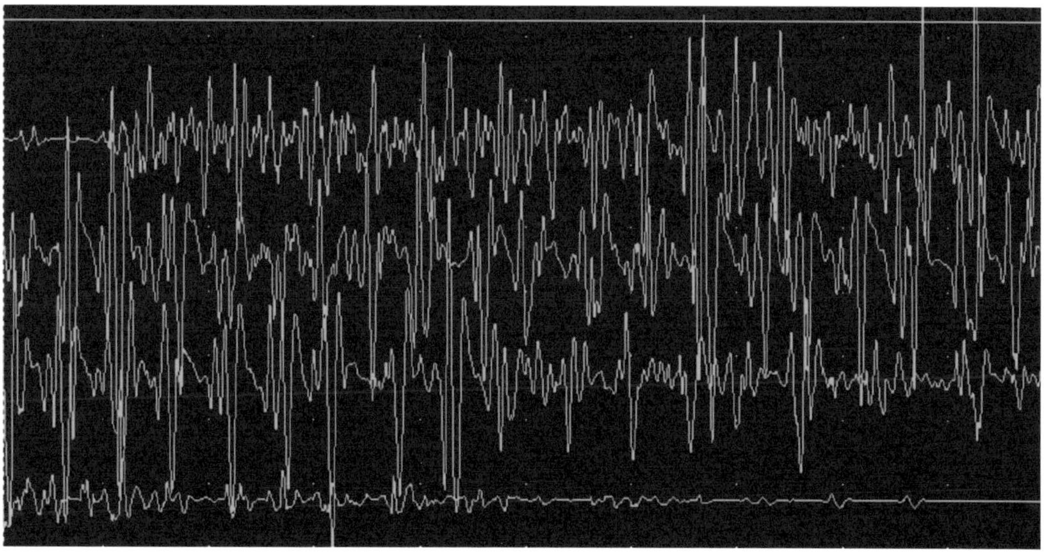

Fig. 18.2 Preoperative electromyography shows action potential bursts in the right temporal muscle and masseter muscle

18.4 Imaging Characteristics

Imaging examination usually indicates no space-occupying lesions. Time-of-flight magnetic resonance angiography (TOF-MRA) suggested the presence of neurovascular conflict or the possible source of blood vessel compression (Fig. 18.3). In addition, magnetic resonance imaging can show significant hypertrophy of the ipsilateral facial muscle.

18.5 Surgical Treatment Strategies

18.5.1 Craniotomy

A retro-mastoid microsurgical approach was performed while the patient was in the lateral decubitus position under general anesthesia. A vertical linear incision was made behind the ear along and medial to the hairline. Anterior edge of bone window to sigmoid sinus, upper edge to transverse sinus. The surgeon will make a curved incision of the dura mater and flip it towards the sigmoid sinus. Cerebrospinal fluid can spontaneously flow out, or gently compress the cerebellum to utilize cerebrospinal fluid outflow (Fig. 18.4).

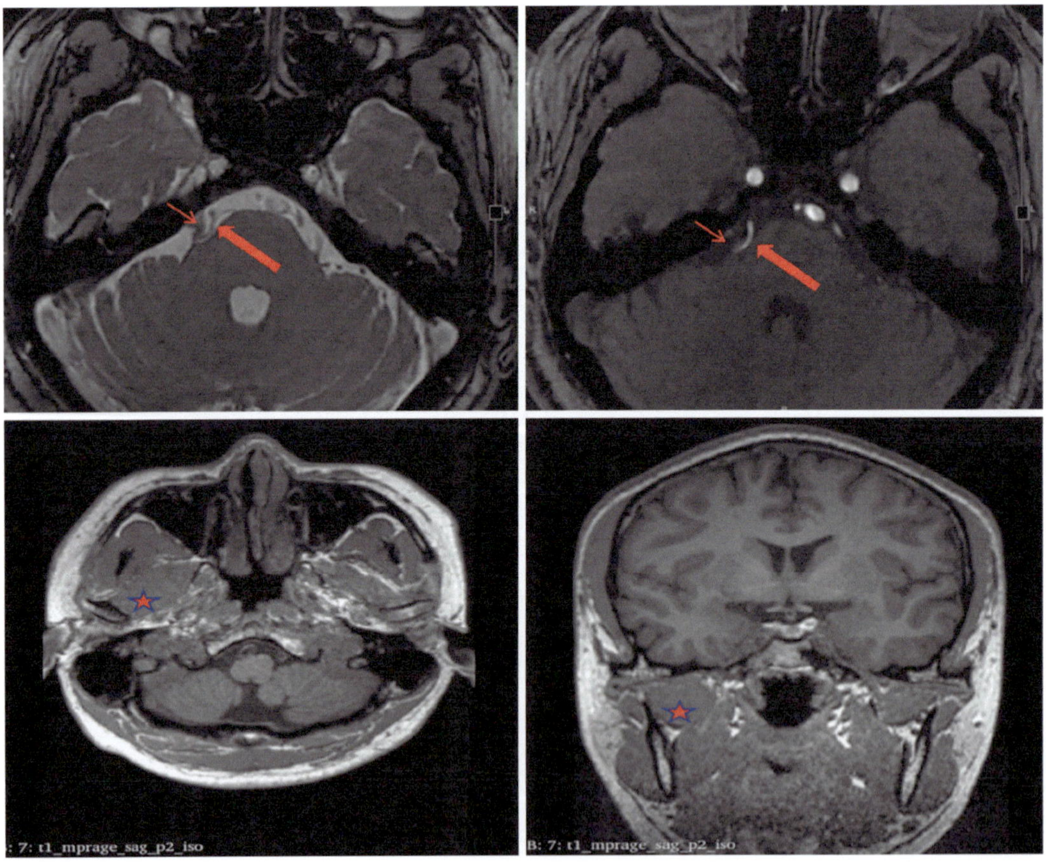

Fig. 18.3 MRI shows a vascular loop (superior cerebellar artery, thick arrow) around the right trigeminal nerve (thin arrow) and significant hypertrophy of the ipsilateral musculus medial pterygoid (☆)

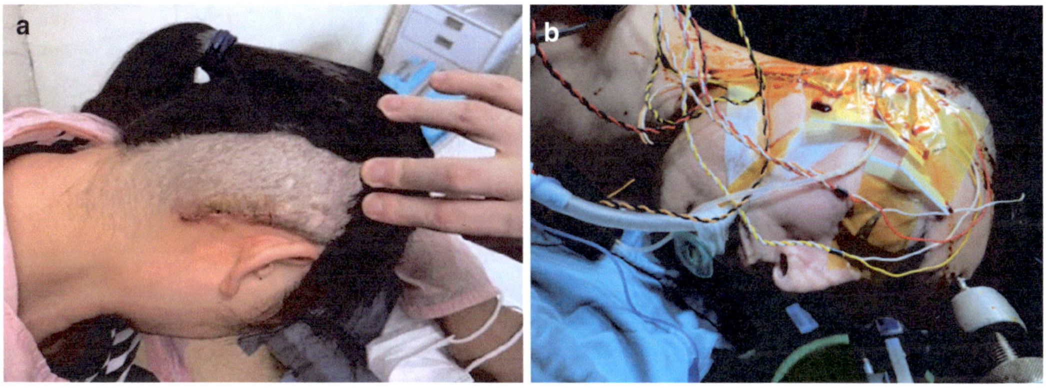

Fig. 18.4 Surgical incision and electrophysiological monitoring. A longitudinal incision of approximately 5 cm in length behind the ear and inside the hairline (**a**). Needle electrodes were inserted into the patient's ipsilateral facial muscle (**b**)

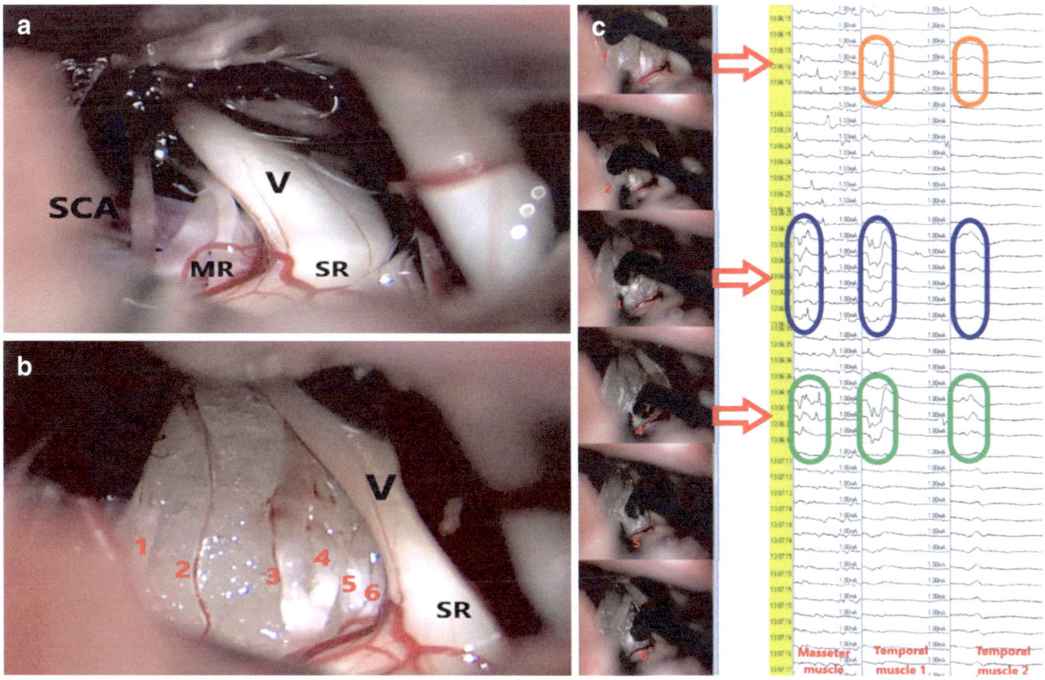

Fig. 18.5 Intraoperative findings. Superior cerebellar artery compresses trigeminal motor root which has six branches. The affected fibers were cut off according to the amplitude of the CMAP from high to low, until CMAP decreased significantly or disappeared. *SCA* superior cerebellar artery, *V* trigeminal nerve, *MR* motor root of trigeminal nerve, *SR* sensory root of trigeminal nerve

18.5.2 Surgical Approach

The surgeon exposes the trigeminal nerve through the cerebellar fissure approach. The entire course of the trigeminal nerve root was exposed after the cerebrospinal fluid was slowly released and the surrounding arachnoidal membrane was dissected. The sensory root was separated from the motor root in the root entry zone (REZ) of the trigeminal nerve (Fig. 18.5).

18.5.3 Microvasscular Decompression and Highly Selective Trigeminal Rhizotomy

Under microscopic inspection, it was noted that the trigeminal motor rootlet was apparently elevated and compressed by superior cerebellar artery, which resulted in high tension of the rootlet. Small pieces of wet gelatin sponge were firstly inserted between the culprit vessels and the motor root of trigeminal nerve to expand the gap. Then suitable of shredded Teflon sponges were interposed between the gelatin sponge and the offending vessels, without direct contact with the potential demyelinating area on the nerve. During surgery, it is often found that there are multiple branches of the trigeminal nerve motor root. At this point, selective trigeminal motor root amputation surgery needs to be performed under the guidance of electrophysiology.

Needle electrodes were inserted into the patient's ipsilateral temporalis muscle, masseter muscle, and external pterygoid muscle. Abnormal discharges of varying degrees in the aforementioned muscles could be recorded during spasms of the masticatory muscles, which was most notable in the temporalis muscle (Fig. 18.5). Highly selective trigeminal rhizotomy (HSTR) was recommended for patients without definite vascular compression. If neurovascular conflict was observed, some Teflon sponges were used to push the involved blood vessels away from the TN motor roots. If no vascular compression was detected, except for trigeminal neurolysis, neurophysiological monitoring was applied to identify the nerve motor branches corresponding to each muscle. Then the branches of motor root of trigeminal nerve were stimulated one by one with nerve probes, and the amplitudes of muscle compound action potential (CMAP) were recorded in the ipsilateral temporalis and masseter muscles. The unaffected nerve fibers were preserved, and the affected fibers were cut off according to the amplitude of the CMAP from high to low, until CMAP decreased significantly or disappeared (Fig. 18.5).

18.5.4 Closure

At the end of the operation, the surgical field should be well irrigated with normal saline to vent air as well as to assure that there is no bleeding. Meanwhile, attention should be paid to make sure the implanted Teflon is stable under the flow of cerebrospinal fluid (CSF). In order to prevent CSF leakage, the dura should be closed tightly. Then, the dura is sealed with glue and covered by an artificial dura plus bone chips to reconstruct the normal anatomy (Fig. 18.6).

18.5.5 Recommend

1. Patients who's TOF-MRA revealed definite vascular compression underwent HSTR assisted by intraoperative EMG plus MVD.
2. Preoperative TOF-MRA revealed that neurovascular conflict was absent at the root of the TN in some patients, in this condition, HSTR, assisted by intraoperative EMG was recommend.

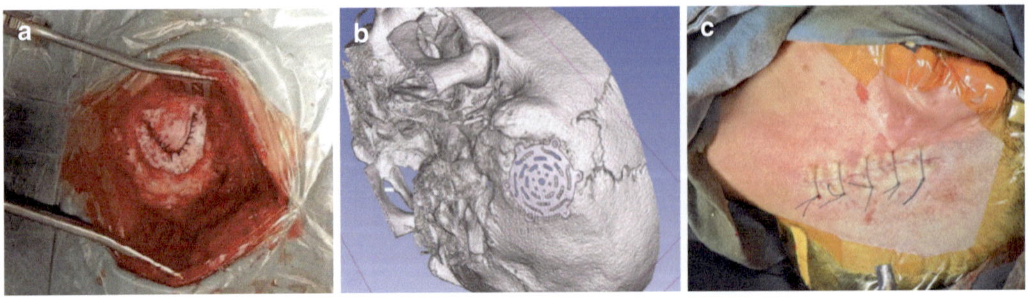

Fig. 18.6 Clouse. Dural membrane should be always stitched in a watertight pattern

References

1. Chen L. Microvascular decompression of trigeminal motor root: a considerable surgical cure for hemimasticatory spasm. J Neurosurg Sci. 2020;64:488–9.
2. Christie C, Rodriguez-Quiroga SA, Arakaki T, Rey RD, Garretto NS. Hemimasticatory spasm: report of a case and review of the literaturedagger. Tremor Other Hyperkinet Mov (N Y). 2014;4:210.
3. Panda AK, Gopinath G, Singh S. Parry-Romberg syndrome with hemimasticatory spasm in pregnancy; a dystonia mimic. J Neurosci Rural Pract. 2014;5:184–6.
4. Sinha R, Chattopadhyay PK, Roychowdhury SK, Bennur S. Hemimasticatory spasm: a case report with a new management strategy. J Maxillofac Oral Surg. 2011;10:170–2.
5. Woo KA, Kim HJ, Park H, Jeon B. Bilateral hemimasticatory spasm in a patient with hypereosinophilic syndrome. Parkinsonism Relat Disord. 2021;93:55–7.
6. Cruccu G, Inghilleri M, Berardelli A, et al. Pathophysiology of hemimasticatory spasm. J Neurol Neurosurg Psychiatry. 1994;57:43–50.
7. Gunduz A, Karaali-Savrun F, Uluduz D. Hemimasticatory spasm following pontine infarction. Mov Disord. 2007;22:1674–5.
8. Xu H, Xu B, Huang X, Zhang D, Cai X. Treatment of hemimasticatory spasm secondary to parry-romberg syndrome via partial resection of the trigeminal nerve motor branch under intraoperative neurophysiological monitoring: a case report and literature review. Front Surg. 2023;10:1146163.
9. Cersosimo MG, Bertoti A, Roca CU, Micheli F. Botulinum toxin in a case of hemimasticatory spasm with severe worsening during pregnancy. Clin Neuropharmacol. 2004;27:6–8.
10. Kim JH, Han SW, Kim YJ, et al. A case of painful hemimasticatory spasm with masseter muscle hypertrophy responsive to botulinum toxin. J Mov Disord. 2009;2:95–7.
11. Teive HA, Piovesan EJ, Germiniani FM, et al. Hemimasticatory spasm treated with botulinum toxin: case report. Arq Neuropsiquiatr. 2002;60:288–9.
12. Chon KH, Lee JM, Koh EJ, Choi HY. Hemimasticatory spasm treated with microvascular decompression of the trigeminal nerve. Acta Neurochir. 2012;154:1635–9.
13. Wang YN, Dou NN, Zhou QM, et al. Treatment of hemimasticatory spasm with microvascular decompression. J Craniofac Surg. 2013;24:1753–5.
14. Dou NN, Zhong J, Zhou QM, Zhu J, Wang YN, Li ST. Microvascular decompression of trigeminal nerve root for treatment of a patient with hemimasticatory spasm. J Craniofac Surg. 2014;25:916–8.
15. Sun H, Wei Z, Wang Y, Liu C, Chen M, Diao Y. Microvascular decompression for hemimasticatory spasm: a case report and review of the literature. World Neurosurg. 2016;90:703.e5–703.e10.
16. Chen L, Wu G, Wang H, Guo X, Chitkara N. Hemimasticatory spasm: does microvascular decompression of trigeminal motor root work? Neurol India. 2021;69:757–8.
17. Auger RG, Litchy WJ, Cascino TL, Ahlskog JE. Hemimasticatory spasm: clinical and electrophysiologic observations. Neurology. 1992;42:2263–6.

19 Microvascular Decompression for the Treatment of Non-Aneurysmal Vascular Compression-Induced Oculomotor Nerve Paralysis

Yinda Tang and Shi-Ting Li

19.1 Introduction

After Professor Peter Jannetta's pioneering success in 1966 with microvascular decompression (MVD) on the facial and trigeminal nerves in the posterior fossa [1–3], this procedure has become the established treatment for hemifacial spasm and trigeminal neuralgia. Its surgical indications have gradually expanded to include glossopharyngeal neuralgia, intractable dizziness, tinnitus, and neurogenic hypertension among various cranial nerve diseases involving neurovascular conflicts, termed "neurovascular compression syndrome" (NVCS) [4, 5]. The oculomotor nerve, responsible for eye movement and pupil reflexes as the third cranial nerve originating from the midbrain, traverses through the heavily vascularized subarachnoid cisterns. Consequently, one might associate neurovascular conflicts with oculomotor nerve palsy (ONP), presenting clinically as diplopia, ophthalmoplegia, and anisocoria. However, beyond well-recognized causes such as posterior communicating artery (PCom) aneurysms leading to compressive ONP, little is known about ONP solely caused by non-aneurysmal vascular compression (nAVC) [6–8]. Cases treated with MVD for nAVC-induced ONP (nAVC-ONP) are exceedingly rare, with sporadic reports [9–23]. Yet, with advancements in high-resolution MRI and 3D post-processing techniques, the relationship between nAVC and ONP seems to be gradually unveiled [17, 24–26]. Consequently, the therapeutic value of MVD in such diseases is progressively emerging. This chapter presents five cases of MVD-treated nAVC-ONP from our center [27], accompanied by a preliminary discussion informed by existing literature on similar cases, aiming to explore this field further.

19.2 Case Reports from Our Center

Between October 2022 and October 2023, our center performed MVD surgery on five cases pre-diagnosed with nAVC-ONP. The cases are reported as follows (Table 19.1):

Case 1
A 65-year-old male was admitted on October 31, 2022, complaining of diplopia and progressive left upper eyelid ptosis for 4 years. His medical history included residual sequelae of left peripheral facial palsy for 11 years and hypertension, with no specific treatment received previously.

Y. Tang
XinHua Hospital, Shanghai JiaoTong University School of Medicine, Shanghai, China

S.-T. Li (✉)
Department of Neurosurgery, XinHua Hospital, Shanghai JiaoTong University School of Medicine, Shanghai, China
e-mail: lsting66@164.com

S.-T. Li et al. (eds.), *Microvascular Decompression Surgery*,
https://doi.org/10.1007/978-981-96-0767-9_19

Table 19.1 Case Reports from Our Center

	Case Item	1	2	3	4	5
General information	Sex	Male	Male	Female	Male	Female
	Age	65 years	44 years	64 years	44 years	61 years
	Duration	4 years	1 year	8 years	1 month	6 days
	Side	Left	Right	Right	Left	Right
	Nonsurgical treatment	None	Citicoline, mecobalamin, and methylprednisolone	Pyridostigmine and prisms	None	None
	Past medical history	Sequelae of left peripheral facial palsy for 11 years	Hypertension	None	None	Sequelae of left peripheral facial palsy for 1.5 years
Preoperative symptoms	Diplopia	Have	Have	Have	Have	Have
	Ptosis	Complete	Partial	None	Partial	Complete
	Eye movement disorder	Partial, inability to move upward	None	Partial, restricted medial movement	None	Complete, fixed lateral gaze
	Dilated pupil	Have	None	None	None	Have
Preoperative imaging	Source of compression	PCA, SCA	PCA, SCA, uncus	SCA	PCA, SCA	PCA
	Signs of nerve compression	Sandwich-like compression	Sandwich-like compression	Nerve deformation	Sandwich-like compression	Nerve deformation
	Compression site	Proximal	Proximal and distal	Proximal	Proximal	Proximal
Assessment scale	Symptom scale	2	1	1	1	2
	Imaging scale	2	2	2	2	2
	Total scale	4	3	3	3	4
Operation	Approach	Anterior subtemporal	Pterional-transsylvian-transuncal	Pterional-transsylvian-transuncal	Pterional-transsylvian-transuncal	Pterional-transsylvian-transuncal
	Offending vessels	PCA, SCA	PCA, SCA	SCA	PCA, SCA	PCA
	Other responsibilities for compression	None	Uncus, PPCFD	None	None	Arachnoid band and a small artery
	Compression site	Proximal	Proximal and distal	Proximal	Proximal	Proximal
	Decompression methods	Teflon plus gelatin sponge	Teflon plus gelatin sponge	Teflon	Teflon plus gelatin sponge	Teflon plus gelatin sponge

Postoperative outcomes	Added dysfunction	None	None	None	None	None
	Immediate postoperative effect	Mild improvement in upward eye movement function one week after surgery	Within a day, the symptom of upper eyelid ptosis completely resolved, diplopia improved	No change	Two days after surgery, the symptoms of upper eyelid ptosis began to alleviate. Complete resolution of ptosis was observed by 2 weeks	At 1-month post-surgery, the complete upper eyelid ptosis had progressed to partial, the pupil returned to normal, and partial eye movement recovery occurred
	Long-term postoperative results	After 5 months, slight improvement in eyelid lifting and upward gaze function	After 8 months, diplopia disappeared	After 6 months, partial relief of diplopia and partial internal movement restrictions	Diplopia completely resolved by 6 months after surgery	By 4 months post-surgery, all oculomotor nerve functions had completely recovered, and the diplopia had disappeared
	Follow-up time	12 months	8 months	6 months	6 months	4 months
	Total effect	Slightly resolved	Completely resolved	Partially resolved	Completely resolved	Completely resolved

PCA posterior cerebral artery, *SCA* superior cerebellar artery; sandwich-like compression: simultaneous compression from above and below, *PPCFD* posterior petroclinoid dural fold

Physical examination revealed oculomotor nerve dysfunction: dilation of the pupil on the affected side, complete left upper eyelid ptosis, and inability of the eye to move upward. Thin-layer MRI (FIESTA, 3D TOF fusion, 3D reconstruction) indicated compression of the left oculomotor nerve root exit zone (REZ) by the posterior cerebral artery (PCA) and superior cerebellar artery (SCA) from above and below, with evident compression observed in imaging, displaying a sandwich-like compression pattern. On November 3, 2022, surgery was performed using an anterior subtemporal approach, extensively freeing the arachnoid membrane near the oculomotor nerve REZ. During the procedure, PCA and SCA were found compressing the nerve, consistent with preoperative imaging findings. Decompression of SCA and PCA was conducted using the "Teflon plus gelatin sponge techniques" (see Sect. 19.4). Postoperatively, no new oculomotor nerve dysfunction was observed. After 1 week, there was a mild improvement in upward eye movement function. Follow-up examinations at 5 months and 1 year post-surgery showed slight improvement in eyelid lifting and upward gaze function, with no changes in the pupil and no further improvement in upward eye movement function.

Case 2

A 44-year-old male was admitted on March 6, 2023, complaining of diplopia and progressive right upper eyelid ptosis worsening over a year, with no response to previous treatment with citicoline, mecobalamine, and methylprednisolone. On examination, partial right-sided upper eyelid ptosis was observed, the pupil was normal, and eye movement was intact. Thin-layer MRI suggested contact between the PCA and SCA with the proximal segment of the oculomotor nerve, resulting in a sandwich-like compression. Additionally, there was significant prominence of the uncus, distinctly bulging out of the tentorial edge, closely abutting the distal part of the interpeduncular cisternal segment of oculomotor nerve on the affected side. Surgery was performed on March 16, 2023, utilizing the pterional transsylvian fissure approach. During the procedure, upon extensive opening of the fissure, the uncus was observed invading the interpeduncular cisternal segment from the lateral aspect, compressing the distal oculomotor nerve. This was excised subpially. Subsequent meticulous arachnoid dissection revealed compression of the proximal oculomotor nerve by PCA from above. These two compressions from the superior direction caused the oculomotor nerve to bend downward, constrained at its distal end by the inferiorly located posterior petroclinoid dural fold (PPCDF), creating a third constriction from below, with visible grayish changes in the nerve at this site. Finally, SCA was seen compressing the nerve from below to above at the proximal end, forming the fourth compression site. The "Teflon plus gelatin sponge technique" was used to decompress PCA and SCA. Following decompression, the nerve's deformation was improved and the PPCDF was detached. Postoperatively, there were no new oculomotor nerve dysfunctions. Within a day, the symptom of upper eyelid ptosis completely resolved, diplopia improved, and after 8 months, diplopia disappeared, with sustained normal eyelid function (Fig. 19.1).

Case 3

A 64-year-old female was admitted on May 22, 2023, reporting progressive diplopia worsening over 8 years with no significant medical history. She had previously been diagnosed with myasthenia gravis and treated with pyridostigmine, which proved ineffective. Subsequently, she visited an ophthalmologist and used prisms initially, which provided initial relief but showed a progressive increase in prism diopters due to worsening symptoms. On examination, it was found that the right eye had restricted medial movement, while other directions were normal. The pupil was normal, and there was no upper eyelid ptosis. Thin-layer MRI revealed significant inferior-to-superior compression of the proximal oculomotor nerve by the SCA, causing nerve deformation and bending. Surgery was performed on May 25, 2023, utilizing the pterional transsylvian fissure approach. Intraoperatively, SCA's compression from below on the proximal oculomotor nerve was

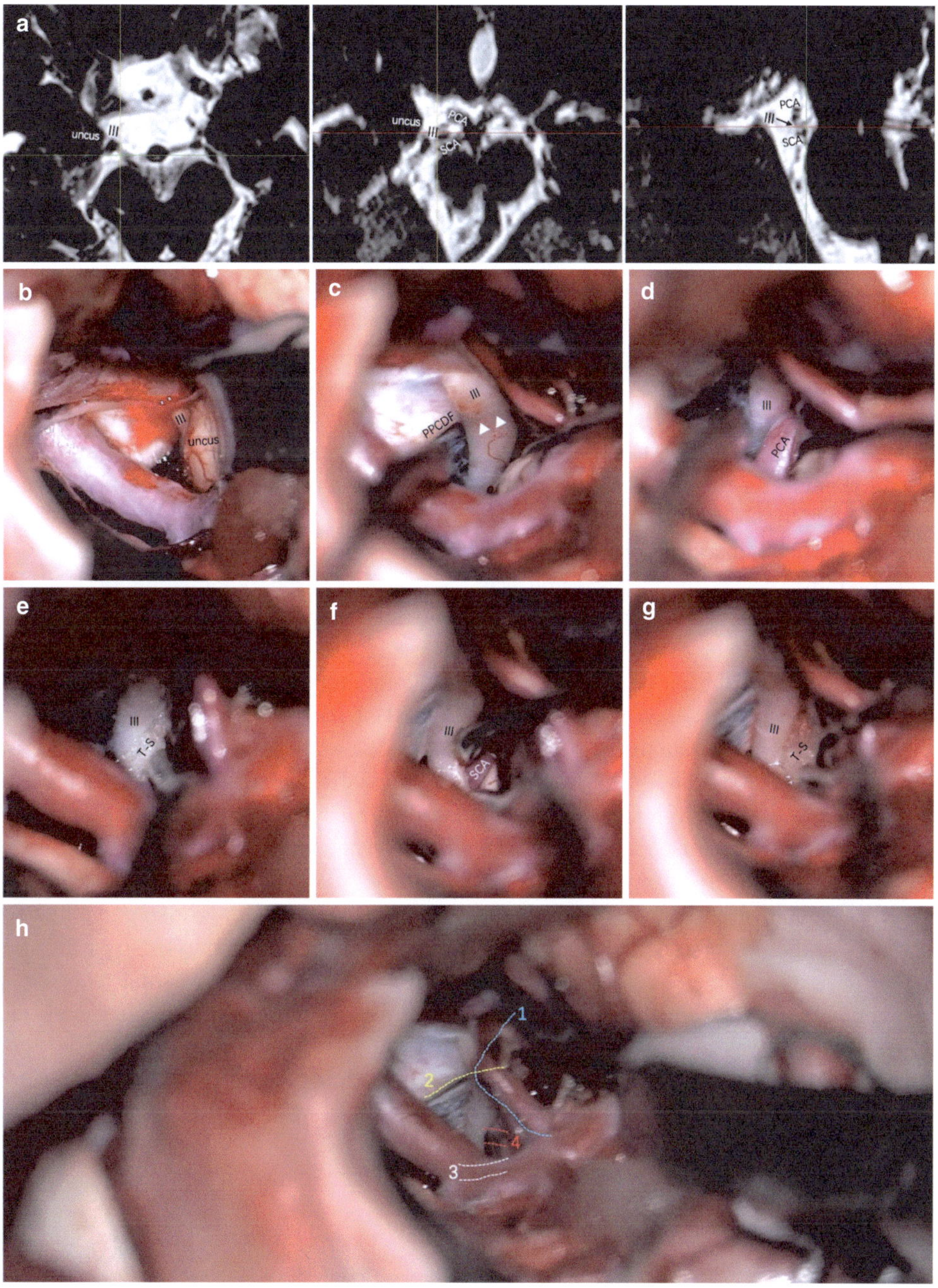

Fig. 19.1 Preoperative imaging and intraoperative findings of case 2. (**a**) Preoperative MRI (FIESTA sequence) demonstrated a "sandwich-like" compression pattern involving the oculomotor nerve, posterior cerebral artery (PCA), and superior cerebellar artery (SCA). (**b**) Upon elevation of the planum polare, the uncus was observed compressing the distal oculomotor nerve (III). (**c**) Partial resection of the uncus provided improved visibility of the oculomotor nerve and revealed the posterior petroclinoid dural fold (PPCDF) exerting pressure from below on the distal segment of the interpeduncular cistern, where grayish discoloration of the nerve was noted (white triangles). (**d**) Proximal exposure revealed further compression by the PCA from above. (**e**) Teflon and gelatin sponge (T-S) were inserted to isolate the PCA from the nerve. (**f**) Compression of the oculomotor nerve by the SCA from below was also identified. (**g**) The SCA was similarly isolated from the nerve using Teflon and gelatin sponge. (**h**) An overview of the four points of compression: 1-uncus, 2-PPCDF, 3-PCA, 4-SCA. *PCA* posterior cerebral artery, *SCA* superior cerebellar artery

confirmed, and decompression was performed using Teflon. Due to high vascular tension, there was inadequate space for the insertion of gelatin sponge. Postoperatively, there were no new oculomotor nerve dysfunctions. At the 6-month follow-up, the patient still exhibited partial internal movement restrictions, but subjectively reported partial relief of diplopia. She continued to require prism glasses, but there was no increase in diopter strength post-surgery.

Case 4

A 44-year-old male was admitted on June 20, 2023, complaining of diplopia for 1 month accompanied by fatigue, with no significant medical history. On examination, partial left-sided upper eyelid ptosis was observed, the pupil was normal, and eye movement was intact. Thin-layer MRI indicated compression of the proximal oculomotor nerve by PCA from above and SCA from below. Surgery was conducted on June 27, 2023, using the pterional transsylvian fissure approach. Intraoperatively, compression of the proximal oculomotor nerve by SCA from below and PCA from above was confirmed. Decompression procedures using Teflon and gelatin sponge were performed for both arteries. Postoperatively, there were no new oculomotor nerve dysfunctions. Two days after surgery, the symptoms of upper eyelid ptosis began to alleviate. Complete resolution of ptosis was observed by 2 weeks, and diplopia completely resolved by 6 months after surgery.

Case 5

A 61-year-old female was admitted on August 21, 2023, with a sudden onset of right-sided upper eyelid ptosis lasting 6 days. She had a history of left peripheral facial palsy 1.5 years prior, which had residual effects despite acupuncture treatment. Examination revealed complete right-sided upper eyelid ptosis, a dilated pupil, and a fixed lateral gaze, indicating complete oculomotor nerve paralysis. Thin-layer MRI showed compression of the proximal oculomotor nerve by the PCA and its branch from above, resulting in nerve deformation. Surgery was performed on August 23, 2023, using the pterional transsylvian fissure approach. During the procedure, significant traction of the arachnoid band was observed on the ventral side of the oculomotor nerve's REZ, causing twisting and deformation of the proximal rootlets. Sharp dissection of the arachnoid band restored the nerve's morphology, and further exploration confirmed compression of the dorsal aspect of the REZ by the PCA. Decompression was achieved using Teflon and gelatin sponge. Additionally, a small artery closely adjacent to the nerve's rootlets on the ventral aspect of the REZ was isolated with gelatin sponge. Postoperatively, no new oculomotor nerve dysfunctions were observed. At 1 month post-surgery, the complete upper eyelid ptosis progressed to partial, the pupil returned to normal, and partial recovery of eye movement occurred, though residual diplopia remained. By 4 months post-surgery, all oculomotor nerve functions had completely recovered, and the diplopia had resolved (Fig. 19.2).

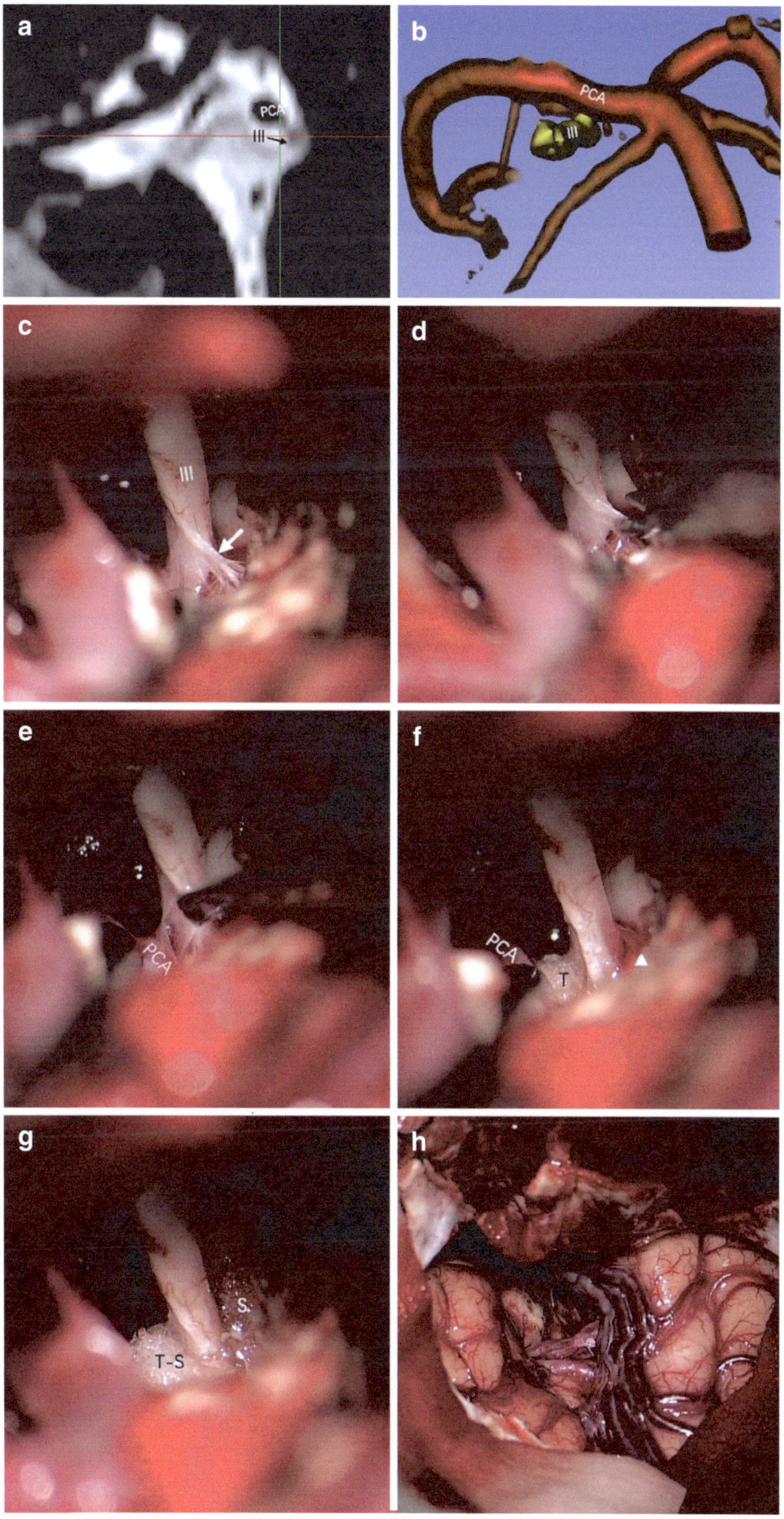

Fig. 19.2 Preoperative imaging and intraoperative findings for case 5. (**a**) Preoperative sagittal MRI (FIESTA sequence) showed the proximal portion of the oculomotor nerve (III) being compressed by the PCA and one of its branches from above, resulting in deformation. (**b**) A 3D reconstruction from DICOM data (FIESTA and 3D-TOF sequences) further illustrated the anatomical relationship at the compression site. (**c**) A significant arachnoid band (white arrow) was seen exerting tension on the ventral side of the nerve's root entry zone (REZ), causing twisting and deformity of the proximal rootlets. (**d**) The arachnoid band was sharply cut to relieve this tension. (**e**) Subsequent exploration confirmed dorsal compression of the REZ by the PCA from above. (**f**) Decompression was performed using Teflon and gelatin sponge. (**g**) Additionally, a small artery in close proximity to the nerve rootlets on the ventral REZ was identified. (**h**) This artery was isolated using gelatin sponge. The final intraoperative view revealed the superficial region via the noninvasive transsylvian approach. *PCA* posterior cerebral artery

19.3 Review of Literature Cases

In chronological order, we reviewed 15 reported cases (16 surgeries) as follows (Table 19.2).

Kojo (1988) [23] was the first to report the case of MVD-treated nAVC-ONP in the literature. A 47-year-old woman, with a 17-year history of migraines, presented with sudden left ocular muscle paralysis, including diplopia, left blepharoptosis, enlarged pupil, and limited left eye movement. Imaging revealed a small PCom aneurysm in the left side, which was considered as a potential cause of ONP. However, during surgery, the aneurysm was confirmed not in direct contact with the oculomotor nerve; rather, the enlarged PCom itself compressed the nerve approximately 1–2 mm from the midbrain. A sponge was used to separate the PCom from the nerve to relieve the compression. Within 5 days post-surgery, ptosis and diplopia improved, and after 28 days, only unequal pupil size remained. Complete recovery occurred after 2 years. This was the first historical case that confirmed the presence of nAVC in the interpeduncular cisternal segment of oculomotor nerve, leading to ONP, which was cured by MVD.

Nakagawa (1991) [22] reported a 59-year-old male presenting with sudden left oculomotor nerve paralysis. Imaging revealed a small PCom aneurysm, a fetal-type PCom, and a forward-bending left P2 segment of the PCA, possibly associated with arteriosclerosis. During surgery using a left frontotemporal approach, the aneurysm was found unrelated to the oculomotor nerve, but compression was evident from the anterior curve of the P2 segment of PCA. Surgical intervention involved the insertion of a sponge and the occlusion of the small aneurysm. Within 1 month post-surgery, complete eye movement recovery occurred, and ptosis improved after 2 weeks, leaving minor residual diplopia. However, 2 months after the first surgery, the patient experienced recurrent diplopia and right-sided ptosis. A second surgery revealed the oculomotor nerve's traction by dense arachnoid bands at the tentorial margin, compressed by the P2 segment of the PCA. The nerve decompression procedure involved loosening the arachnoid bands and inserting a sponge between the nerve and PCA. Three months post-surgery, significant symptom relief occurred, and after a year, all symptoms disappeared, except for unequal pupil size. The author suggested that vascular compression in the oculomotor nerve induced neuropathy, resulting in rapidly progressing oculomotor nerve paralysis, which could be effectively treated by MVD.

Mulderink (2001) [21] reported a 69-year-old male with a history of chronic headaches experiencing sudden left oculomotor nerve paralysis. Imaging revealed an aneurysm in the cavernous sinus segment of the internal carotid artery (ICA) and an infundibular dilatation (ID) at the beginning of the PCom. Surgery within 1 week of onset utilized a frontotemporal approach. Intraoperatively, the PCom's starting point was dilated, but compression on the oculomotor nerve originated from the PCom itself. Decompression involved suspending the PCom using a periostial sling. After 3 months, symptoms and headaches were completely relieved. The authors suggested MVD for oculomotor nerve paralysis of unknown origin.

Noji and Hadaka (2003) [20] reported a 74-year-old male with preoperative left eye pain and complete oculomotor nerve paralysis. Imaging showed an ICA-PCom aneurysm. During surgery, arteriosclerotic curved PCom was identified, compressing the oculomotor nerve rather than the aneurysm. Decompression by releasing the arachnoid led to partial symptom relief within 7 weeks.

Babbitz (2005) [19] reported a 36-year-old male experiencing progressive left retro-orbital pain and left eye paralysis for 2 months. MRI revealed a small meningeal tumor on the lateral wall of the left cavernous sinus and tentorium, multiple lesions on the left optic nerve, and a fetal-type PCA. High-dose steroid treatment improved eye movement but not the pain. Surgery exposed an ectatic PCom compressing the oculomotor nerve in the interpeduncular cisternal segment. Post-surgery, diplopia, ptosis, and headaches vanished after 8 days.

Suzuki (2008) [18] reported a 78-year-old male with complete left oculomotor nerve paral-

Table 19.2 Review of historical literature cases

	Case Item	1	2		3	4	5	6	7	8	9	10	11	12	13	14	15
General information	Author	Kojo	Nakagawa		Mulderink	Noji and Hadaka	Babbitz	Suzuki	Inoue	Fukushima	Kheshaifati	Fukami	Haider	Pomeraniec	Onuma	Zhang	Dowlati
	Year	1988	1991		2001	2003	2005	2008	2012	2013	2016	2018	2019	2020	2021	2022	2023
	Sex	Female	Male		Male	Male	Male	Male	Female	Female	Male	Female	Female	Female	Male	Male	Female
	Age	47 years	59 years		69 years	74 years	36 years	78 years	62 years	60 years	16 years	70 years	76 years	71 years	70 years	54 years	53 years
	Duration	Sudden onset	Sudden onset	Sudden onset	Sudden onset	NA	Sudden onset	NA	4 years	2 years	3 weeks	Sudden onset	3 weeks	1 year	2 weeks	5 years	3 weeks
	Side of symptom	Left	Left	Right	Left	Left	Left	Left	Left	Left	Right	Left	Left	Left	Left	Right	Left
	Non-surgical preoperative treatment	None	None	None	None	None	High-dose hormone therapy for 2 weeks with recovery of eye movements	None	None	None	None	None	None	None	None	Neostigmine intravenous injection and ophthalmic strabismus surgery	Left ptosis, double vision, and orbital pain for 3 weeks. Self-resolved before surgery
	Past medical history	Migraine 17 years	None	2 months after surgery	Chronic headache	Oph-thalmalgia	Progressively severe left retro-orbital headache	NA	None	NA	Transient right ptosis that developed 1 year previously.	Left headache 1 month	Hyper-tension, hyper-cholester-olemia	Cushing's disease, previously treated with two trans-sphenoidal resections and subsequent gamma knife radiosurgery	None	Hyper-cholester-olemia	Hyper-cholester-olemia
Pre-operative symptoms	Diplopia	Have	NA	Have	NA	Have	Have	Have	Brief spells of left vertical diplopia	NA	Have	None	None	NA	Have	Have	None
	Ptosis	Have	Have	Have	NA	Have	Have	Have	NA	Partial	Have	Have	Partial	Have	Have	Have	None
	Eye movement disorder	Total	NA	Total	NA	Total	None	Total	Involuntary downward eye movements	None	Have	None	None	Partial	Have	Have	None
	Dilated pupil	Have	NA	Have	NA	Have	Have	Have	None	None	Have	Have	None	Have	None	Have	None
Pre-operative imaging	Source of compression	Pcom aneurysm	Pcom aneurysm	NA	Pcom-ID	Pcom aneurysm	Small meningioma along the tentorium and the lateral wall of the cavernous sinus	Pcom aneurysm	PCA, SCA	Pcom-ID	PCA	Pcom-ID	Pcom aneurysm	SCA, PCA	Pcom-ID	PCA	Pcom aneurysm

(continued)

Table 19.2 (continued)

	Case Item	1	2		3	4	5	6	7	8	9	10	11	12	13	14	15
Operation	Approach	NA	Frontotemporal	Sub-temporal	Fronto-temporal-transSylvian	NA	Combined transSylvian and subtemporal	Pterional	Subtemporal	Fronto-temporal	Subtemporal	NA	Sub-temporal	Modified orbito-zygomatic and transSylvian	NA	Subtemporal	Fronto-temporal
	Offending vessels	Pcom	PCA	PCA	Pcom	Pcom	Pcom	PCA, SCA	PCA, SCA	Pcom-ID	PCA	Pcom-ID	Pcom	PCA	Pcom-ID	PCA	Pcom-ID
	Other responsibilities for compression	None	None	Dense arachnoid bands at the tentorial margin	None	None	None	None	None	None	None	None	None	Tentorial edge	None	None	None
	Compression site	Proximal	NA	NA	NA	NA	Distal	NA	Proximal	NA	Proximal	NA	NA	NA	NA	NA	NA
	Decompression methods	Gelatin sponge	Gelatin sponge	Gelatin sponge	Periosteal sling	Releasing the arachnoid	Releasing the arachnoid	Releasing the arachnoid	Teflon suspension	Clipping of ID	Teflon	Oxidized cellulose and fibrin glue	Teflon	Teflon	Oxidized cellulose and fibrin glue suspension	Teflon	Teflon
Post-operative outcomes	Added dysfunction	None	None	None	None	None	None	None	Slight left-sided oculomotor nerve palsy, resolving in 1 week	None	None	None	None	Complete oculomotor nerve paralysis but reverted to preoperative conditions within two days after a short course of steroids	None	None	Slight ptosis
	Postoperative effect	Ptosis and diplopia resolved at 5 days, only pupil inequality present at 28 days, complete recovery at 2 years	Complete recovery of eye move-ments at 1 month, recovery of ptosis at 2 weeks, residual slight diplopia	One year after the operation, the symptoms had completely dis-appeared, and only unequal pupils remained	Symptoms completely relieved in 3 months, headaches also relieved	Symptoms mostly relieved 7 weeks after surgery	Headache and diplopia and ptosis were completely relieved 8 days after surgery	Symptoms signi-ficantly relieved 1 month after surgery	Symptoms disappeared immediately after surgery and were completely normal at 6 months follow-up	Symptoms relieved 1 month after surgery	Improve-ment in 3 months after surgery, complete remission in 6 months	Pupil dilation relief in the immediate post-operative period and ptosis relief at 3 months post-operati-vely	Complete post-operative remission (exact duration unknown)	No improvement 1 year after surgery	Complete remission within 1 month after surgery, maintained for 10 years of follow-up	No relief in the immediate postoperative period, and at 3 months the symptoms had significantly improved, with only mild upward visual weakness present	Complete remission at 1-year follow-up
	Total effect	Completely resolved	Basically resolved	Basically resolved	Completely resolved	Partially resolved	Completely resolved	Basically resolved	Completely resolved	Completely resolved?	Completely resolved	Comp-letely resolved?	Comp-letely resolved	No recovery	Completely resolved	Partially resolved	Com-pletely resolved

NA means information in the original article is not accessible
? means uncertainty of information from the original article
Pcom posterior communicating artery, *Pcom-ID* infundibular dilatation of the posterior communicating artery, *PCA* posterior cerebral artery, *SCA* superior cerebellar artery

ysis. Imaging revealed an ICA-PCom aneurysm. Surgery revealed the aneurysm was unrelated to the oculomotor nerve but found compression from the PCA and SCA on the oculomotor nerve. After arachnoid release, symptoms significantly improved within a month.

Inoue (2012) [17] described another clinical condition different from ONP, ocular neuromyotonia (ONM), which was also the first report to confirm the vascular compression theory of this disease through preoperative image reconstruction and surgical evidence. The patient was a 62-year-old female with no previous history. She had paroxysmal and transient vertical diplopia in the left eye in the past 4 years, involuntary downward movement of the eye, normal pupil, and no predisposition factors. Preoperative MRI reconstruction indicated compression on the oculomotor nerve from the P2 segment of PCA and S1 segment of SCA. The subtemporal approach was adopted. Using Teflon suspension technique, the PCA and SCA were displaced respectively. Post-surgery, immediate relief occurred, followed by temporary mild oculomotor nerve paralysis, resolving within a week. Symptoms remained completely relieved at a 6-month follow-up.

Fukushima (2013) [16] reported a 60-year-old female with progressive left-sided partial blepharoptosis for 2 years. Preoperative imaging revealed PCom-ID compressing the oculomotor nerve. Surgery indicated ID compression; however, due to difficulty in decompression, only ID clipping was performed. Symptoms improved after a month.

Kheshaifati (2016) [15] described a 16-year-old male with intermittent right-sided blepharoptosis for a year, lasting 3 weeks with pain, diplopia, eye muscle paralysis, and pupil dilation. Imaging revealed asymmetric bilateral PCAs, with the right side showing P2 segment compression on the oculomotor nerve REZ. With the subtemporal approach, P2-PCA compression of the oculomotor nerve REZ was demonstrated. MVD was performed by placing a piece of Teflon between the artery and the nerve. After surgery, significant improvement was noted at 3 months, and complete relief occurred at 6 months.

Fukami (2018) [14] presented a case of a 70-year-old female with left-sided headaches and blepharoptosis, slightly dilated pupil, but no eye movement or diplopia issues. MRI and imaging indicated PCom-ID on the left side. Surgery confirmed ID compression on the oculomotor nerve and the PcomA and ID were moved from the oculomotor nerve using oxidized cellulose and fibrin glue. Pupil dilation immediately resolved post-surgery, and blepharoptosis improved after 3 months.

Haider (2019) [13] reported a 76-year-old female with a history of hypertension and hyperlipidemia, presenting with progressive left-sided partial blepharoptosis over 3 weeks. Preoperative imaging showed an ICA-PCom aneurysm on the left side. During surgery, the aneurysm was clipped, but the compression on the oculomotor nerve was from a fetal-type PCom. MVD was performed with a Teflon felt between the PCom and nerve. Post-surgery, symptoms completely resolved.

Pomeraniec (2020) [12] detailed a 71-year-old female with Cushing's disease, who underwent two transsphenoidal surgeries and Gamma Knife treatments. She developed progressive left-sided blepharoptosis, eye movement issues, and pupil inequality for a year. MRI suggested compression on oculomotor nerve by the SCA and PCA. A left-sided modified orbitozygomatic craniotomy was performed, showing the PCA pushing the nerve against the tentorial edge. Cottonoid buffers were placed between the PCA and nerve. Early post-surgery, symptoms worsened to complete oculomotor nerve paralysis but reverted to preoperative conditions within 2 days. At 1 year, the symptoms persisted, suggesting the need for early intervention and caution for previous history of sellar irradiation.

Onuma (2021) [11] presented a 70-year-old male with sudden onset diplopia, left-sided blepharoptosis, and eye muscle paralysis. Imaging showed PCom-ID compressing the oculomotor nerve, which was confirmed during surgery. The offending ID was transposed and adhered to the dura mater of the sphenoidal bone with oxidized cellulose and fibrin glue to successfully relieved the compression, and within a month, symptoms completely resolved, maintained over 10 years.

Zhang (2022) [10] reported a 54-year-old male with progressive right-sided blepharoptosis, diplopia, eye muscle paralysis, and pupil dilation over 5 years, who had once undergone treatment with neostigmine injection and ophthalmic strabismus surgery. MRI showed the right PCA contacting the oculomotor nerve. Subtemporal craniotomy was utilized, and surgery confirmed PCA compression on the oculomotor nerve and Teflon cotton was used for decompression. Post-surgery, symptoms gradually improved over 3 months, with mild residual weakness in upward gaze.

Dowlati (2023) [9] described a 53-year-old female with left-sided diplopia and retro-orbital pain for 3 weeks, accompanied by blepharoptosis. Symptoms had resolved on their own at the time of visit. Imaging indicated an ICA-PCom aneurysm. Intraoperatively, there was no aneurysm, but acturally the PCom-ID compressing the oculomotor nerve. MVD was done with a piece of Teflon placed between the ID and nerve. Post-surgery, mild residual blepharoptosis developed, but it completely resolved a year later.

19.4 Discussion

Based on aforementioned 20 cases (21 surgeries) of MVD-treated nAVC-ONP/ONM in our center and reported in the literature, there is reason to believe that MVD can serve as an effective surgical approach for nAVC-ONP/ONM. However, there still exist several uncertainties regarding preoperative assessment, surgical indications, and operational details. The following are preliminary discussions regarding these relevant issues.

19.4.1 Preoperative Diagnosis and Evaluation: Symptomatology

When presented with a patient whose chief complaints are diplopia, ptosis, or ocular motility disturbances, it is often easy to arrive at a symptomatic diagnosis of external ophthalmoplegia. However, distinguishing this from the ultimate diagnosis of nAVC-ONP involves multiple levels of differentiation, requiring a comprehensive analysis based on medical history, clinical presentation, and imaging studies.

Firstly, it's crucial to identify the involvement of the ocular motor nerve as the oculomotor nerve, rather than the trochlear or abducens nerves. When ocular motility impairment or diplopia involves outward or inferolateral movement, this can often be attributed to abducens or trochlear nerve paralysis rather than ONP. Pure limitation in inward ocular movement sometimes needs to rule out internuclear ophthalmoplegia, which involves the medial longitudinal fasciculus of the affected brainstem side, rather than ONP. In cases where both eyes are unable to gaze towards one side horizontally, indicating simultaneous paralysis on that side's abduction and contralateral adduction, it may indicate a brainstem lesion affecting the abducens nucleus on that side, known as internuclear ophthalmoplegia combined with abducens nerve root damage. When there's unilateral ocular adduction and abduction paralysis along with contralateral eye's adduction limitation, it's termed as a one-and-a-half syndrome, essentially an expansion of the abducens nucleus lesion mentioned earlier, involving the contralateral medial longitudinal fasciculus, often seen in a more extensive pontine lesion on that side. When symptoms primarily manifest as mild ptosis, if associated symptoms include pupil constriction, enophthalmos, and facial anhidrosis, consideration should be given to Horner's syndrome resulting from sympathetic pathway damage rather than ONP.

For patients whose affected nerve is specifically identified as the oculomotor nerve, further exclusion of intraorbital structural lesions is necessary. Clinical indications such as a history of orbital trauma, redness, swelling, warmth, or inflammatory manifestations in the orbital area, exophthalmos, or enophthalmos all support the possibility of external ophthalmoplegia due to intraorbital lesions. Ocular myopathies, which involve the eye muscles themselves, are diagnostically challenging but typically affect only certain extraocular muscles and leave the pupil unaffected. When patients have a history of aging, vascular diseases like hypertension, diabetes, rheumatic immune diseases, or malignancies, it supports the diagnosis of neuropathic external ophthalmoplegia, i.e., ONP. However, it's still crucial to rule out well-known common neurological disorders such as myasthenia gravis, thyroid eye disease, Miller-Fisher syndrome, and congenital ONP cases, in order to establish the diagnosis of acquired ONP (aONP). Even with these steps in place, differentiating among these diagnoses may still be challenging. Some patients may need to undergo ineffective "diagnostic therapy" to exclude a misdiagnosis. For instance, in the case of Zhang (2022) [10], ineffective treatments with neostigmine and ophthalmic surgeries were necessary to rule out myasthenia gravis and ophthalmic-related diseases. Also, in case 2 and case 3 of our center, the corresponding diagnosis was excluded only after the ineffective treatments with glucocorticoids and nutraceutical drugs, or brompyrsmine and ophthalmic prism therapy.

aONP itself is rare. According to a study by Fang et al. [7] published in JAMA Ophthalmology in 2017, the annual incidence rate was 4.2 per 100,000. This research, based on 145 newly diagnosed aONP cases in a single center over 37 years, found the etiological breakdown as follows: microvascular issues (42%), trauma (12%), tumor compression (11%), post-neurosurgery (10%), aneurysm compression (6%), other causes (5%), stroke (4%), idiopathic (4%), pituitary stroke (2%), Tolosa-Hunt syndrome (2%), and giant cell arteritis (1%). The "other" category (5%) included singular instances of carotid-cavernous fistula, herpes zoster, carcinomatous meningitis, ophthalmoplegic migraine, cavernous sinus thrombosis, and post-viral paralysis. The most common cause was microvascular issues, defined as significant self-recovery within 4 months without aberrant regeneration, while excluding other known causes; diabetes is typically considered the most common underlying condition leading to microvascular issues. Compressive causes accounted for 17%, among which aneurysmal compression was only 6%, and even the discussed nAVC was not found in this study. Despite the small number of reported cases, it is evident that nAVC-ONP is indeed rare. However, there is reason to suspect that the incidence of nAVC-ONP may be underestimated. For instance, among cases defined as idiopathic or microvascular in this study, there may have been cases of nAVC-ONP; furthermore, in cases where angiography diagnosed ONP as PCom artery aneurysms, the actual source of compression was not the aneurysm but PCom-ID [9] or PCom itself [13, 20, 23], or even adjacent blood vessels [18, 22], suggesting that certain nAVC-ONP cases may have been misclassified as aneurysmal ONP due to imaging examinations. How then can nAVC-ONP be further differentiated from cases of aONP?

Pupillary involvement is considered an essential clinical sign supporting a compressive etiology. The oculomotor nerve contains both the large somatic motor fibers that supply the extraocular muscles and the smaller parasympathetic fibers that control the pupil. In the cisternal segment, there is a clear distribution pattern: somatic motor fibers are located in the core, while parasympathetic fibers are in the superficial dorsomedial area. Thus, it's generally believed that conditions such as microvascular issues related to diabetes primarily affect the blood supply to the neural core, sparing the superficially located pupil fibers; however, compressive factors are more likely to impact the superficial regions, often resulting in ipsilateral pupil dilation [28, 29]. However, this clinical presentation is not constant. For example, in the case reported by Fukushima (2013) [16], confirmed to be due to nAVC during surgery, the pupil was not affected. The authors suggested that although parasympathetic fibers are superficially located, they are situated medially, whereas in this case, the compressive source was from lateral. Fang's study [7] also statistically examined pupil involvement, reporting rates of 16% in microvascular ONP and 64% in compressive ONP. Despite significant differences, relying solely on unequal pupil size cannot differentiate between the two. Therefore, for aONP patients with unequal pupils, suspicion of nAVC-ONP is heightened, but the absence of pupil involvement cannot entirely rule out nAVC-ONP.

Anatomical studies among different species, including humans, have confirmed specific spatial distributions of oculomotor nerve cell bodies and their axons, which control different extraocular muscles, from the oculomotor nucleus in the midbrain to the fibers in the peripheral segments located from the cisternal segment to the intraorbital region [29]. However, based on reported cases, there are significant and uncertain individual differences in extraocular muscle movement symptoms, even among cases of nAVC compression. Fang's large-scale study [7] further indicates that the involvement of extraocular muscles, including ptosis and external third nerve dysfunction, showed no significant differences in occurrence rates among different etiological groups. Eye pain and headaches, as the most common accompanying symptoms, have almost identical occurrence rates in microvascular and compressive ONP cases (61% vs. 60%). Thus, these clinical presentations do not provide reliable information helpful in diagnosing nAVC-ONP.

Regarding clinical symptom assessment, it's worth noting that while ONP presents as a loss of oculomotor nerve function, typical NVCS such as facial spasms and trigeminal neuralgia manifest as signs of neural excitement. From this perspective, it's challenging to categorize ONP under NVCS. However, is there a form of oculomotor nerve pathology that presents with signs of excitement? Oculomotor neuromyotonia (OMN) is a rare acquired disorder reported in only 57 cases [30]. Its characteristic clinical feature is transient diplopia caused by episodic, brief, sustained contractions of at least one eye muscle, lasting from 30 s to several minutes. The oculomotor nerve is most commonly affected, followed by the trochlear and abducens nerves, and is typically attributed to paroxysmal neuronal excitation. Potential causes of OMN include cranial irradiation (55%–80%), thyroid eye disease (4%–20%), cavernous sinus lesions, intracranial masses, vitamin deficiencies, and NVC (0%–12%), and rare idiopathic cases. Inoue's case (2012) [17] is the only reported case in the literature diagnosed preoperatively with nAVC through 3D imaging reconstruction and successfully treated with MVD surgery for OMN associated with nAVC, serving as the best evidence for the existence of nAVC-OMN. Regarding the relationship between nAVC-OMN and nAVC-ONP, Inoue believes that they are not contradictory; changes in demyelination and pseudo-synaptic effects caused by vascular compression may be associated with excitatory symptoms, but excessive compression can lead to nerve paralysis and resulting functional deficits. Thus, it is speculated that nAVC-OMN might be an earlier stage of nAVC-ONP. However, this inference has limitations since all other previously mentioned nAVC-ONP cases did not initially present with excitatory symptoms. In conclusion, significant differences in symptoms can clearly distinguish between OMN and ONP. However, both seem to be attributable to nAVC, and further evaluation is required for diagnosis establishment.

19.4.2 Preoperative Diagnosis and Evaluation: Imaging

Imaging examinations, including MRI, CT, DSA, among others, are essential routine diagnostic tools. Many scholars and our center strongly recommend performing specialized thin-slice MRI sequence scans and subsequently conducting multimodal fusion and 3D reconstruction of imaging data. This approach might currently offer the most valuable means to establish the etiological diagnosis of nAVC-ONP preoperatively, providing anatomical evidence for devising surgical strategies. The specific implications include: (1) Determining the presence of common compressive causes like aneurysms or tumors; (2) Clarifying the specific anatomical characteristics of nAVC; (3) Establishing the existence of other potential anatomical variations causing compression; (4) Assessing the surgical approach-related risk factors.

Although aneurysmal and tumorous compressions are relatively uncommon causes of ONP, aneurysms can potentially lead to life-threatening subarachnoid hemorrhage, while tumors may result in more severe neurological dysfunction. Therefore, they have historically received widespread attention from clinicians and serve as the foremost etiological differential diagnoses of ONP. Modern neuroimaging techniques, including routine MRI/MRA, CT/CTA, and DSA, usually enable the diagnosis of intracranial aneurysms and tumors. Among the previously reported 15 cases of nAVC-ONP, 10 were identified preoperatively through routine imaging as having an aneurysm or a PCom-ID related to the cisternal segment of oculomotor nerve, while one case revealed a skull base tumor. Surgical interventions were conducted based on these identified organic lesions, underscoring the importance of conventional imaging techniques in nAVC-ONP. However, among these 11 cases considered to have an aneurysm, ID, or tumor causing compression preoperatively, only 3 cases were consistent with the preoperative considerations after surgical exploration [11, 14, 16]; in 6 cases, the compression of the oculomotor nerve was confirmed to be from adjacent vessels rather than an aneurysm [13, 18, 22, 23], PCom ID [21], or a tumor [19]; in 2 cases, no aneurysm was found [9, 20], indicating false-positive limitations of routine imaging techniques in diagnosing nAVC-ONP.

Hashimoto and his team detected relationships between the extraocular nerves (oculomotor, trochlear, abducens) and adjacent arteries that might lead to corresponding extraocular movement disorders using special thin-slice spoiled-gradient recalled acquisition (SGRA) sequences (1.6–2 mm thick), not visualized by conventional MRI (10 mm thick) [26, 31, 32]. The Yousry team observed a close relationship between the trochlear nerve and surrounding vessels in six cases of superior ophthalmic myokymia (SOM) using three-dimensional Fourier transform constructive interference in steady-state (3D CISS) and 3D time-of-flight (3D TOF) sequences [33, 34]. With the advancement of modern MRI technology, an increasing number of high-resolution thin-slice sequences are applied clinically. Through post-processing of original data, free-angle 3D reconstructions of neurovascular anatomy can be achieved to assist in devising surgical plans, increasingly common in preoperative imaging diagnoses of hemifacial spasms and trigeminal neuralgia [35, 36]. These techniques are also employed in the preoperative diagnosis of nAVC-ONP or nAVC-OMN. In Inoue's reported case of nAVC-OMN, the use of fast imaging employing steady-state acquisition (FIESTA) sequences (0.8 mm thick) allowed for 3D reconstruction of the oculomotor nerve and surrounding PCA, SCA, and BA vascular structures, aiding in selecting the subtemporal approach over the pterional approach, and successful decompression [17]. In Zhang's reported nAVC-ONP cases, thin-slice MRI sequences and 3D reconstruction were used to establish the relationship between the oculomotor nerve and the PCA preoperatively, followed by postoperative imaging comparisons after MVD surgery [10]. In all cases of nAVC-ONP in our center, thin-slice scans using FIESTA and 3D TOF sequences were conducted preoperatively, providing excellent visualizations of the oculomotor nerve in the cisternal segment and the posterior cranial fossa vessels, respectively. These were fused, reconstructing clear 2D images and 3D models displaying both nerves and vessels distinctly. This facilitated the observation of the anatomical relationship between the oculomotor nerve and adjacent vessels, including responsible vessels, compressed areas, and potential nerve deformations, aiding in establishing the diagnosis and surgical plan (Fig. 19.3).

One of our cases (case 2) was quite unique. Routine MRI showed a suspected lesion adjacent to the tentorial edge, in close contact with the ipsilateral oculomotor nerve. Further FIESTA sequences clarified that this protrusion abutting the oculomotor nerve was not a tumor but a self-protruded temporal uncus. Fusion and reconstruction of 3D TOF sequences simultaneously revealed signs of compression on the oculomotor nerve by both the PCA and SCA. Intraoperatively, the aforementioned rare radiographic findings were confirmed. The patient's oculomotor nerve from REZ to the entry of the roof of the cavernous sinus was successively compressed by the SCA from below to above, PCA from above to below, and the uncus from superolateral to inferomedial, ultimately compressing the twisted

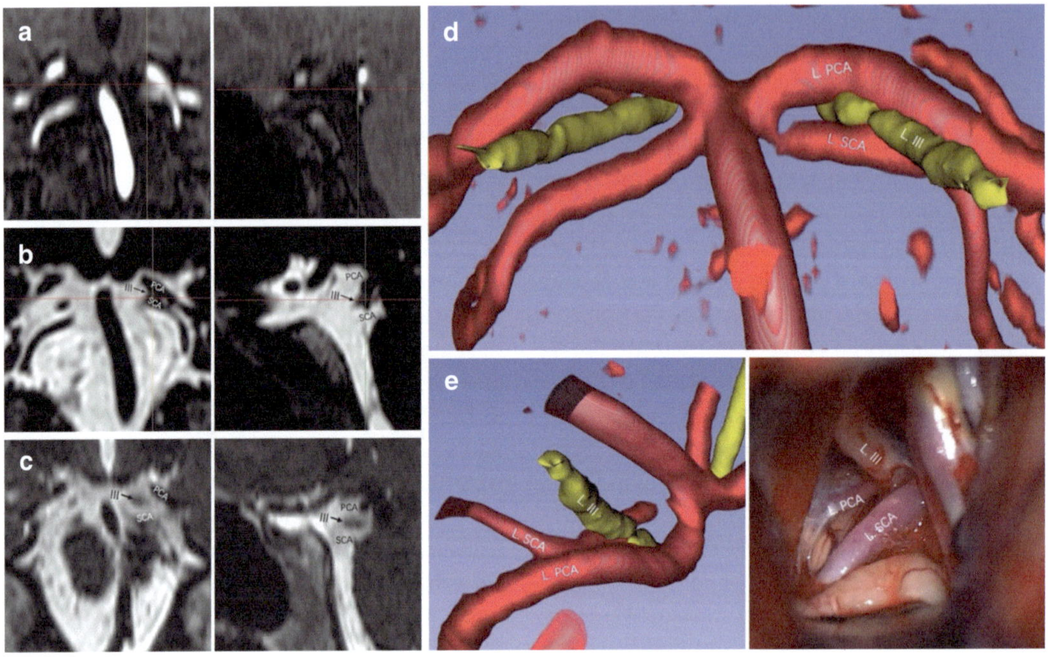

Fig. 19.3 An example of application of the thin-slice MRI scans using 3D-TOF and FIESTA sequences, and 3D reconstruction for preoperative and postoperative assessment in our center. (**a**) In preoperative coronal and sagittal images of 3D-TOF sequence, the arteries are evident while the nerves are invisible; (**b**) When combined with FIESTA sequence, both artery and nerve can be clearly identified. As in this patient (case 1), a sandwich-like compression pattern in which the oculomotor nerve was compressed simultaneously by PCA from above and SCA from below was evident; (**c**) The postoperative scan using FIESTA sequence demonstrated isolation of the oculomotor nerve from both PCA and SCA after MVD surgery; (**d**) Preoperative 3D reconstruction facilitated the observation of the anatomical relationship between the oculomotor nerve and adjacent vessels; (**e**) The reconstructed 3D model (left)was rotated to simulate the anatomical condition in operation (right), further demonstrating it aiding in establishing the diagnosis and surgical plan

nerve against the sharp edge of the PPCDF, causing multiple compressions. We safely resected the protruding uncus and performed decompressions of the SCA and PCA, resulting in significant symptom relief in the early postoperative period without new oculomotor nerve functional deficits, with a definite long-term follow-up effect. Idiopathic herniation or protrusion of the temporal uncus is rarely reported in the literature [37, 38], and cases of prominent uncus compressing the oculomotor nerve causing ONP are exceedingly rare, with only one such case reported in imaging literature without surgical confirmation [39]. Thus, our case represents the first reported instance confirming the self-protruded temporal uncus as a compressive etiology of nAVC-ONP through preoperative imaging, intraoperative findings, and postoperative efficacy. Additionally, in this case, the oculomotor nerve was ultimately pushed and ridden onto the sharp edge of the PPCDF, a dural structure forming the posteromedial margin of oculomotor trigon of the roof of the cavernous sinus, closely related to the distal cisternal oculomotor nerve. When the nerve is pushed and displaced, this dural structure might potentially become a "passive" source of oculomotor nerve compression. Similar findings were also found in Pomeraniec's cases, where PCA compression displaced the oculomotor nerve towards the tentorial edge [12]. This ligament itself exhibits ossification variations [40], suggesting that for ONP patients, if skull base high-resolution CT (HRCT) reveals this ossification variation, it should be fused with thin-slice MRI sequences to clarify its relationship with the oculomotor nerve.

For patients considering surgery, imaging examinations carry another essential significance, that is evaluating surgical risks. Surgical approaches exposing the cisternal oculomotor nerve usually adopt the subtemporal or frontotemporal approaches, necessitating necessary traction on the temporal or frontal lobes to access deeper basal brain areas. Therefore, our center performs preoperative assessments of the superficial cerebral venous systems, including the superficial sylvian veins and Labbe veins, using MRV, CTV, or DSA to guide the selection of the surgical approach. This is crucial in avoiding serious surgical approach-related complications, such as venous damage due to intraoperative traction, which will be further discussed in the following section. Additionally, routine CT bone window settings can evaluate the degree of aeration of the frontal sinus and the skull base bones, aiding surgeons in preventing cerebrospinal fluid leaks.

Despite the numerous advantages of imaging examinations, particularly high-resolution thin-slice imaging techniques, it's crucial to remember that for the diagnosis of nAVC-ONP, imaging remains a useful tool rather than a gold standard. In fact, for all NVCS, including hemifacial spasms and trigeminal neuralgia, there exists such an uncertain relationship between positive findings on imaging and established diagnoses [41]. Liang et al. performed 3D CISS sequence thin-slice MRI scans on 196 healthy volunteers (392 oculomotor nerves), finding a high proportion of imaging contact between these completely functional oculomotor nerves and PCA and SCA, reaching 55.1% and 58.9%, respectively. The number of cases with nerve bending caused by PCA, SCA, and PCom compression was 7, 5, and 7, respectively. Liang also conducted the same imaging examination on seven patients with explicit ONP symptoms and without aneurysmal or tumorous compression, all showing evident oculomotor nerve compression by vessels, comprising 4 cases of PCA, 2 cases of PCom, and 1 case of BA compression. Thus, finding the presence of neurovascular contact or even significant compression solely through imaging is highly sensitive but lacks specificity. It cannot serve as a diagnostic criterion for oculomotor nerve NVCS with clinical significance (existence of ONP/-ONM symptoms) and must be combined with clinical symptoms while excluding all other possible causes. In cases where both symptomatic and imaging evidence exist, can we be 100% certain of the aforementioned diagnosis? Onuma [11] reviewed 18 cases from the literature of nonsurgical treated nAVC-ONP patients with evidence of neurovascular contact in imaging, where 13 cases showed effectiveness, with a treatment effectiveness rate of 72%. This suggests that these 13 patients might not have been under vascular compression, while the remaining 5 patients might have benefited from MVD surgery. Therefore, the diagnosis and evaluation of oculomotor nerve NVCS require higher-level clinical research in the future to provide satisfactory resolutions.

19.4.3 Recommended Diagnostic and Treatment Process in Our Center

As mentioned above, clinical presentations of oculomotor nerve neurovascular compression syndromes (NVCS) manifest as a rare set of clinical syndromes with no clear diagnostic and treatment standards currently established. Based on existing literature and the clinical and imaging features known to our center, we have proposed an oculomotor nerve NVCS assessment scale (S-T Evaluation Scale) [27] to guide diagnosis and corresponding treatment plans (Table 19.3).

This scale is applicable to patients where common causes in neuro-ophthalmology and neurology have been ruled out, along with definitive compressive etiologies such as aneurysms or tumors. The aim is to identify the truly clinically significant NVCS of the oculomotor nerve, i.e., those exhibiting oculomotor nerve pathology in the presence of ONP/ONM symptoms and evidence of neurovascular compression on imaging studies. The scale is divided into clinical symptomatology (S) and topography (T) of NVC based on imaging (using sub-2 mm thin-section sequences, such as FIESTA, CISS, and 3D TOF MRI scans), each graded on a scale of 0, 1, or 2. The final score is the sum of both parts.

Table 19.3 The scoring details of "S-T Evaluation Scale"

Score Two domains	0	1	2
Clinical symptoms(s)	No abnormality related to the oculomotor nerve, eye movements, or pupillary anomalies	Any oculomotor nerve-related abnormalities, such as diplopia or ptosis, and dysfunction or hyperactivity of vertical, downward, or inward eye movements without any pupil anomalies	Any oculomotor nerve-related abnormalities with pupil anomalies including pupillary dilation on the affected side (with a diameter at least 0.5 mm greater than the contralateral side) and diminished or absent light reflex
Topography (T) of NVC based on MRI	No imaging contact between the cisternal segment of the oculomotor nerve and adjacent vessels or neural structures	Imaging contact between the cisternal segment of the oculomotor nerve and adjacent vessels or neural structures, but without evident compression signs	Imaging contact with evident compression signs, including oculomotor nerve deformation or sandwich-like compression pattern (simultaneous compression from above and below)
Total score	Total score = S + T		

NVC neurovascular compression

In terms of symptomatology (S):

- A score of 0 indicates no abnormality related to the oculomotor nerve, eye movements, or pupillary anomalies.
- A score of 1 indicates any oculomotor nerve-related abnormalities, such as diplopia complained by the patient, or clinically evident ptosis, and dysfunction or hyperactivity of vertical, downward, or inward eye movements without any pupil anomalies.
- A score of 2 is assigned when pupil anomalies are present, including pupillary dilation on the affected side (with a diameter at least 0.5 mm greater than the contralateral side) and diminished or absent light reflex.

In terms of topography (T):

- A score of 0 indicates no imaging contact between the cisternal segment of the oculomotor nerve and adjacent vessels or neural structures.
- A score of 1 indicates imaging contact between the cisternal segment of the oculomotor nerve and adjacent vessels or neural structures, but without evident compression signs.
- A score of 2 indicates imaging contact with evident compression signs, including oculomotor nerve deformation or sandwich-like compression pattern (simultaneous compression from above and below).

As the assessed patients already present oculomotor nerve-related complaints and signs, scoring 0 in symptomatology carries no clinical value. Similarly, when topography scores 0, suggesting no clear evidence of neurovascular compression, NVCS should be ruled out. Therefore, total scores of 0 (S = 0, T = 0) or 1 (S = 0, T = 1; S = 1, T = 0) exclude clinically significant (presence of ONP/ONM symptoms and imaging evidence of NV compression) oculomotor nerve NVCS. Total scores of 2–4 are interpreted as follows:

- A total score of 2 (S = 1, T = 1), where the pupils are not affected, and the imaging shows only nerve-vessel contact, indicates a "suspected" nAVC-ONP/-ONM.
- A total score of 3 has two scenarios: (1) S = 1, T = 2; (2) S = 2, T = 1. Here, either symptoms or imaging shows a more typical compression of the oculomotor nerve (pupil involvement or nerve deformation), suggesting a higher likelihood of NVCS as the actual cause, which indicates a "probable" nAVC-ONP/-ONM.
- A total score of 4 (S = 2, T = 2) presents typical signs of oculomotor nerve compression, indicating the highest likelihood of NVCS as the actual cause and was termed as "confirmed" nAVC-ONP/-ONM.

The established scoring helps guide treatment options. As the score increases, the likelihood of NVCS being the actual cause increases, with a higher possibility of benefiting from MVD surgery. Conversely, conservative or medicinal treatments should be prioritized. Since the effectiveness of conservative or medicinal treatment requires time for evaluation, the course characteristics and treatment history also play crucial roles in treatment selection. Simultaneously, considering the risks of general anesthesia, craniotomy, and nerve decompression procedures, assessing the timing and indications for surgery requires comprehensive evaluation. As reported, Kojo [23], Mulderink [21], Haider [13], and Onuma's [11] cases were operated within 1 month of onset, showing definite improvement post-surgery. Onuma suggested operating within 21 days of onset. However, most reported surgical cases and the first 3 of our 5 patients underwent surgery after a considerable time from onset. On the other hand, cases like Babbitz's [19] and Dowlati's [9] had substantial symptom improvement following conservative or medicinal treatment, with exploratory surgery done due to suspected tumors or aneurysms. Furthermore, considering other cases where conservative treatment resulted in satisfactory outcomes, it cannot be ruled out that some patients might benefit equally from conservative treatment, challenging the recommendation for early surgery.

Therefore, we recommend that for patients scoring 2 and 3, if the symptoms are of recent onset, medical treatment and follow-ups should be initially recommended. Steroids may be given to ONP patients to alleviate acute nerve edema, vasodilators to improve microcirculation, and prism for temporary diplopia relief. For ONM patients, carbamazepine can be used to suppress nerve excitability. As per Fang's extensive study [7], conservative treatment follow-up should be at least 4 months since microcirculation impairment is defined as resolving within 4 months spontaneously. Patients with a score of 2 or 3, after 4 months without improvement, or for those with a duration exceeding 4 months, may undergo MVD surgery after a thorough risk assessment and patient consent.

For patients scoring 4, due to the high probability of nAVC being the actual cause, prompt surgical intervention is suggested. Referring to cases of ONP caused by aneurysmal compression, Leivo [8] summarized the relationship between surgery timing and recovery, suggesting better recovery with earlier surgery. Hence, for patients scoring 4, early MVD is recommended for better outcomes.

In our 5 cases, based on the aforementioned scoring criteria, 3 scored 3 ($S = 1$, $T = 2$), diagnosable as "probable" nAVC-ONP/-ONM, and 2 scored 4, diagnosable as "confirmed" nAVC-ONP/-ONM. Among the 3 cases scoring 3, 2 (case 2 and case 3) had a duration of more than 4 months with no improvement, justifying the timing of MVD. Case 4 had symptoms for only 1 month and showed significant improvement after MVD; however, the possibility of nonsurgical treatment being equally effective cannot be excluded. The 2 cases scoring 4 had durations of 4 years (case 1) and 6 days (case 5), with case 1 showing insignificant improvement post-surgery and case 5 having satisfactory outcomes, suggesting that early decompression surgery benefits patients scoring 4, while delayed surgery is not conducive to symptom relief. The reasonableness of the S-T Evaluation Scale system and treatment selection process requires further validation through high-quality future clinical studies.

19.4.4 Key Points Related to Surgery

MVD is a definitive surgical method commonly used for the causative treatment of common cranial nerve NVCS. Limited data from existing reports and cases in our center suggest its considerable efficacy in managing nAVC-ONP/-ONM. Similar to routine MVD procedures, the MVD for the oculomotor nerve should adhere to the principles of adequate exposure and effective decompression, raising core concerns about the surgical approach and decompression techniques.

The anatomical location of the oculomotor nerve is deep and divided into several segments: intramesencephalic, interpeduncular cisternal, petroclinoid, trigonal, cavernous, fissural, and orbital [42]. The interpeduncular cisternal segment, where the compression typically occurs, lies between PCA above and SCA below. This segment is adjacent and just inferomedial to the temporal uncus. The PPCDF is the boundary between the cisternal segment and the petroclinoid segment, and runs transversely below the nerve. The cisternal segment is anchored to the Liliequist's membrane, linking the nerve to adjacent vessels, uncus, and the tentorial edge. All these structures forming the anatomical basis for oculomotor nerve NVCS. Therefore, the surgical approach for oculomotor nerve MVD focuses on exposing its interpeduncular cisternal segment.

There are various approaches to reach the interpeduncular cistern, ventrolateral midbrain, and basilar apex regions. The most commonly used are the frontotemporal/pterional and the subtemporal approaches. The operative details and differences between these approaches and their variants have been extensively elaborated in neurosurgical literatures [43–45]. Similarly, in 16 reported oculomotor nerve MVD surgeries (15 patients underwent unilateral surgery, and 1 patient had bilateral surgery), the most frequent approaches were the frontotemporal/pterional approach (5 cases) [9, 16, 18, 21, 22] and the subtemporal approach (5 cases) [10, 13, 15, 17, 22], with 1 case utilizing a combined transsylvian and subtemporal approach [19], 1 case using modified orbitozygomatic transsylvian approach [12], while details for the other 4 cases were unspecified. Among our five cases, the initial case (case 1) used the subtemporal approach, while the subsequent 4 cases utilized the frontotemporal/pterional transsylvian approach. Both approaches adequately exposed the interpeduncular cisternal segment of oculomotor nerve, but our preference leaned toward the frontotemporal/pterional approach due to considerations such as brain lobe traction, vein handling, and uncus removal.

The subtemporal approach, more specifically the anterior subtemporal or pretemporal approach [46–48], provides a lateral view along the middle cranial fossa and lateral wall of the cavernous sinus to access the area above and medial to the tentorial edge. This approach involves lifting the anterior part of the temporal lobe upward and backward, making it operationally convenient but risks more aggressive temporal lobe retraction compared to the conventional subtemporal transtentorial approach, as the latter exposes the ventrolateral pontine area below the oculomotor nerve level. Extensive temporal lobe retraction increases the risk of temporal lobe contusions and bleeding. The frontotemporal approach by opening the Sylvian fissure allows a direct route to the interpeduncular cistern area through the shortest anterolateral trajectory without significant retraction of the temporal and frontal lobes, reducing corresponding risks. While dissecting the Sylvian fissure is time-consuming and carries a risk of damaging vessels and the operculum cortex, mature microneurosurgical techniques can overcome these challenges.

Retraction of the anterior temporal lobe often requires detaching the superficial Sylvian vein on the temporal side with drainage into the sphenoparietal sinus, posing risks of temporal lobe ischemic bleeding in cases with predominant venous return through this route [49]. Variations exist in the Labbe vein's early drainage into the basal temporal dura, also risking retraction-induced vein damage [50]. Techniques like translocation of the sphenoparietal sinus or Labbe vein [51–53], and extradural temporal polar approach via the cavernous sinus [49, 54, 55] are available but are complex skull base procedures with high technical thresholds, less amenable to widespread application. Therefore, for cases planned for the subtemporal approach, we recommend thorough preoperative venous imaging. If high-risk venous factors such as those mentioned above are present, consider switching to the frontotemporal craniotomy.

When preoperative imaging suggests medial protrusion of the uncus, which potentially compressing the oculomotor nerve, we suggest frontotemporal/pterional transsylvian transuncal approach [56, 57] instead of the subtemporal approach. This approach safely and effectively removes the uncus under direct vision. Even if preoperative imaging does not confirm significant contact between the uncus and the oculomotor nerve, partial uncal removal might be necessary during surgery to enhance the exposure and space for subsequent decompression procedures. In facial spasm MVD surgeries, we sometimes perform subpial resection of the flocculus to increase the facial nerve REZ exposure and operating freedom and the uncal removal is a derivation of this concept. Among our 5 cases, except for 1 case (case 1) using the anterior subtemporal approach, the remaining 4 utilized the frontotemporal/pterional transsylvian transuncal approach. In one case (case 2) the uncus was considered as the compressive factor, and in the other three cases (case 3, case 4, case 5) it was aimed to increase the visual field and space for decompression by removing parts of the uncus. None of the patients experienced memory or language function impediments or seizures postoperatively, preliminarily indicating the safety of this technique.

Regarding the operative details of the frontotemporal/pterional transsylvian approach, extensive literature discusses them [58–60], hence not elaborated here. However, due to the need to fully expose the interpeduncular cisternal segment of oculomotor nerve, including its emergence from the brainstem (REZ area), some specific details require mention. The head's position should have the forehead lower than the chin, positioning the zygomatic prominence highest, allowing an inferior-to-superior view from the skull base. Rotation should not exceed 30 degrees, ensuring natural downward sagging of the frontal and temporal lobes on both sides of the Sylvian fissure. Using interfascial/subfascial techniques, retract the temporal muscle backward and downward until adequately exposing the zygoma and lateral orbital rim. This prevents temporal muscle accumulation that might obstruct the posterosuperior view, crucial in male patients with well-developed temporal muscles. The sphenoidal ridge removal should extend to the lateral end of the superior orbital fissure, and the orbital part of the greater sphenoidal wing and frontal bone should be shaved until the roof and lateral wall of the orbit is skeletonized, also for the unobstructed view from anteroinferolateral to posterosuperomedial. The opening of Sylvian fissure should start from the anterior Sylvian point, anteriorly dissecting the frontotemporal arachnoid fold along the sphenoidal ridge, through the Sylvian stem and the sphenoidal part of the fissure into the carotid cistern. It is still necessary to open the posterior branch of the Sylvian fissure and the proximal 2–3 cm region of the operculoinsular compartment of the fissure. This posterior opening of the Sylvian fissure is conducive to increasing the scope of posterior frontotemporal separation, that is, to add a direct surgical view and angle along the limen insula and the anterior surface of it to the proximal end of the interpeduncular segment of the oculomotor nerve. Coupled with the above-mentioned inferior-to-superior view along the skull base, it maximizes controlling the entire interpeduncular cistern segment of the oculomotor nerve. Sylvian fissure dissection should be performed under high magnification, protecting all vessels and the operculum cortex inside the fissure using various microneurosurgical techniques [61–64]. The self-retaining retractors assist in securing and fixing both sides of the frontotemporal lobes after sufficiently loosening the sylvian fissure without tension. After gently pulling down the planum polare, the uncus becomes visible medially. In cases where the uncus compresses against the oculomotor nerve, adhering to the principle of subpial resection is necessary, thus one should retain the arachnoid and pia surrounding the nerve to prevent direct contact between instruments and the nerve, avoiding potential damage.

The essential step in MVD surgery is safely and effectively relieving vascular compression on the oculomotor nerve, which is crucial for determining surgical efficacy. Comprehensive exploration and decompression, targeting all potential compression sites and compressing vessels, is the decompression principle proposed by our center for facial and trigeminal nerve MVDs, widely recognized in this field [65–68]. Similarly, for oculomotor nerve MVD, we adhere to this principle, ensuring full-length decompression of the interpeduncular cisternal segment of oculomotor nerve and relieving all related compressive factors.

Initially, a thorough sharp release of the Liliequist's membrane around the oculomotor nerve aims to reduce subsequent nerve retraction. These membranes can form bands, contributing to abnormal nerve traction. Nakagawa [22] reported findings of abnormally dense Liliequist's membranes causing late-onset right ONP in a bilateral surgery case. Our case 5 revealed evident Liliequist's membrane band traction, distorting the nerve's proximal area, which normalized after sharp release.

Subsequently, we sequentially explored the PCA, PCom, SCA, and PPCDF and their relations with the oculomotor nerve. When these structures made contact with the oculomotor nerve, suspected compression was indicated. Changes in nerve coloration and/or deformation indicated responsible compression. Both responsible and suspected compression received decompression. In our 5 cases, three (case 1, case 2 and case 4) confirmed preoperative imaging findings with PCA and SCA simultaneously contacting the oculomotor nerve, one of the three involving simultaneous responsible compression of both vessels, while the other two having PCA as responsible compression and SCA as suspected compression. In all these three cases, simultaneous decompression of PCA and SCA was performed. Another two cases with isolated responsible compression of PCA (case 5) or SCA (case 3) underwent decompression accordingly. No compression involving the PCom was found. In the case (case 2) with PPCDF compression, after completing vascular decompression, the nerve naturally disengaged from the dural fold, relieving the compression. Among the reported 16 surgeries, 2 cases identified simultaneous compression of both PCA and SCA on the oculomotor nerve [17, 18], while the rest presented single compression factors: 5 cases with PCom [13, 19–21, 23], 5 cases with PCA [10, 12, 15, 22], and 4 cases with the PCom-ID [9, 11, 14, 16]. Concerning compression sites, three cases in the reported surgeries were near the proximal end of the oculomotor nerve [15, 17, 23], and one was near the distal end adjacent to the cavernous sinus entrance [19], with unclear descriptions for the others. In our cases, all vascular compressions were located proximally, except for one case (case 2) with simultaneous distal compression by the uncus and PPCDF. Cases reported with ONP caused by compression from aneurysms [8, 69], pituitary adenomas [70, 71], and other space-occupying lesions [72] predominantly featured compressions not at the nerve's proximal interpeduncular cistern segment but at the distal part of this segment or adjacent to the cavernous sinus entrance. These results suggest that compression can occur at any point along the interpeduncular cisternal segment of oculomotor nerve, thus mandating comprehensive exploration and decompression throughout the surgery.

The technical details of decompression vary widely in the literature. Among the 16 surgeries reported, 9 utilized isolation techniques, implanting materials at the NVC sites: 5 used Teflon [9, 10, 12, 13, 15], 3 employed sponge [22, 23], and 1 used oxidized cellulose and fibrin glue [14]; 3 cases employed suspension techniques to relocate and secure vessels near the skull base dura, which included autologous fascial strips [21], Teflon strips [17], and oxidized cellulose plus fibrin glue adhering [11]; 3 cases involved only releasing the arachnoid membrane [18–20]; and in 1 case, due to difficulties in decompression, only the clipping of the PCom-ID was performed [16]. It's evident that isolation techniques, particularly using Teflon, were the most commonly used. All the five cases in our center, the Teflon isolation method was utilized. In four cases (case 1, case 2, case 4, and case 5), a refinement of technique utilized in trigeminal and facial nerve MVD was employed, involving placing moistened gelatin sponge between the Teflon cushion and the nerve to prevent potential adverse effects of direct contact between them [73]. In the remaining case (case 3), gelatin sponge wasn't used due to the narrow space between the nerve and the culprit SCA. In terms of specific details, considering that the force applied during the procedure was more directed away from the surgeon, the technique employed had slight variations in addressing the compression of the PCA and SCA. In cases involving the SCA, as the vessel positioned deeper beneath the nerve, the process initially involved placing Teflon to push the SCA away from the nerve's depth, followed by placing gelatin sponge between the cushion and the nerve. Conversely, when dealing with the PCA, which is positioned superficially above the nerve, the method first involved placing a softer gelatin sponge between the nerve and the vessel to avoid excessive pressure on the deeper located nerve. Additionally, utilizing the expanding property of the gelatin sponge helped maintain separation between the vessel and the nerve. Subsequently, a Teflon cushion was placed between the gelatin sponge and the vessels, effectively protecting the nerve. We believe this Teflon plus gelatin sponge decompression technique is simple, safe, and effective and should be considered the primary choice for MVD procedure.

19.4.5 Postoperative Complications and Surgical Outcomes

In the 15 cases reported in the literature and the 5 cases from our center, there were no occurrences of common complications associated with intracranial surgery such as intracranial hemorrhage, stroke, intracranial infection, cerebrospinal fluid leakage, or epilepsy. Within the literature's 15 cases, 3 presented with new-onset functional impairment of the oculomotor nerve, all of which were early, transient manifestations. None of the cases from our center experienced oculomotor nerve-related complications.

Of the 15 cases in the literature, 4 showed partial improvement or complete recovery of oculomotor nerve function as early as about 1 week postoperatively. During the 6-month follow-up, among the literature's cases, 10 experienced complete recovery, 5 showed partial recovery, and 1 displayed no improvement. Within our center's 5 cases, 3 (case 2, case 4, case 5) experienced complete remission, 1 showed partial remission (case 3), and 1 exhibited mild improvement (case 1).

Factors affecting postoperative outcomes, aside from the decompression procedures during surgery, may be related to preoperative disease progression, clinical presentations, and other variables. Future high-quality clinical research is required to elucidate these associations.

19.5 Conclusion

nAVC-ONP/ONM is a group of oculomotor nerve-related NVCS that currently lack comprehensive clinical understanding and diagnosis. A meticulous analysis of symptoms and imaging is necessary to establish a diagnosis. We proposed a novel clinical assessment scale that holds certain significance in guiding the diagnosis and treatment protocols for this condition. Based on the existing limited case data, MVD surgery appears to be a safe and effective means of treating nAVC-ONP/ONM.

References

1. Jannetta PJ. The history of microvascular decompression surgery. In: Li ST, Zhong J, Sekula R, editors. Microvascular decompression surgery. Berlin: Springer; 2016. p. 1–7.
2. Jannetta PJ. Arterial compression of the trigeminal nerve at the pons in patients with trigeminal neuralgia. J Neurosurg. 1967;26(1):159–62.
3. Jannetta PJ, Rand RW. Transtentorial retrogasserian rhizotomy in trigeminal neuralgia by microneurosurgical technique. Bull Los Angel Neuro Soc. 1966;31(3):93–9.
4. McLaughlin MR, et al. Microvascular decompression of cranial nerves: lessons learned after 4400 operations. J Neurosurg. 1999;90(1):1–8.
5. Barker FG 2nd, et al. The long-term outcome of microvascular decompression for trigeminal neuralgia. N Engl J Med. 1996;334(17):1077–83.
6. Belotti F, et al. The oculomotor neurovascular conflict: literature review and proposal of management. Clin Neurol Neurosurg. 2020;195:105920.
7. Fang C, et al. Incidence and etiologies of acquired third nerve palsy using a population-based method. JAMA Ophthalmol. 2017;135(1):23–8.
8. Leivo S, et al. Early surgery improves the cure of aneurysm-induced oculomotor palsy. Surg Neurol. 1996;45(5):430–4.
9. Dowlati E, et al. Posterior communicating artery infundibulum with oculomotor nerve palsy treated with microvascular decompression: a case report and 2-dimensional technical operative video. Br J Neurosurg. 2023;37(3):405–8.
10. Zhang J, et al. Microvascular decompression for a patient with oculomotor palsy caused by posterior cerebral artery compression: a case report and literature review. World J Clin Cases. 2022;10(20):7138–46.
11. Onuma K, et al. Microvascular decompression for oculomotor nerve palsy due to nonaneurysmal vascular compression. World Neurosurg. 2021;145:102–6.

12. Pomeraniec IJ, et al. Microvascular decompression of the posterior cerebral artery for treatment of oculomotor nerve palsy. J Cerebrovasc Endovasc Neurosurg. 2020;22(2):85–9.
13. Haider AS, et al. Acute oculomotor nerve palsy caused by compression from an aberrant posterior communicating artery. Cureus. 2019;11(1):e3920.
14. Fukami S, et al. Microvascular decompression for oculomotor nerve palsy due to compression by infundibular dilatation of posterior communicating artery. World Neurosurg. 2018;119:142–5.
15. Kheshaifati H, Al-Otaibi F, Alhejji M. Microvascular decompression for oculomotor nerve palsy: a case report and literature review. World Neurosurg. 2016;88:695e1–3.
16. Fukushima Y, et al. Ptosis as partial oculomotor nerve palsy due to compression by infundibular dilatation of posterior communicating artery, visualized with three-dimensional computer graphics: case report. Neurol Med Chir (Tokyo). 2014;54(3):214–8.
17. Inoue T, et al. Ocular neuromyotonia treated by microvascular decompression: usefulness of preoperative 3D imaging: case report. J Neurosurg. 2012;117(6):1166–9.
18. Suzuki K, et al. Oculomotor palsy treated by microvascular decompression. Surg Neurol. 2008;70(2):210–2.
19. Babbitz JD, Harsh GR. Concomitant ectatic posterior communicating artery and tentorial meningioma as a source of oculomotor palsy: case report. Neurosurgery. 2005;57(6):E1316; discussion E1316.
20. Noji M, Hidaka K. Ophthalmalgia and oculomotor nerve palsy associated with compression of an atherosclerotic and tortuous posterior communicating artery: a case report. Jpn J Neurosurg. 2003;12:623–6.
21. Mulderink TA, et al. Third nerve paresis caused by vascular compression by the posterior communicating artery. J Stroke Cerebrovasc Dis. 2001;10(3):139–41.
22. Nakagawa H, et al. Bilateral oculomotor nerve palsies due to posterior cerebral arterial compression relieved by microvascular decompression—case report. Neurol Med Chir (Tokyo). 1991;31(1):45–8.
23. Kojo N, et al. A case of ophthalmoplegic migraine with cerebral aneurysm. No Shinkei Geka. 1988;16(5 Suppl):503–7.
24. Tan T, Tee JW, Wang YY. Oculomotor nerve palsy secondary to aberrant posterior cerebral artery. BMJ Case Rep. 2014;2014:bcr2014205063.
25. Silva EB Jr, et al. Bilateral oculomotor nerve palsies due to vascular conflict. Arq Neuropsiquiatr. 2010;68(5):819–21.
26. Hashimoto M, et al. Vascular compression of the oculomotor nerve disclosed by thin-slice magnetic resonance imaging. Am J Ophthalmol. 1998;125(6):881–2.
27. Zhao H, Tang Y, Li S. Microvascular decompression for oculomotor nerve palsy due to non-aneurysmal neurovaslur conflict: 5 cases report and literature review. World Neurosurg. 2024;191:e356. https://doi.org/10.1016/j.wneu.2024.08.130.
28. Liang C, et al. Anatomical features of the cisternal segment of the oculomotor nerve: neurovascular relationships and abnormal compression on magnetic resonance imaging. J Neurosurg. 2009;111(6):1193–200.
29. Ksiazek SM, et al. Fascicular arrangement in partial oculomotor paresis. Am J Ophthalmol. 1994;118(1):97–103.
30. Stockman AC, et al. Ocular neuromyotonia: case reports and literature review. Strabismus. 2018;26(3):133–41.
31. Hashimoto M, Ohtsuka K, Hoyt WF. Vascular compression as a cause of superior oblique myokymia disclosed by thin-slice magnetic resonance imaging. Am J Ophthalmol. 2001;131(5):676–7.
32. Ohtsuka K, et al. Vascular compressive abducens nerve palsy disclosed by magnetic resonance imaging. Am J Ophthalmol. 1996;122(3):416–9.
33. Yousry I, et al. MR anatomy of the proximal cisternal segment of the trochlear nerve: neurovascular relationships and landmarks. Radiology. 2002;223(1):31–8.
34. Yousry I, et al. Superior oblique myokymia: magnetic resonance imaging support for the neurovascular compression hypothesis. Ann Neurol. 2002;51(3):361–8.
35. Liao CC, Wu KH, Chen G. Application of preoperative multimodal image fusion technique in microvascular decompression surgery via suboccipital retrosigmoid approach. World Neurosurg. 2023;173:e37–47.
36. Naraghi R, et al. Classification of neurovascular compression in typical hemifacial spasm: three-dimensional visualization of the facial and the vestibulocochlear nerves. J Neurosurg. 2007;107(6):1154–63.
37. Yavarian Y, Bayat M, Brondum Frokjaer J. Herniation of uncus and parahippocampal gyrus: an accidental finding on magnetic resonance imaging of cerebrum. Acta Radiol Short Rep. 2015;4(1):2047981614560077.
38. Horowitz M, et al. Misinterpretation of parahippocampal herniation for a posterior fossa tumor: imaging and intraoperative findings. J Neuroimaging. 2002;12(1):78–9.
39. Kiss-Bodolay D, et al. The use of diffusion magnetic resonance imaging tractography in supporting anatomical conflict between an uncal protrusion and the oculomotor nerve: a case report of isolated inferior rectus palsy. Surg Neurol Int. 2023;14:194.
40. Kimball D, et al. Ossification of the posterior petroclinoid dural fold: a cadaveric study with neurosurgical significance. J Neurol Surg B Skull Base. 2015;76(4):272–7.
41. Boecher-Schwarz HG, et al. Sensitivity and specificity of MRA in the diagnosis of neurovascular compression in patients with trigeminal neuralgia. A correlation of MRA and surgical findings. Neuroradiology. 1998;40(2):88–95.
42. Park HK, et al. Microsurgical anatomy of the oculomotor nerve. Clin Anat. 2017;30(1):21–31.
43. Zhao X, et al. Tailoring the surgical corridor to the basilar apex in the pretemporal transcavernous approach: morphometric analyses of different neurovascular mobilization maneuvers. Acta Neurochir. 2020;162(11):2731–41.
44. Tayebi Meybodi A, et al. Comparative analysis of orbitozygomatic and subtemporal approaches to the

basilar apex: a cadaveric study. World Neurosurg. 2018;119:e607–16.
45. Tayebi Meybodi A, et al. Comprehensive anatomic assessment of the Pterional, orbitopterional, and orbitozygomatic approaches for basilar apex aneurysm clipping. Oper Neurosurg. 2018;15(5):538–50.
46. Wen HT, et al. The pretemporal approach: surgical anatomy, operative technique, and rationale. Oper Tech Neurosurg. 2001;4(2):73–81.
47. de Oliveira E, et al. The pretemporal approach to the interpeduncular and petroclival regions. Acta Neurochir. 1995;136(3–4):204–11.
48. Heros RC, Lee SH. The combined pterional/anterior temporal approach for aneurysms of the upper basilar complex: technical report. Neurosurgery. 1993;33(2):244–50; discussion 250–1.
49. Day JD, Giannotta SL, Fukushima T. Extradural temporopolar approach to lesions of the upper basilar artery and infrachiasmatic region. J Neurosurg. 1994;81(2):230–5.
50. Koperna T, Tschabitscher M, Knosp E. The termination of the vein of "Labbe" and its microsurgical significance. Acta Neurochir. 1992;118(3–4):172–5.
51. Kyoshima K, Oikawa S, Kobayashi S. Preservation of large bridging veins of the cranial base: technical note. Neurosurgery. 2001;48(2):447–9.
52. Sugita K, Kobayashi S, Yokoo A. Preservation of large bridging veins during brain retraction. Technical note. J Neurosurg. 1982;57(6):856–8.
53. Katsuno M, et al. A modified anterior temporal approach for low-position aneurysms of the upper basilar complex. Surg Neurol Int. 2015;6:10.
54. Krisht AF, Kadri PA. Surgical clipping of complex basilar apex aneurysms: a strategy for successful outcome using the pretemporal transzygomatic transcavernous approach. Neurosurgery. 2005;56(2 Suppl):261–73; discussion 261–73.
55. Seoane E, et al. The pretemporal transcavernous approach to the interpeduncular and prepontine cisterns: microsurgical anatomy and technique application. Neurosurgery. 2000;46(4):891–8; discussion 898–9.
56. Delaunois J, Vaz G, Raftopoulos C. Transsylvian transuncal approach for an anterior midbrain cavernous malformation resection: a case report. Oper Neurosurg. 2018;14(3):E38–43.
57. Post N, Russell SM, Jafar JJ. Role of uncal resection in optimizing transsylvian access to the basilar apex: cadaveric investigation and preliminary clinical experience in eight patients. Neurosurgery. 2005;56(2 Suppl):274–80; discussion 274–80.
58. Wen HT, et al. The pterional approach: surgical anatomy, operative technique, and rationale. Oper Tech Neurosurg. 2001;4(2):60–72.
59. Vishteh AG, et al. The pterional approach. Oper Tech Neurosurg. 1998;1(1):39–49.
60. Yasargil MG, Reichman MV, Kubik S. Preservation of the frontotemporal branch of the facial nerve using the interfascial temporalis flap for pterional craniotomy. Technical article. J Neurosurg. 1987;67(3):463–6.
61. Cohen-Gadol AA. Atraumatic Sylvian fissure split: nuances and pitfalls. Oper Neurosurg. 2020;18(2):217–24.
62. Hafez A, Bucard JB, Tanikawa R. Integrated multimaneuver dissection technique of the Sylvian fissure: operative nuances. Oper Neurosurg. 2017;13(6):702–10.
63. Kazumata K, et al. Operative anatomy and classification of the sylvian veins for the distal transsylvian approach. Neurol Med Chir (Tokyo). 2003;43(9):427–33; discussion 434.
64. Wen HT, et al. Microsurgical anatomy of the temporal lobe: part 2–Sylvian fissure region and its clinical application. Neurosurgery. 2009;65(6 Suppl):1–35; discussion 36.
65. Li Y, et al. Surgical treatment of hemifacial spasm with zone-4 offending vessel. Acta Neurochir. 2013;155(5):849–53.
66. Feng BH, et al. Microvascular decompression for trigeminal neuralgia: zone exploration and decompression techniques. J Craniofac Surg. 2015;26:2381.
67. Zhong J, et al. Microvascular decompression surgery: surgical principles and technical nuances based on 4000 cases. Neurol Res. 2014;36(10):882–93.
68. Zhong J, et al. A clinical analysis on microvascular decompression surgery in a series of 3000 cases. Clin Neurol Neurosurg. 2012;114(7):846–51.
69. Hall S, et al. The resolution of oculomotor nerve palsy caused by unruptured posterior communicating artery aneurysms: a cohort study and narrative review. World Neurosurg. 2017;107:581–7.
70. Ferrareze Nunes C, et al. Endoscopic endonasal transoculomotor triangle approach for adenomas invading the parapeduncular space: surgical anatomy, technical nuances, and case series. J Neurosurg. 2018;130:1304–14.
71. Wu X, et al. Pituitary adenoma with oculomotor cistern extension: membranous anatomy and clinical application. Acta Neurochir. 2023;165(10):2985–93.
72. Nonaka Y, et al. Surgical management of nonvascular lesions around the oculomotor nerve. World Neurosurg. 2014;81(5–6):798–809.
73. Chang B, et al. A new application of gelatin sponge in the treatment of hemifacial spasm by microvascular decompression: a technical note. J Neurol Surg A Cent Eur Neurosurg. 2021;83:183.

20 Microvascular Decompression for Superior Oblique Myokymia

Shusaku Noro, Bunsho Asayama, and Hirohiko Nakamura

Key Points

Question: Does superior oblique myokymia (SOM) really result from vascular compression of the trochlear nerve, and is it cured by microvascular decompression (MVD)?

Findings: We performed a literature review to identify seven patients (including our 2 cases) who were successfully treated with MVD of the trochlear nerve for SOM without serious and persistent complications. This study also revealed a higher prevalence of compression than previously reported, suggesting that fusion imaging may be particularly useful for identifying this condition.

Meaning: MVD should be more frequently considered as a potential treatment option when patients present with SOM.

20.1 Introduction

Superior oblique myokymia (SOM), as termed by Hoyt and Keane in 1970 [1], is an acquired abnormality of the innervation of the superior oblique muscle, with no known risk factors, that causes episodic torsional oscillations of the eye [2]. These symptoms can be quite severe and even incapacitating, causing significant impairment of daily activities [2–5].

S. Noro (✉) · B. Asayama · H. Nakamura
Nakamura Memorial Hospital,
SAPPORO, Hokkaido, Japan
e-mail: shusaku@med.nmh.or.jp

Several strategies have been used to treat this condition, including antiepileptic drugs, such as carbamazepine, beta-blocker eye drops, and surgery of the superior oblique muscle or tendon; however, all harbor the possibility of recurrence [2, 6]. SOM may result from vascular compression of the trochlear nerve [2, 7], and it has been suggested that MVD surgery could completely resolve symptoms [2, 5].

In 1983, Bringewald [7] first suggested that SOM may result from vascular compression of the trochlear nerve, and Samii et al. [8] later reported that microvascular decompression surgery of this nerve could completely resolve symptoms [2]. Few other reports, however, have documented the use of MVD for the treatment of SOM [2, 8–12]. Hence, many physicians are unaware that vascular compression of the root exit zone (REZ) of the trochlear nerve, defined as the first ~1.2 mm peripheral portion of the nerve from its exit point [13], may play an important role in SOM pathogenesis [7] and that this disorder is potentially curable by MVD [2]. In fact, even if ophthalmologists are well informed about SOM, they are less likely to consult neurosurgeons due to perceived morbidity risk, such as stroke or contusion, after MVD.

Ruttum [6] suggested that preventative trochlear nerve decompression surgery is probably unnecessary because no neurologic sequelae of SOM, other than myokymic symptoms, have been reported. However, for some patients, these myo-

S.-T. Li et al. (eds.), *Microvascular Decompression Surgery*,
https://doi.org/10.1007/978-981-96-0767-9_20

kymic symptoms can be quite severe and even incapacitating, with significant impairment to quality of life (QOL) [3–5]. Tenotomy and tenectomy of the superior oblique tendon have been more commonly used for the management of the condition; however, these surgeries carry a risk of iatrogenic superior oblique palsy that generally necessitates weakening of the ipsilateral inferior oblique muscle [6]. In contrast, MVD has been demonstrated to be the only definitive therapy [7–13]. Furthermore, potential risks, such as death or stroke, associated with MVD have been shown to be extremely low for skillful neurosurgeons.

We experienced performing MVD on six patients with SOM using a lateral supracerebellar infratentorial (SC-IT) approach. Postoperatively, all patients had immediate and complete resolution of symptoms without recurrence during extended follow-up [2]. Herein, we report the clinical characteristics of 2 of these cases with a review of related literature and present a caveat in the lateral SC-IT approach to treat SOM [2].

20.2 Methods

The patients underwent 3.0-T MRI (MAGNETOM Skyra, Siemens, Germany) of the cerebellopontine angle cistern with T2 sampling perfection with application-optimized contrast using different flip angle evolution (SPACE) and true fast imaging with steady precession (FISP), using the following parameters: for T2 SPACE, voxel size: 0.53 × 0.53 × 0.5 mm, slice thickness: 0.5 mm, echo time (TE): 187 ms, repetition time (TR): 1500 ms; for true FISP, voxel size: 0.49 × 0.49 × 0.35 mm, slice thickness: 0.35 mm, TE: 3.33 ms, TR: 7.33 ms. 3D fusion imaging was performed preoperatively using Workstation (SYNAPSE VINCENT ver. 5.2, Fujifilm, Tokyo, Japan) [2].

All surgical procedures were performed by a lateral SC-IT approach.

Case 1

History and Examination

A 37-year-old man presented with an intermittent fluttering sensation in his left eye lasting for several seconds per episode and repeatedly occurring for 4 years [2]. Aside from the left eye abnormality, he had no significant medical history [2]. The patient was initially evaluated by an ophthalmologist [2]. Slit-lamp examination revealed an intermittent intorsional microtremor in the left eye, diagnosed as left SOM [2]. Visual acuity, visual fields, color vision, and extraocular muscle movements were all normal, consistent with the diagnosis [2]. Conventional MRI of the brain showed no abnormalities. However, medical treatment with the anticonvulsants carbamazepine and gabapentin provided no symptomatic relief, and his symptoms gradually worsened, eventually preventing him from performing his job [2]. To evaluate the brainstem in more detail, T2 SPACE and true FISP were used to yield high-resolution images of the very small structures surrounded by cerebrospinal fluid [2]. Fusion images (Fig. 20.1) showed compression of the trochlear nerve by a branch of the superior cerebellar artery (SCA) [2]. The ophthalmologist recommended MVD, and the patient eventually underwent neurosurgical treatment [2].

Operation

MVD of the left trochlear nerve was performed via a left lateral SC-IT approach [2]. After intubation, the patient's head was placed in a Mayfield head holder, and the patient was positioned in the lateral park-bench position with the head turned 45° towards the floor with slight flex-

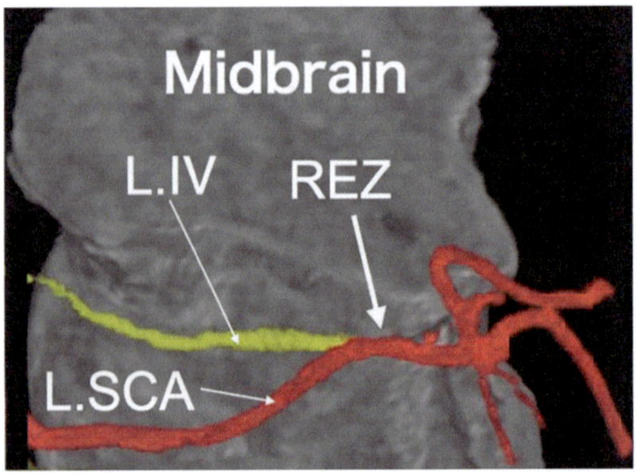

Fig. 20.1 Preoperative fusion imaging is shown. The REZ of the left trochlear nerve is compressed by the superior cerebellar artery. *REZ* root exit zone, *L.IV* left cranial nerve IV, *L.SCA* left superior cerebellar artery

ion to allow easy exposure of the supracerebellar window [2]. A curved "L"-shaped skin incision was performed along the transverse sinus and the sigmoid sinus [2]. The suboccipital muscles were dissected using monopolar cautery [2]. The transverse sinus, transverse-sigmoid junction, and proximal part of the sigmoid sinus were exposed, and a dura opening was performed [2]. Cerebrospinal fluid was released from the cerebellopontine cistern [2]. By dissecting along the superior edge of the cerebellum, the superior petrosal vein, branches of the SCA, and a distal portion of the trochlear nerve were identified [2].

The REZ of the trochlear nerve was compressed on both the ventral and dorsal surfaces by the SCA [2]. Initially, the portion of the SCA compressing the dorsal side was transposed far from the trochlear nerve using Teflon felt. The SCA compressing the dorsal part was wrapped in Teflon felt, transposed far from the trochlear nerve, and adhered to the surface of the cerebellum using fibrin glue [2]. A small branch of the SCA, not identified preoperatively, was then confirmed to be compressing the ventral side [2]. This vessel was similarly wrapped, gradually transposed toward the distal portion of the trochlear nerve, and attached to the surface of the midbrain using Teflon felt [2]. No other vessels were found around the REZ of the trochlear nerve (Fig. 20.2) [2].

Postoperative Course

Immediately following surgery, involuntary rotatory eye movements ceased completely [2]. No medication was provided after surgery, and the patient was discharged on the seventh postoperative day (standard recovery period for trigeminal neuralgia and hemifacial spasm in Japan), satisfied with the treatment [2]. In addition, the intermittent intorsional microtremor revealed by slit-lamp examination ceased completely [2]. His condition improved after surgery, although he had mild left trochlear nerve palsy with diplopia on downgaze [2]. This complication completely resolved within 9 months following surgery,

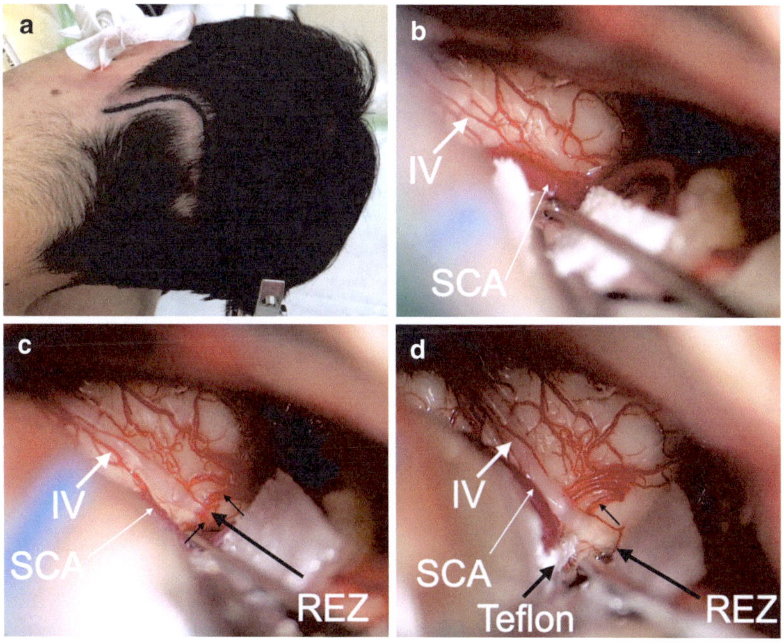

Fig. 20.2 Microvascular decompression of the trochlear nerve. (**a**) Skin incision. (**b**) The trochlear nerve (cranial nerve IV) was compressed by the superior cerebellar artery (SCA) on the rostral surface. (**c**) After displacing the SCA, the trochlear nerve was also compressed by a small branch (short black arrows) of the SCA on the ventral surface. (**d**) The vessels were attached to the surface of the midbrain using Teflon felt and fibrin glue, and absence of vessels around the root exit zone (REZ) of the trochlear nerve was confirmed

without evidence of recurrence as of the 60-month follow-up [2]. No further neurological deficit was observed [2].

Case 2

History and Examination

A 56-year-old man presented with a 3-year history of intermittent diplopia that started spontaneously and gradually increased in frequency [2]. He reported a pulsating sensation in his right eye and a flickering movement in his right field of vision [2]. This symptom was described as, "the vision jumps up and down," and it worsened when he looked down and was particularly disabling while driving [2]. The patient reported no relevant medical history, and conventional MRI of the brain showed no abnormalities [2]. However, fusion images (Fig. 20.3) showed right trochlear nerve compression by an SCA branch [2]. The results of slit-lamp examination indicated a diagnosis of right SOM [2]. Slit-lamp examination demonstrated high-frequency and low-amplitude episodes of spasmodic intrusion and depression of the right eye [2]. Visual acuity, visual fields, color vision, and extraocular muscle movements were all normal, providing a clinical picture consistent with SOM showed right SOM [2].

Prior to referral to our neurosurgical service, the patient underwent treatment with carbamazepine, clonazepam, and acupuncture for 3 years with virtually no response [2].

Operation

MVD was performed via a right lateral SC-IT approach [2]. After a small suboccipital craniotomy, bridging veins on the tentorial surface of the cerebellum were found, which obstructed the view of the REZ from the lateral side [2]. Therefore, we extended the exposure more medially for better visualization of the REZ without sacrificing the bridging veins [2]. We made a possible space to approach deeper carefully, so as not to damage the bridging veins [2]. The SCA branch was found to be close to the origin of the nerve in the ambient cistern [2]. The trochlear nerve was kinked by a small branch of the SCA on the ventral side, which was not identified preoperatively; however, no vessels compressed the rostral side [2]. The vessel was wrapped in Teflon felt, gradually transposed toward the distal portion of the trochlear nerve, and adhered to the surface of the midbrain using fibrin glue [2]. No other vessels were identified around the REZ of the trochlear nerve (Fig. 20.4) [2].

Postoperative Course

The patient reported full resolution of symptoms and had no neurological deficit [2]. No medication was prescribed after surgery, and he was discharged on the seventh postoperative day, satisfied with his treatment outcome [2]. No evidence of recurrence was found throughout a 53-month follow-up period.

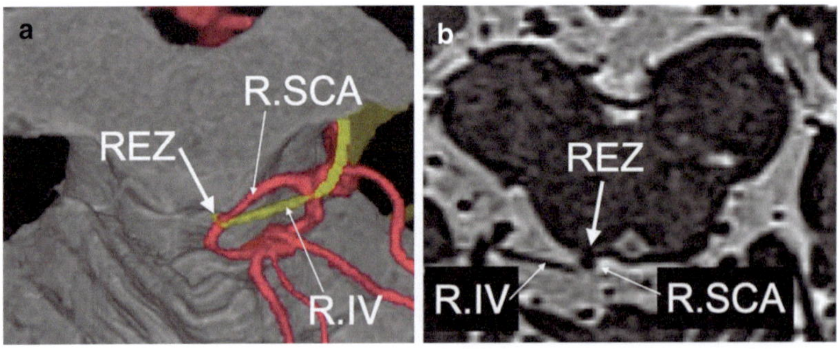

Fig. 20.3 Preoperative magnetic resonance (MR) imaging and fusion imaging. (**a**) Fusion imaging and (**b**) true fast imaging with steady-state precession (FISP) are shown. The REZ of the right trochlear nerve is compressed by a branch of the superior cerebellar artery. *REZ* root exit zone, *R.IV* right cranial nerve IV, *R.SCA* right superior cerebellar artery

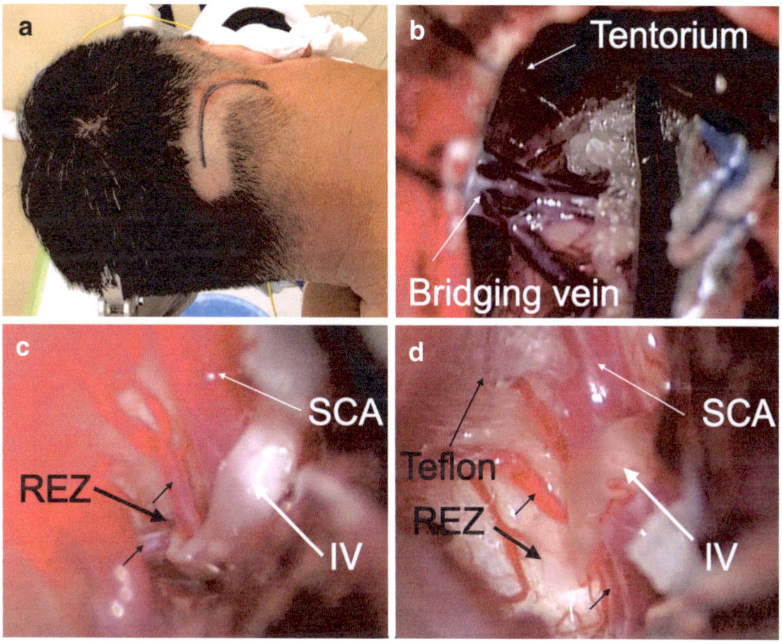

Fig. 20.4 Microvascular decompression of the trochlear nerve. (**a**) Skin incision. (**b**) Large bridging veins at the superior cerebellar surface were preserved. (**c**) The trochlear nerve (cranial nerve IV) was compressed by a small branch (short black arrows) of the superior cerebellar artery (SCA) on the ventral surface, although there were no vessels compressing the rostral side. (**d**) The vessel was attached to the surface of the midbrain using Teflon felt and fibrin glue, and absence of vessels around the root exit zone (REZ) of the trochlear nerve was confirmed

20.3 Literature Review

Previously reported cases of SOM treated via neurosurgery are listed in Table 20.1. In addition, we searched PubMed using the key terms "superior oblique myokymia" and "microvascular decompression" to identify published articles related to MVD surgery of the trochlear nerve [2].

Only 5 reported cases of SOM were treated with MVD [2]. Four of them received some medication preoperatively, but their symptoms were not alleviated. Vascular contact occurred on either or both the dorsal and ventral surfaces of the trochlear nerve [2]. In terms of the approach, retrosigmoid approach was used in 3, lateral supracerebellar approach in 1, and interhemispheric transtentorial approach in 1. In all 5 reported cases, symptoms were relieved after MVD, although a transient trochlear nerve palsy occurred in 3 of the 5 cases [2, 8–10]. No deaths were associated with this procedure [2].

20.4 Discussion

Similar to vascular facial nerve compression as a cause of hemifacial spasm [2, 14], vascular compression of the trochlear nerve may cause SOM. In 1983, Bringewald [7] first suggested that SOM may result from vascular compression of the trochlear nerve [2]. Both conditions have progressive episodic symptoms and can be cured by MVD of the compressed nerve [2]. Indeed, Samii et al. [8] reported that MVD surgery could completely resolve symptoms [2]. Similar pathophysiology likely underpins both conditions and may involve pressure-induced demyelination with an ectopic generation of ephaptic impulse transmissions along the compressed nerve [2, 15]. Arguably, the strongest support for this neurovascular hypothesis comes from an MRI study performed by Yousry et al. [16] in 2002 in which vascular compression of the trochlear nerve was confirmed in all 6 included right SOM patients [2, 11].

Table 20.1 Neurosurgical case reports of superior oblique myokymia

Reference	Age (years)	Sex	Offending vessel	Disease duration (years)	Pre-MVD treatment	Result	F/U period (months)	Complications	Location
Samii et al. (1998) [8]	50	M	Small artery	>17	CBZ, PHT, VPA, PRM, BTX	Cured (immediately)	22	Trochlear nerve palsy for 5 months	Ventral
Hashimoto et al. (2004) [10]	49	M	SCA branch	8	CBZ, BAC	Cured (immediately)	12	Trochlear nerve palsy for 3 months	Ventral and dorsal
Mikami et al. (2005) [11]	67	M	SCA branch	>11	CBZ, PHT, BAC	Cured (immediately)	18	–	Ventral and dorsal
Fam et al. (2014) [12]	47	M	SCA branch	6	CBZ, GBP, BAC, timolol eye drops	Cured (immediately)	18	–	Dorsal
Kawasaki et al. (2019) [9]	77	F	SCA branch	2	–	Cured (immediately)	24	Trochlear nerve palsy for 2 weeks	Ventral and dorsal
Present cases [2]	37	M	SCA branch	4	CBZ, GBP	Cured (immediately)	60	Trochlear nerve palsy for 9 months	Ventral and dorsal
	56	M	SCA branch	3	CBZ, GBP, BAC, timolol eye drops	Cured (immediately)	53	–	Ventral

BAC baclofen, *BTX* botulinum toxin, *CBZ* carbamazepine, *F/U* follow-up, *GBP* gabapentin, *MVD* microvascular decompression, *PHT* phenytoin, *PRM* primidone, *SCA* superior cerebellar artery, *VPA* valproic acid

Previously reported treatments for SOM include several pharmacological therapies yielding variable results [2, 17]. Patients with SOM most commonly receive anticonvulsants or eye drops as palliative therapies that may not dramatically improve patient outcomes [2]. Although such therapies are not invasive, they can occasionally cause severe side effects such as vertigo or unsteady gait without improvement of oscillopsia [3, 9]. In addition, these palliative therapies may not dramatically improve patient outcomes, as a recurrence rate as high as 50% has been reported [12]. To ameliorate postoperative diplopia [18], simultaneous inferior oblique myectomy has also been performed in some cases with variable results [1, 4, 19]. Brazis et al. [20] reported the disappearance of oscillopsia in 4 patients who underwent tenectomy combined with inferior oblique myectomy [2]. Tenotomy and tenectomy of the superior oblique tendon are more commonly used for managing SOM; however, these surgeries carry a risk of iatrogenic superior oblique palsy that generally weakens the ipsilateral inferior oblique muscle [2, 6]. In contrast, MVD has been demonstrated to be the only definitive cure [2, 7–12, 14]. Furthermore, potential risks associated with MVD such as death or stroke are extremely low for skilled neurosurgeons [2].

Five previous reports [8–12] described the complete resolution of SOM and improved functioning after MVD. While 4 of the 7 total reported patients with this condition (including our 2 cases) experienced a transient trochlear nerve palsy, this complication resolved within 2 weeks to 9 months after MVD [2]. No recurrence was reported [2]. In our report, the 2 patients experienced neurovascular conflict caused by trochlear nerve impaction by branches of the SCA, which were not identified preoperatively [2]. In 1 patient, vascular contact occurred on both the dosal and ventral surfaces of the trochlear nerve, while the ventral surface was exclusively involved in the other case [2]. A branch of the SCA may be impossible to identify by imaging, even considering the remarkable advances in imaging technology [2]. Had preoperative 3D fusion imaging not revealed trochlear nerve REZ compression by the proximal SCA, the patient might not have elected to receive MVD [2]. Nevertheless, 3D fusion imaging can be very helpful for supporting the decision to take a surgical approach and ultimately improves the safety of the procedure [2]. Furthermore, the intraoperative findings allowed us to expand our knowledge of the trochlear nerve and midbrain structure [2].

In the previous literature, there are no reports regarding the tentorial bridging veins in MVD for SOM. In the lateral SC-IT approach, it is difficult to confirm the trochlear nerve REZ if large tentorial bridging veins of the surface of the cerebellum are present [2]. Sacrificing these veins has been considered relatively safe [2, 21–24]. Kodera et al. [23] reported that these veins could be sacrificed if the collateral circulation of each vein is preserved [2]. However, Jakola et al. [25] reported that sacrificing even a limited number of tentorial bridging veins might cause venous infarction or hemorrhage in the cerebellum [2, 26]. It is impossible to determine which veins can be sacrificed during surgery, although the anatomical relationship of the venous system of the cerebellum and tentorium has been well investigated [2, 26–30].

In our study, the large bridging veins were preserved, although they obstructed the REZ of the trochlear nerve from the lateral side [2]. Consequently, we extended the exposure more medially to visualize the REZ [2]. The keyhole approach is usually recommended in MVD surgery; however, we feel it was a good strategy to make a skin incision on the medial side as a precaution [2].

Fortunately, both our patients were cured following MVD, though the first patient did experience transient and mild trochlear nerve palsy [2]. Although we initially recognized that trochlear nerve palsy was the most likely postoperative complication and could potentially impact daily activities, the patient was genuinely satisfied with his treatment at discharge and reported improved ability to function after the complication was resolved [2]. In fact, this experience encouraged us to such an extent that we recommended this treatment approach to the second patient [2]. The neurosurgical treatment of SOM requires experience with MVD, and our team has completed over 700 such operations without patient death or stroke [2]. When this surgical technique is used, exposure of the trochlear nerve is conducted in a similar manner as exposure of the trigeminal nerve; however, it is redirected medially and superiorly [2]. Using this approach, the REZ of the trochlear nerve is identified at the dorsal aspect of the brainstem in the transverse-sigmoid sinus angle [2, 9].

The diagnosis of SOM can be relatively straightforward if a patient presents with an intermittent ocular fluttering sensation lasting for several seconds [2]. At this time, we recommend MVD surgery in patients with medically refractory symptoms who have been diagnosed by an ophthalmologist well-informed about SOM [2]. Without knowledge of the efficacy and safety of this procedure, ophthalmologists may be less likely to consult neurosurgeons due to perceived morbidity risks, such as stroke or cranial nerve disturbance, after MVD [2].

The high rates of patient satisfaction and treatment response recorded in this study are clinically meaningful and encouraging [2].

20.5 Conclusion

In summary, we have described two rare cases involving patients who underwent neurosurgical treatment for SOM [2]. Preoperative fusion images created by T2 SPACE and true FISP were critical in understanding the affected neurovascular structures [2].

Ophthalmologists and neurologists whose patients present with an intermittent fluttering ocular sensation should perform an MRI investigation for ipsilateral vascular compression of the trochlear nerve [2]. Furthermore, in the lateral SC-IT approach, neurosurgeons should be aware that sacrificing the tentorial bridging veins might cause venous infarction or hemorrhage in the cerebellum [2]. The final indication that SOM is curable by MVD will require the recognition of the condition and its successful treatment [2].

References

1. Hoyt WF, Keane JR. Superior oblique myokymia. Report and discussion on five cases of benign intermittent uniocular microtremor. Arch Ophthalmol. 1970;84(4):461–7.
2. Noro S, Seo Y, Honjo K, et al. Lateral supracerebellar infratentorial approach for superior oblique myokymia: a case. Oper Neurosurg. 2022;22(3):101–5.
3. Borgman CJ. Topical timolol in the treatment of monocular oscillopsia secondary to superior oblique myokymia: a review. J Optom. 2014;7(2):68–74.
4. Susac JO, Smith JL, Schatz NJ. Superior oblique myokymia. Arch Neurol. 1973;29(6):432–4.
5. Frens DB. Superior oblique myokymia: a treatable cause of monocular diplopia. Wis Med J. 1980;79(4):30–1.
6. Ruttum MS, Harris GJ. Superior oblique myectomy and trochlear resection for superior oblique myokymia. Am J Ophthalmol. 2009;148(4):563–5.
7. Bringewald PR. Superior oblique myokymia. Arch Neurol. 1983;40(8):526.
8. Samii M, Rosahl SK, Carvalho GA, Krzizok T. Microvascular decompression for superior oblique myokymia: first experience. Case report. J Neurosurg. 1998;89(6):1020–4.
9. Kawasaki T, Fujitsu K, Ichikawa T, et al. Superior oblique myokymia: a case report of surgical treatment, review of the literature, and consideration of surgical approach. World Neurosurg. 2019;131(17):197–9.
10. Hashimoto M, Ohtsuka K, Suzuki Y, Minamida Y, Houkin K. Superior oblique myokymia caused by vascular compression. J Neuroophthalmol. 2004;24(3):237–9.
11. Mikami T, Minamida Y, Ohtsuka K, Houkin K. Resolution of superior oblique myokymia following microvascular decompression of trochlear nerve. Acta Neurochir. 2005;147(9):1005–6.
12. Fam MD, Scott C, Forster A, Kamel MH. Microvascular decompression for superior oblique myokymia: case report. Br J Neurosurg. 2014;28(4):552–5.
13. Yousry I, Moriggl B, Dieterich M, Naidich TP, Schmid UD, Yousry TA. MR anatomy of the proximal cisternal segment of the trochlear nerve: neurovascular relationships and landmarks. Radiology. 2002;223(1):31–8.
14. Jannetta PJ, Abbasy M, Maroon JC, Ramos FM, Albin MS. Etiology and definitive microsurgical treatment of hemifacial spasm. Operative techniques and results in 47 patients. J Neurosurg. 1977;47(3):321–8.
15. Nielsen VK. Electrophysiology of the facial nerve in hemifacial spasm: ectopic/ephaptic excitation. Muscle Nerve. 1985;8(7):545–55.
16. Yousry I, Dieterich M, Naidich TP, Schmid UD, Yousry TA. Superior oblique myokymia: magnetic resonance imaging support for the neurovascular compression hypothesis. Ann Neurol. 2002;51(3):361–8.

17. Sathyan S, Antony RC. Superior oblique myokymia: some novel observations. Middle East Afr J Ophthalmol. 2017;24(3):162–4.
18. Kommerell G, Schaubele G. Superior oblique myokymia. An electromyographical analysis. Trans Ophthalmol Soc UK. 1980;100(4):504–6.
19. De Sa LC, Good WV, Hoyt CS. Surgical management of myokymia of the superior oblique muscle. Am J Ophthalmol. 1992;114(6):693–6.
20. Brazis PW, Miller NR, Henderer JD. The natural history and results of treatment of superior oblique myokymia. Arch Ophthalmol. 1994;112(8):1063–7.
21. Hart MG, Santarius T, Kirollos RW. How I do it—pineal surgery: supracerebellar infratentorial versus occipital transtentorial. Acta Neurochir. 2013;155:463–7.
22. Hernesniemi J, Romani R, Albayrak BS, et al. Microsurgical management of pineal region lesions: personal experience with 119 patients. Surg Neurol. 2008;70:576–83.
23. Kodera T, Bozinov O, Surucu O, Ulrich NH, Burkhardt JK, Bertalanffy H. Neurosurgical venous considerations for tumors of the pineal region resected using the infratentorial supracerebellar approach. J Clin Neurosci. 2011;18:1481–5.
24. Rey-Dios R, Cohen-Gadol AA. A surgical technique to expand the operative corridor for supracerebellar infratentorial approaches: technical note. Acta Neurochir. 2013;155:1895–900.
25. Jakola AS, Bartek J Jr, Mathiesen T. Venous complications in supraerebellar infratentorial approach. Acta Neurochir. 2013;155:477–8.
26. Matsushima T, Fukui M, Suzuki S, Rhoton AL Jr. The microsurgical anatomy of the infaratentorial lateral supracerebellar approach to the trigeminal nerve for tic douloureux. Neurosurgery. 1989;24:890–5.
27. Muthukumar N, Palaniappan P. Tentorial venous sinuses: an anatomic study. Neurosurgery. 1998;42:363–71.
28. Rhoton AL Jr. The posterior fossa veins. Neurosurgery. 2000;47(3 Suppl):S131–53.
29. Ueyam T, Al-Mefty O, Tamaki N. Bridging veins on the tentorial surface of the cerebellum: a microsurgical anatomic study and operative considerations. Neurosurgery. 1998;43:1137–45.
30. Matsuo S, Baydin S, Güngör A, et al. Midline and off-midline infratentorial supracerebellar approaches to the pineal gland. J Neurosurg. 2017;126:1984–94.

Microvascular Decompression for Trigeminal Neuralgia Secondary to Vertebrobasilar Dolichoectasia

21

Francesco Signorelli, Fabio Zeoli,
and Massimiliano Visocchi

21.1 Introduction

Trigeminal neuralgia (TN) due to vasculonervous conflict is a common chronic pain disorder characterized by recurrent episodes of electric shock-like or stabbing pain affecting the dermatomal distribution of trigeminal nerve [1–3]. This condition is almost always unilateral [4]; it manifests more commonly on the left side and within the territories of the maxillary (V2) and mandibular (V3) branches of the trigeminal nerve [5]. The incidence of TN is higher in women and increases with age [6]. The mostly implicated blood vessels responsible for compression of the trigeminal root are the superior cerebellar artery, in about 75% of cases, the anterior inferior cerebellar artery, in 10%, or a vein, in 7% [1, 7]. Less commonly, TN may be secondary to vertebrobasilar dolichoectasia (VBD).

21.2 Trigeminal Neuralgia Secondary to Vertebrobasilar Dolichoectasia

Vertebrobasilar dolichoectasia (VBD; from the Greek *dolicho*, "elongation," and *ectasia*, "dilatation") is an uncommon cause of trigeminal neuralgia (TN).

VBD, as originally described by Smoker et al., is a rare cerebrovascular disease characterized by ectatic, elongated, and tortuous vertebrobasilar arteries (VBA) [8]. The abnormal arteries may sometimes compress, directly or indirectly—thorough displacements of adjacent vessels [6]—the root of the trigeminal nerve resulting in TN [9].

Diagnostic criteria, firstly proposed by Ubogu et al. [10], include basilar artery (BA) or vertebral artery (VA) diameter > 4.5 mm, deviation of any portion >10 mm from the shortest expected course, BA length > 29.5 mm or intracranial VA length > 23.5 mm; also, for the BA, when bifurcation is above the suprasellar cistern or if any segment lies adjacent to the margin of the clivus or dorsum sellae, elongation is considered to be present [11].

F. Signorelli · F. Zeoli · M. Visocchi (✉)
Institute of Neurosurgery, Fondazione Policlinico Universitario A. Gemelli IRCCS, Catholic University, Rome, Italy

S.-T. Li et al. (eds.), *Microvascular Decompression Surgery*,
https://doi.org/10.1007/978-981-96-0767-9_21

According to recent studies, VBD-induced TN accounts for 2% to 7.7% of all cases of TN [1, 12–15].

In TN secondary to VBD, pain occurs more commonly, but not exclusively, on the left side, and left predominance may be related to hemodynamic and anatomical factors. VA arises from the subclavian artery; since the right subclavian artery originates from the brachiocephalic trunk, while the left originates directly from the aortic arch, and blood flow and shear stress are higher in the left VA than the right one [9]. As with other forms of classical TN, medical therapy—mainly with carbamazepine [16] or oxcarbazepine—is the first-line treatment in VBD-associated TN. When medical therapy fails, surgical options such as trigeminal rhizotomy, percutaneous thermocoagulation, mechanical balloon compression, microvascular decompression (MVD), and gamma knife radiosurgery (GKRS) can be considered [15, 17]. Among these, MVD is currently proposed as the first surgical choice for the treatment of TN caused by VBD [6, 18–20], as it is nondestructive and addresses the vascular etiology.

This technique, firstly described by Jannetta in 1967 [21], aims at isolating the trigeminal nerve from the vessel responsible for compression by placing a piece of material between the vessel and the nerve. However, when the artery involved is a dolichoectatic VBA, the usual procedure is technically more challenging; dolichoectatic arteries presents with atherosclerosis, abnormal course, increased diameter, low elasticity, and limited mobility. These factors significantly amplify the complexity of the surgery, particularly during vessel displacement, posing potential risks such as plaque dislodgement, rupture of branch vessels, and vasospasm [22]. Consequently, achieving a precise and clear dissection between the VBA and the arachnoid surrounding the trigeminal nerve is not only crucial for the safety of the surgical procedure but is also essential in determining a complete relocation of the VBA away from the trigeminal nerve. Several studies have demonstrated the superiority of MVD over alternative surgical procedures in ensuring a longer pain-free period (without medication) while keeping a low rate of complications [1, 23–25]. However, there are few reports on the efficacy and safety of MVD in case of VBD. In a random-effects meta-analysis by Di carlo et al. [26], which included 167 patients with TN attributed to VBD, the immediate postsurgery pain relief rate was notably high at approximately 97%, with a very slight decrease to 92.9%, at the last follow-up (55 months). Comparable results were found in the retrospective analysis by Yu et al. [9] and Inoue et al. [18].

Recent advancements in radiosurgery have revolutionized traditional surgical approaches, with GKRS emerging as a promising minimally invasive procedure for TN, whether associated with VBD or not. However, studies have indicated that the pain control rates achieved with GKRS were inferior compared to MVD [27, 28]. Over the past decades, several variations of surgical decompression have been investigated to separate the offending dolichoectatic VBA from the compressed trigeminal nerve. These can be broadly classified into the interposition and transposition technique. The former, which is the traditional method and is widely used in patients with neurovascular compression syndrome due to small vessels such as the superior cerebellar artery (SCA) and the anterior inferior cerebellar artery (AICA), involves the insertion of an implant between the offending vessel and the nerve; the latter method involves repositioning the VBA away from the nerve using biomedical glue [29], Teflon slings or pads [30, 31], and aneurysm clips [32]. The interposition technique remains a simpler and safer option but might inadequately address severe pulsatile compression in case of dolichoectatic VBA. On the other hand, the transposition method, while potentially more effective in reducing pulsatile pressure from the offending artery, demands meticulous care to avoid complications such as brainstem infarction or injury to perforator arteries [33]. A recent meta-analysis reviewed 14 studies comprising 306 patients, emphasizing the high efficacy of both approaches. Immediate postoperative pain relief (BNI I-II) was achieved in 97% of cases with interposition and 98% with transposition, with comparable long-term outcomes (96% vs. 95% at last follow-up). However, the transposition technique demonstrated a higher rate of postoperative complications, such as permanent facial hypoesthesia and hearing impairment, likely due to the intricate manipulation required for vessel repositioning [34].

21.3 Illustrative Case

A 62-year-old male patient presented to our department with a 7-year history of paroxysmal, lancinating right-sided trigeminal neuralgia in maxillary (V2) and mandibular (V3) territories.

Brain magnetic resonance imaging (MRI) with gadolinium contrast revealed the presence of an abnormality of the right vertebral artery (VA) (with no visualization of V4 segment) and a dolichoectatic basilar artery (BA) with a tortuous course causing at the right cerebellopontine angle (CPA) a mechanical compression on the trigeminal nerve (Fig. 21.1).

A right retrosigmoid approach was performed under general anesthesia, with the patient placed in a left park bench position. After CPA and trigeminal nerve exposition, arachnoid dissection revealed the dolichoectatic BA compressing the right anterolateral region of brainstem and the trigeminal nerve root. Microvascular decompression of the dolichoectatic BA was obtained using the interposition technique: Two layers of Teflon, held with fibrin glue, were placed between the artery and the nervous structures. Particular care was taken to avoid injury of the artery during the vascular microdissection, given the potentially fragile vessel walls in VBD. Then we performed internal neurolysis of V2 and V3. Dandy vein was preserved (Fig. 21.2). Pain completely resolved

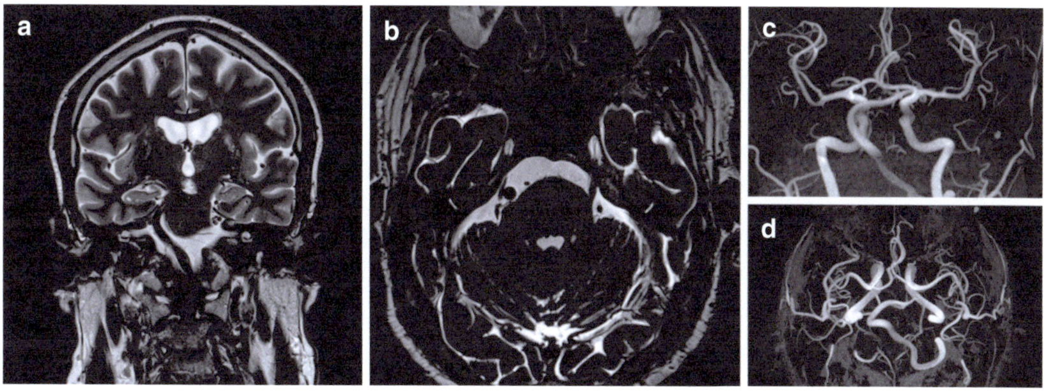

Fig. 21.1 Magnetic resonance imaging showing the neurovascular conflict (**a**, **b**) and the vertebrobasilar dolichoectasia (**c**, **d**). **a**: coronal plane, T2-weighted sequence; **b**: axial plane, 3D-CISS sequence; **c**: coronal plane, MR angiogram; **d**: sagittal plan, MR angiogram

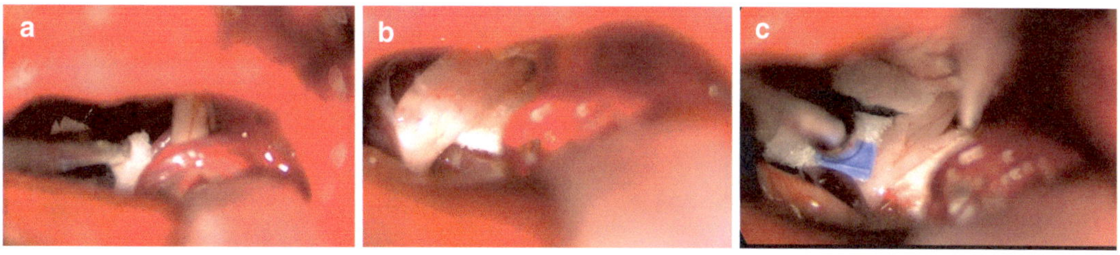

Fig. 21.2 Intraoperative images showing vascular compression (**a**), decompression by means of teflon (**b**) and neurolysis (nerve "combing") (**c**)

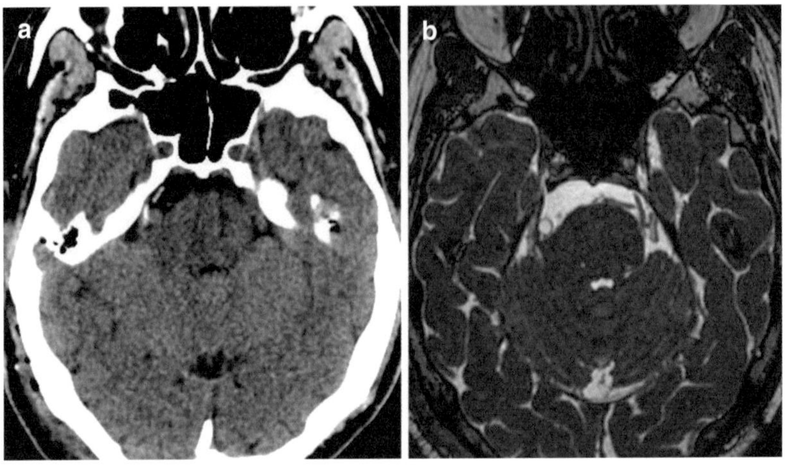

Fig. 21.3 Postoperative CT scan (**a**) and MRI T2-weighted sequence, axial plane (**b**)

after surgery and no neurological deficits were reported. Postoperative brain computed tomography imaging and MRI (Fig. 21.3) showed satisfactory surgical outcomes and excluded bleeding complications. The patient was discharged on day 6 after surgery. The patient reported satisfactory pain control at 1-month follow-up. Four weeks after surgery, medication was completely and definitively stopped. No pain recurrence and/or sensory abnormalities were found at 3–/6–/12-months follow-up, and the patient is still on a medication-free status.

21.4 Conclusions

Vascular compression is a frequent and treatable cause of essential trigeminal neuralgia. Even in the rare and complex case of a dolichoectatic vertebrobasilar artery, microsurgical decompression method can provide excellent long-term outcomes in patients with TN who do not respond to medication.

References

1. Apra C, Lefaucheur JP, Le Guerinel C, Caroline A, Jean-Pascal L, Guérinel CL. Microvascular decompression is an effective therapy for trigeminal neuralgia due to dolichoectatic basilar artery compression: case reports and literature review. Neurosurg Rev. 2017;40(4):577. https://hal.sorbonne-universite.fr/hal-01992001.
2. Sindou M, Keravel Y, Abdennebi B, Szapiro J. Neurosurgical treatment of trigeminal neuralgia. Direct approach of percutaneous method? Neurochirurgie. 1987;33(2):89–111.
3. Leland Rogers C, Shetter AG, Fiedler JA, Smith KA, Han PP, Speiser BL, et al. Gamma knife radiosurgery for trigeminal neuralgia: the initial experience of The Barrow Neurological Institute. Int J Radiat Oncol Biol Phys. 2000;47:1013–9.
4. Headache Classification Committee of the International Headache Society (IHS). The International Classification of Headache Disorders, 3rd edition. Cephalalgia. 2018;38(1):1–211.
5. Cruccu G, Di Stefano G, Truini A. Trigeminal neuralgia. N Engl J Med. 2020;383(8):754–62. https://doi.org/10.1056/NEJMra1914484.
6. Zheng W, Wang L, Wang H, Zhou H, Du Q. Trigeminal neuralgia caused by vertebrobasilar dolichoectasia: efficacy of stepwise decompression technique. Acta Neurochir. 2023;165(10):3019–26.
7. Bašić KV. Accommodation to diagnosis of trigeminal neuralgia. Acta Clin Croat. 2017;56:157–61.
8. Smoker WRK, Corbett JJ, Gentry LR, Keyes WD, Price MJ, McKuske S. High-resolution computed tomography of the basilar artery: 2. Vertebrobasilar dolichoectasia: clinical-pathologic correlation and review. AJNR Am J Neuroradiol. 1986;7:61–72.
9. Yu F, Yin J, Lu PG, Zhao ZY, Zhang YQ, Men XZ. Microvascular decompression by interposition method for treatment of trigeminal neuralgia due to vertebrobasilar dolichoectasia: a retrospective single-center study. Neurosurg Rev. 2022;45(4):2709–15.
10. Ubogu EE, Zaidat OO. Vertebrobasilar dolichoectasia diagnosed by magnetic resonance angiography and risk of stroke and death: a cohort study [internet]. J Neurol Neurosurg Psychiatry. 2004;75:22–6. www.jnnp.com.
11. Stone JL, Lichtor T, Crowell RM. Microvascular sling decompression for trigeminal neuralgia secondary to ectatic vertebrobasilar compression. J Neurosurg. 1993;79(6):943–5.

12. Yang XS, Li ST, Zhong J, Zhu J, Du Q, Zhou QM, et al. Microvascular decompression on patients with trigeminal neuralgia caused by ectatic vertebrobasilar artery complex: technique notes. Acta Neurochir. 2012;154(5):793–7.
13. Park KJ, Kondziolka D, Kano H, Berkowitz O, Ahmed SF, Liu X, et al. Outcomes of gamma knife surgery for trigeminal neuralgia secondary to vertebrobasilar ectasia. J Neurosurg. 2012;116(1):73–81.
14. Ma X, Sun X, Yao J, Ni S, Gong J, Wang J, et al. Clinical analysis of trigeminal neuralgia caused by vertebrobasilar dolichoectasia. Neurosurg Rev. 2013;36(4):573–8.
15. Chai S, Xu H, Wang Q, Li J, Wang J, Wang Y, et al. Microvascular decompression for trigeminal neuralgia caused by vertebrobasilar dolichoectasia: interposition technique versus transposition technique. Acta Neurochir. 2020;162(11):2811–21.
16. Gambeta E, Chichorro JG, W. Zamponi G. Trigeminal neuralgia: an overview from pathophysiology to pharmacological treatments. Mol Pain. 2020;16:1744806920901890.
17. Vanaclocha V, Herrera JM, Martínez-Gómez D, Rivera-Paz M, Calabuig-Bayo C, Vanaclocha L. Is there a safe and effective way to treat trigeminal neuralgia associated with vertebrobasilar dolichoectasia? Presentation of 8 cases and literature review. In: World Neurosurgery, vol. 96. Amsterdam: Elsevier; 2016. p. 516–29.
18. Inoue T, Shitara S, Goto Y, Prasetya M, Fukushima T. Microvascular decompression for trigeminal neuralgia attributable to the vertebrobasilar artery: decompression technique and significance of separation from the nerve root. Acta Neurochir. 2021;163(4):1037–43. https://doi.org/10.1007/s00701-020-04563-8.
19. Honey CM, Kaufmann AM. Trigeminal neuralgia due to vertebrobasilar artery compression. World Neurosurg. 2018;118:e155–60.
20. El-Ghandour NMF. Microvascular decompression in the treatment of trigeminal neuralgia caused by vertebrobasilar ectasia. Neurosurgery. 2010;67(2):330–7.
21. Jannetta PJ. Arterial compression of the trigeminal nerve at the pons in patients with trigeminal neuralgia. J Neurosurg. 2007;107(1):216–37.
22. Shulev 2020.
23. Kraemer JL, de Pereira Filho A, de David G, de Faria MB. Vertebrobasilar dolichoectasia as a cause of trigeminal neuralgia: the role of microvascular decompression. Case report. Arq Neuropsiquiatr. 2006;64(1):128–31.
24. Shi J, Qian Y, Han W, Dong B, Mao Y, Cao J, et al. Risk factors for outcomes after microvascular decompression for trigeminal neuralgia. World Neurosurg. 2020;136:e559–66.
25. Wei Y, Pu C, Li N, Cai Y, Shang H, Zhao W. Long-term therapeutic effect of microvascular decompression for trigeminal neuralgia: Kaplan-meier analysis in a consecutive series of 425 patients. Turk Neurosurg. 2018;28:88–93.
26. Di Carlo DT, Benedetto N, Marani W, Montemurro N, Perrini P. Microvascular decompression for trigeminal neuralgia due to vertebrobasilar artery compression: a systematic review and meta-analysis. Neurosurg Rev. 2022;45(1):285–94.
27. Tripathi M, Mohindra S, Madan R, Ahuja CK, Batish A, Kaur R, et al. Radiosurgery for trigeminal neuralgia secondary to dolichoectatic vessels: case series and review of literature. J Neurosci Rural Pract. 2021;12:455–60.
28. Park KJ, Kondziolka D, Berkowitz O, Kano H, Novotny J, Niranjan A, et al. Repeat gamma knife radiosurgery for trigeminal neuralgia. Neurosurgery. 2012;70(2).
29. Liu J, Wu G, Xiang H, Liu R, Li F, Hei B, et al. Long-Term Retrospective Analysis of Microvascular Decompression in Patients With Recurrent Trigeminal Neuralgia. Front Neurol. 2020;11.
30. Yang XS, Li ST, Zhong J, Zhu J, Du Q, Zhou QM, et al. Microvascular decompression on patients with trigeminal neuralgia caused by ectatic vertebrobasilar artery complex: Technique notes. Acta Neurochir (Wien). 2012;154(5):793–7.
31. Yamahata H, Tokimura H, Hanaya R, Tajitsu K, Hirabaru M, Yamagami M, et al. Microvascular decompression for trigeminal neuralgia due to compression by the vertebral artery: Report of 3 cases. Minimally Invasive Neurosurgery. 2011;54(2):79–82.
32. Lin CF, Chen HH, Hernesniemi J, Lee CC, Liao CH, Chen SC, et al. An easy adjustable method of ectatic vertebrobasilar artery transposition for microvascular decompression. Clin Neurol Neurosurg. 2012;114(7):951–6.
33. Visocchi M, Zeoli F, Signorelli F. Microvascular Decompression for Trigeminal Neuralgia Secondary to Vertebrobasilar Dolichoectasia: Review of the Literature and Illustrative Case. J Clin Med. 2024;13(21):6342.
34. Signorelli F, Zeoli F, Rastegar V, Beccia F, Caronna R, Visocchi M. Interposition versus transposition technique in microvascular decompression for trigeminal neuralgia secondary to vertebrobasilar dolichoectasia: a systematic review and pooled meta-analysis. Front Neurol. 2024;15.

22 Combined Hypoglossal-Facial and Descendens Hypoglossi-Hypoglossal Anastomoses (HFDHHA) in Treating Severe Facial Paralysis: How We Do It

Yinda Tang and Shi-Ting Li

22.1 Overview

Facial paralysis significantly impacts the quality of life and mental well-being of patients. Patients classified as severe (House-Brackmann Grade V–VI) typically require surgical intervention [1, 2]. Several surgical treatment options exist depending on etiology, duration, severity, and patient preferences. Among these, facial nerve substitution/transplantation procedures are suitable for patients with damage closer to the central segment of the facial nerve, with the distal part of the facial nerve still intact and facial muscle motor endplates functionally viable [3, 4].

Common donor nerves include the hypoglossal nerve, accessory nerve, and masseteric nerve. Among these, the hypoglossal-facial anastomosis (HFA) is the most extensively used technique [3, 5–8]. Traditional HFA involves complete severing of the distal end of the hypoglossal nerve and direct end-to-end anastomosis with the extratemporal facial nerve trunk (eFNT) [7]. This method uses the main trunk of the hypoglossal nerve as the donor nerve for reinnervating facial muscles. It offers advantages such as an adequate amount of donor nerve fibers, similarity in thickness between the donor and recipient nerves, and proximity in anatomical locations, ensuring precise facial nerve functional recovery. Recent studies suggest its superiority in central reshaping. However, inevitable disconnection of the hypoglossal nerve leads to functional impairments in the ipsilateral tongue muscles, potentially causing partial tongue atrophy and significantly affecting chewing, swallowing, and speech functions [9, 10].

To address the limitations of traditional HFA, several modified techniques have been proposed. These include: (1) "interpositional-jump graft technique" utilizing a free nerve (such as the sural or great auricular nerve) to bridge between the hypoglossal and facial nerves via end-to-side and end-to-end anastomoses respectively, avoiding complete disconnection of the hypoglossal nerve. However, this technique involves two anastomoses, decreases the quantity of donor fibers, thus affecting the effectiveness of facial nerve function reconstruction and necessitating

Y. Tang
XinHua Hospital, Shanghai JiaoTong University School of Medicine, Shanghai, China

S.-T. Li (✉)
Department of Neurosurgery, XinHua Hospital, Shanghai JiaoTong University School of Medicine, Shanghai, China
e-mail: lsting66@164.com

S.-T. Li et al. (eds.), *Microvascular Decompression Surgery*,
https://doi.org/10.1007/978-981-96-0767-9_22

sacrifice of another nerve for the bridging, resulting in increased surgical trauma [5, 11, 12]; (2) "split technique" involving longitudinal splitting of the hypoglossal nerve to use part of its fibers for anastomosis with the facial nerve, which significantly damages nonlinearly distributed hypoglossal nerve fibers [5, 13, 14]; (3) "reflection method" involves revealing the vertical segment of the facial nerve inside the temporal bone by grinding the mastoid process and then relocating it downward, allowing direct end-to-side anastomosis with the hypoglossal nerve. Although this method overcomes some deficiencies of the interpositional-jump graft technique, it faces challenges due to insufficient donor nerve fibers of the hypoglossal nerve, and the additional difficulty and risk of complications associated with mastoid process drilling [15–18]. Therefore, innovating new modified techniques that ensure optimal effectiveness in restoring facial paralysis from traditional HFA while avoiding tongue muscle functional impairment remains a hot topic in this field.

In 1924, Frazier reported a successful case of repairing the recurrent laryngeal nerve using the superior root of ansa cervicalis, also called the descendens hypoglossi (DH), confirming the safety and feasibility of using the DH as a donor nerve source [19]. Following this, multiple similar reports both domestically and internationally confirmed satisfactory results without related complications of the DH disconnection [20–22]. This success led to exploration in the field of facial paralysis repair. The concept of using the DH as a donor for the facial nerve was proposed as early as 1979 [23]. Subsequently, some scholars conducted clinical practices and explorations [24–28], but the results revealed that the best outcome of this method achieved only grade IV in facial paralysis recovery, with a recovery rate of merely 44.4%, far below traditional HFA [26].

Since 1959, some other scholars have attempted to repair the distal stump of the hypoglossal nerve after HFA with the DH [29–32]. In this approach, the DH, mainly derived from the anterior branch of the C1 nerve, is disconnected and then anastomosed with the distal end of the hypoglossal nerve, thus utilizing the fibers of the cervical plexus to reconstruct the tongue function. Although there seems to be a trend for better results in the more recent studies, likely due to technical advances in microsurgery, nevertheless, the effectiveness and safety of this modification have not been further verified. In this context, the neurosurgical team at Shanghai Xinhua Hospital, led by Dr. Shiting Li, continues to develop and optimize this surgical approach, named combined hypoglossal-facial and descendens hypoglossi-hypoglossal anastomoses (HFDHHA). Over the past 5 years, our team has successfully performed this surgery on over a 100 patients with severe facial paralysis, resulting in excellent recovery of facial paralysis symptoms (House-Brackmann Grade II-III) without noticeable atrophy or functional impairment in the tongue muscles. The results of a recent randomized clinical trial conducted by our team [33] confirmed that this combined procedure not only ensures optimal facial nerve repair but also improves tongue muscle function via the cervical plexus, suggesting its potential for widespread use, thus, the HFDHHA constitutes an innovative modification to the classic HFA technique. In this chapter, we will introduce the relevant anatomy, surgical indications, and details of this procedure, as well as related issues such as perioperative management and postoperative follow-up.

22.2 Surgical Anatomy for the Procedure

The facial nerve, as the seventh cranial nerve, comprises special visceral motor, general visceral motor, general somatic afferent, and special visceral sensory fibers. Among these, the latter three form a small intermediate nerve in the posterior cranial fossa, while the special visceral motor fibers that innervate the facial expression muscles constitute a single trunk. This trunk emerges through the stylomastoid foramen and courses anteriorly between the superficial and deep layers of the parotid gland, branching to supply the facial expression muscles. The eFNT is defined as the segment of the facial nerve from its exit at the stylomastoid foramen to its division into superior and inferior branches upon entering the parotid gland [34, 35]. Although this segment of the facial nerve remains deep, it lacks bony coverage, making it easily exposed using adjacent anatomical landmarks and appropriate dissection techniques, thus being an ideal site for nerve anastomosis.

The hypoglossal nerve, the 12th cranial nerve, comprises general somatic motor fibers. After exiting the hypoglossal canal, the hypoglossal nerve courses posteriorly and laterally, emerging behind the inferior ganglion of the vagus nerve, between the internal carotid artery and internal jugular vein. Subsequently, it travels along the surface of the internal carotid artery and the deep aspect of the posterior belly of the digastric muscle. Based on its extracranial course, it can be divided into a descending segment, a horizontal segment, and an ascending segment [36, 37]. The descending segment refers to the course from the exit of the hypoglossal nerve from the cranium to the anterior margin of the sternocleidomastoid muscle. Afterward, the hypoglossal nerve travels forward horizontally between the styloid process and the posterior belly of the digastric muscle, known as the horizontal segment. Finally, the hypoglossal nerve turns anteriorly to innervate the muscles of the tongue, branching into several divisions. This final portion is known as the ascending segment. During the surgery, the exposure range must include both the descending and horizontal segments to obtain a sufficient length of the hypoglossal nerve for tension-free anastomosis.

The ansa cervicalis is composed of two roots, superior and inferior, typically including fibers from the anterior branches of the C1–C3 spinal nerves [38]. Usually, a portion of the fibers from the anterior branch of the C1 nerve follows the hypoglossal nerve, namely the DH, and then leaves it inside the carotid triangle, running inferiorly along the carotid sheath, constituting the donor nerve for anastomosis with the hypoglossal nerve in the HFDHHA procedure. Although the number of axons in the DH is limited, effective preservation of tongue muscle function can be achieved after anastomosis between the DH and the distal end of the hypoglossal nerve [33].

22.3 Surgical Indications

This procedure is suitable for severe facial paralysis (graded as V–VI in the House-Brackmann scale), caused by various factors, and provided the following conditions are met:

1. The injury site is proximal to the division where the facial nerve branches into upper and lower branches, with no damage to the facial nerve bifurcation and its distal branches.
2. Stable insertion potentials are detectable by electroneurophysiological detection in the affected side's facial muscles.
3. Normal preoperative functionality of both sides of the hypoglossal nerve.
4. The patient expresses a strong desire for treatment.

22.4 Preoperative Evaluation

Similar to all facial rehabilitation surgeries, adequate preoperative evaluation is essential when applying this procedure. This includes gathering medical history, physical examination, imaging studies, and electroneurophysiological examinations. The medical history should emphasize precise disease progression, the course of the disease, and previous treatments. Prolonged disease duration or a history of malignant tumors in the head or face involving radiation or chemotherapy may lead to atrophy and degeneration of the eFNT, making surgery unfeasible. During the physical examination, facial recordings should be performed after obtaining informed consent from the patient, serving as a reference for therapeutic follow-ups. This should encompass static and dynamic facial expressions, recording various facial movements promptly using assessment scales. Imaging studies involve high-resolution temporal bone CT and head-neck MRI to comprehensively depict various regions along the course of the facial nerve. If a specific cause, such as a tumor, is identified as the etiology for facial paralysis, consideration for concomitant causative treatments for facial paralysis is necessary. Electroneurophysiological examinations encompass facial electroneurography (ENoG), electromyography (EMG), insertion potentials, blink reflexes, F-waves, and abnormal muscle response (AMR). Following a comprehensive preoperative assessment, thorough communication with the patient and their family is crucial to understand the patient's preferences before determining the treatment plan.

22.5 Surgical Procedure

22.5.1 Positioning, Incision, and Electroneurophysiological Monitoring

The patient should lie supine with a sandbag under the affected shoulder. The head is turned to the unaffected side, and the neck of the affected side is extended as far as possible and secured with tape. Identifiable bony landmarks include the mastoid tip and the angle of the mandible, while identifiable soft tissue landmarks include the anterior border of the sternocleidomastoid muscle. The superficial course of the external jugular vein crossing the sternocleidomastoid muscle and the projection of the posterior belly of the digastric muscle roughly coincide with a line drawn from the mastoid tip to the angle of the mandible. The eFNT and the main trunk of the hypoglossal nerve are located approximately above and below this line, respectively, and these structures are marked. Needle electrodes are inserted into the frontalis, orbicularis oculi, zygomaticus, orbicularis oris, depressor anguli oris, and tongue muscles for electroneurophysiological monitoring (Fig. 22.1).

22.5.2 Soft Tissue Dissection in the Neck

The skin, subcutaneous tissue, and superficial cervical fascia are incised. The external jugular vein is ligated and dissected while the greater auricular nerve is preserved, typically located about 1 cm above the vein. The investing fascia of the sternocleidomastoid muscle (the superficial layer of the deep cervical fascia) is dissected to reveal the muscle fibers, which are separated forward to the anterior margin of the sternocleidomastoid. A transverse incision of approximately 2 cm is made in the mastoid segment of the sternocleidomastoid tendon, which is then peeled away from the bone, allowing the muscle to be retracted backward. This exposes

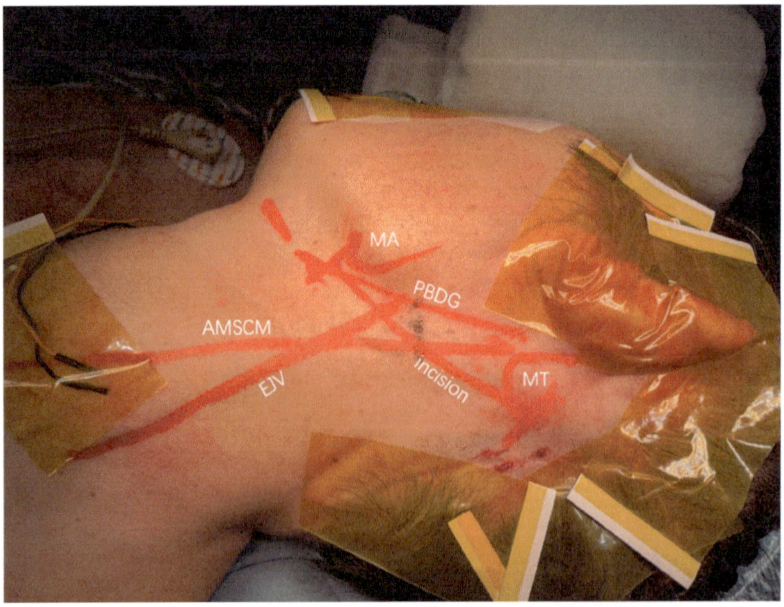

Fig. 22.1 Positioning and incision. *AMSCM* anterior margin of the sternocleidomastoid muscle, *EJV* external jugular vein, *MA* mandibular angle, *MT* mastoid tip, *PBDG* posterior belly of the digastric muscle

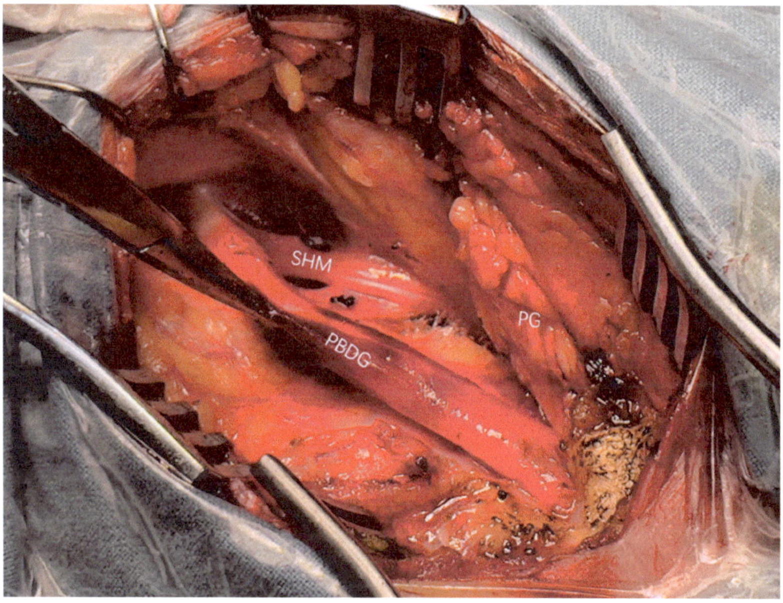

Fig. 22.2 Soft tissue dissection. *PBDG* posterior belly of the digastric muscle, *PG* parotid gland, *SHM* stylohyoid muscle

the upper end of the posterior belly of the digastric muscle along the retromastoid notch. Dissection is continued along its axis until the posterior belly of the digastric muscle is fully exposed and freed. Two mastoid retractors are placed to secure the parotid gland and submandibular gland anteriorly and the sternocleidomastoid muscle posteriorly, centering the posterior belly of the digastric muscle in the surgical field (Fig. 22.2).

22.5.3 Exposure of the Hypoglossal Nerve

The posterior belly of the digastric muscle is pulled forward using a rubber band, which intersects with the stylohyoid muscle at its lower end near the hyoid bone, serving as a relatively fixed landmark for the distal course of the horizontal segment of the hypoglossal nerve. The fascia at this point is separated, allowing for relatively easy exposure of the hypoglossal nerve. If exposure proves difficult, guidance from intraoperative electroneurophysiology may be beneficial. It should be noted that several veins might crisscross in this area, which should be preserved as much as possible. Exposure is continued approximately 1 cm distally to observe the horizontal segment of the hypoglossal nerve's main trunk, which branches into the various tongue muscles, marking the furthest end of the harvested hypoglossal nerve main trunk (Fig. 22.3).

22.5.4 Exposure of the DH

Dissection is reversed along the main trunk of the hypoglossal nerve until its proximal descending segment is reached, exposing the origin of the DH. This point marks the nearest end of the harvested hypoglossal nerve main trunk and serves as the starting point for continued anterograde exposure of the DH. The DH is relatively delicate, running posteriorly to the main trunk of the hypoglossal nerve at an angle of about 30°, with variations in the coursing plane, requiring a combination of blunt and sharp dissection. Nerve fibers and surrounding blood vessels are protected. The length of the exposed DH should be sufficient for tension-free anastomosis with the distal end of the hypoglossal nerve. Therefore, based on the length of the hypoglossal nerve determined in previous steps, the exposure range of the DH should be increased by approximately 1 to 2 cm (Fig. 22.4).

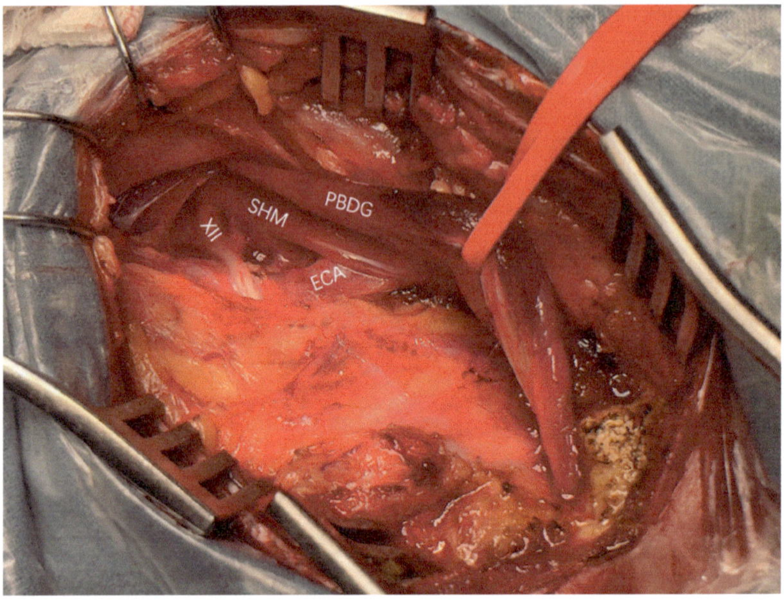

Fig. 22.3 Exposure of the hypoglossal nerve. *ECA* external carotid artery, *PBDG* posterior belly of the digastric muscle, *SHM* stylohyoid muscle, *XII* hypoglossal nerve

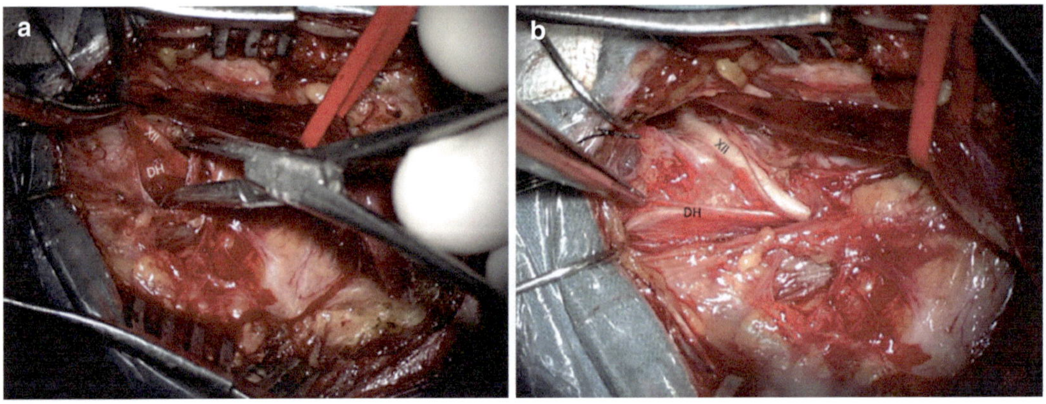

Fig. 22.4 Exposure of the DH. (**a**) Reverse dissection to expose the origin of the DH; (**b**) Continued anterograde exposure of the ansa cervicalis. *DH* descendens hypoglossi, *XII* hypoglossal nerve

22.5.5 Exposure of the eFNT

The posterior belly of the digastric muscle is pulled backward, focusing the surgical field on the mastoid tip and the upper end of the posterior belly of the digastric muscle near the posterior wall of the parotid gland. Low-power coagulation and dissection of the parotid fascia in this area reveal the posterior auricular artery, which usually crosses superficially over the facial nerve trunk, serving as a reliable anatomical landmark. This exposure reveals the eFNT. Subsequently, the surrounding parotid tissue is dissected bluntly along the long axis of the facial nerve to increase the length of exposure. The surrounding parotid tissue is trimmed to enhance the freedom of downward flipping of the facial nerve. The accompanying posterior auricular artery should be preserved as much as possible. In some cases where the eFNT is relatively short, partial drilling of the mastoid tip and removal of the fascial soft tissue around the stylomastoid foramen may be performed to increase its length (Fig. 22.5).

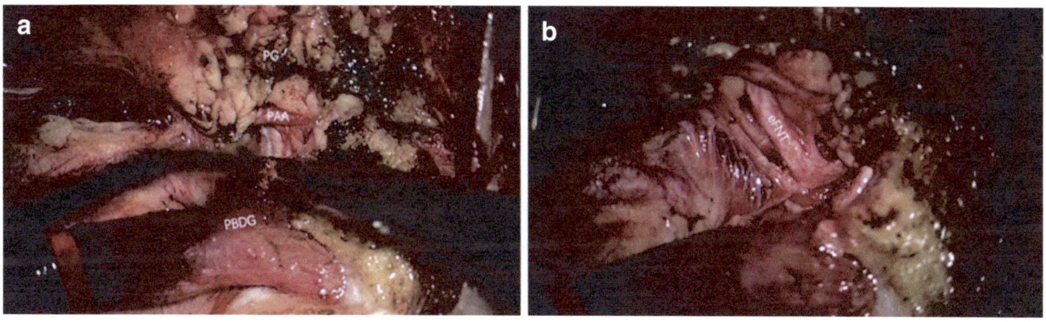

Fig. 22.5 Exposure of the facial nerve. (**a**) opening the parotid gland to expose the facial nerve; (**b**) Increasing the length of exposed facial nerve trunk. *eFNT* extratemporal facial nerve trunk, *PAA* posterior auricular artery, *PBDG* posterior belly of the digastric muscle, *PG* parotid gland

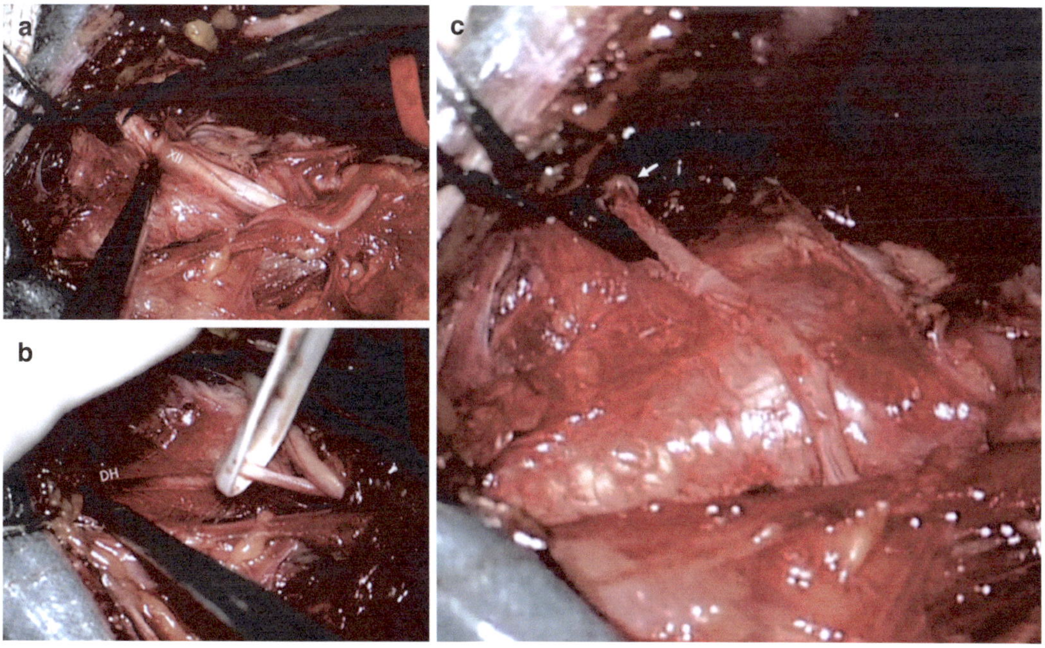

Fig. 22.6 End-to-end anastomosis of the DH—hypoglossal nerve. (**a**) transection of the distal end of the hypoglossal nerve; (**b**) transection of the distal end of the DH; (**c**) end-to-end anastomosis of the DH to the hypoglossal nerve. *DH* descendens hypoglossi, *XII* hypoglossal nerve; the arrow indicates the anastomosis site

22.5.6 End-to-End Anastomosis of the DH: Hypoglossal Nerve

The distal end of the DH is sharply transected and flipped forward toward the hypoglossal nerve. Subsequently, the distal segment of the hypoglossal nerve is marked and fixed with a 6-0 Prolene suture to prevent retraction of the distal end into soft tissues. The hypoglossal nerve is sharply transected proximal to the marked location. Under high magnification, the nerve ends are trimmed, and excessive connective tissue is removed to achieve a smooth interface. End-to-end anastomosis of the DH to the hypoglossal nerve is performed using a 9-0 Prolene suture, typically with 2 to 3 stitches to ensure a smooth joining of the nerve sections. Finally, the anastomosis site is wrapped with an artificial nerve sheath (GI 5X30, Tech Thinkful, Beijing, China) (Fig. 22.6).

22.5.7 End-to-End Anastomosis of the Hypoglossal Nerve: Facial Nerve

The freed main trunk of the hypoglossal nerve is flipped upward from the deep plane of the posterior belly of the digastric muscle toward the parotid area, ensuring that it remains within its original plane to avoid length loss due to superficially located vessels, fascia, and muscle bundles. Close to the stylomastoid foramen, the facial nerve is sharply transected and flipped downward. The ends of the two nerves are approximated, supported by moistened gelatin sponge or rubber. Under high magnification, the nerve ends are trimmed, and excessive connective tissue is removed to achieve a smooth interface. The epineurium of the nerves is sutured with 6 to 8 stitches using 9-0 Prolene sutures, with efforts made to ensure tension-free anastomosis. An artificial nerve sheath is also used to envelop the anastomotic sites to prevent postoperative adhesion (Fig. 22.7).

22.5.8 Closure of the Incision

After confirmation of a bloodless surgical field, the fascia and muscle layers are closed layer by layer, the sternocleidomastoid muscle is repositioned, and finally, the subcutaneous tissue and skin are closed (Fig. 22.8).

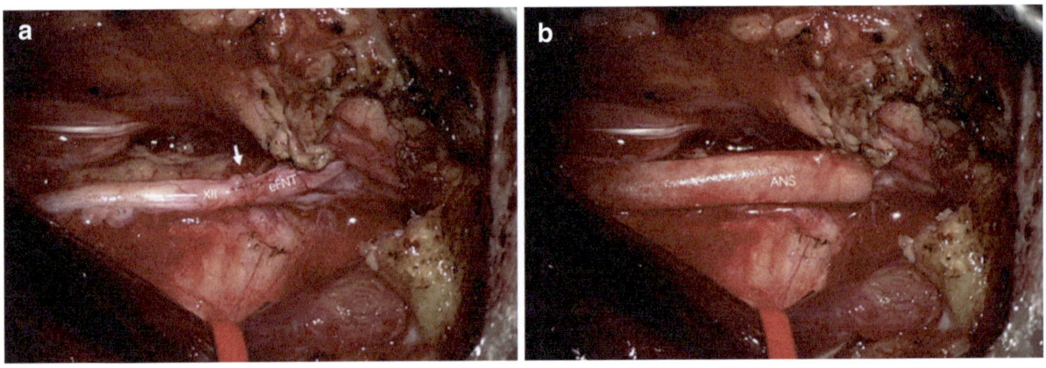

Fig. 22.7 End-to-end anastomosis of the hypoglossal nerve—facial nerve. (**a**) The anastomosis is completed; (**b**) The anastomotic sites is enveloped using an artificial nerve sheath. *ANS* artificial nerve sheath, *eFNT* extratemporal facial nerve trunk, *XII* hypoglossal nerve; the arrow indicates the anastomosis site

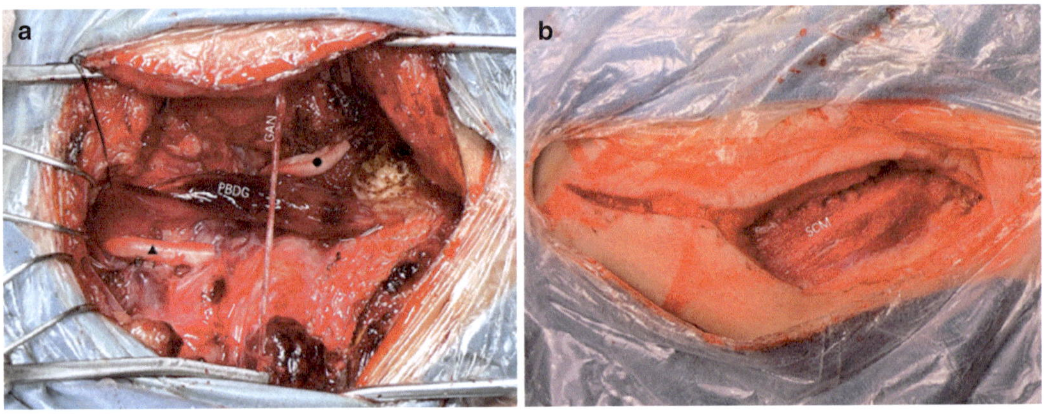

Fig. 22.8 (**a**) The final surgical field; (**b**) Incision closure. *GAN* greater auricular nerve, *PBDG* posterior belly of the digastric muscle, *SCM* sternocleidomastoid muscle; the triangle indicates the DH—hypoglossal anastomosis; the circle indicates the hypoglossal nerve—facial anastomosis

22.6 Key Technical Points of Surgery

The critical aspect of this surgery lies in achieving tension-free and accurate alignment of nerve axons. Adequate, but not excessive, anatomical exposure is essential for this purpose.

For the exposure of the hypoglossal nerve, the intersection of the distal end of the posterior belly of the digastric muscle and the stylohyoid muscle serves as an anatomical landmark. A combination of direct dissection and electroneurophysiological detection is employed. Dissection is performed from either the proximal end to the distal end or vice versa to ensure adequate length of the hypoglossal nerve is exposed. In terms of the facial nerve, the anterior edge of the upper end of the posterior belly of the digastric muscle is used as an anatomical landmark, with incision of the posterior parotid wall adjacent to it reliably locating the eFNT. The posterior auricular artery can also serve as a useful landmark within the parotid gland. Further dissection toward both ends is conducted to reveal sufficient length.

Once the nerves are exposed, maximizing their freedom of movement is crucial for ensuring tension-free alignment. The anastomotic sites require wrapping with artificial nerve sheaths and fixation using fibrin glue to prevent displacement.

22.7 Perioperative Management

Postoperative management includes medication and wound care. The medication regimen primarily consists of neurotrophic drugs, such as methylcobalamin, adenosylcobalamin, and vitamin B1. Regarding wound care, maintaining cleanliness and regularly changing dressings are crucial. During the first month post-surgery, excessive neck movements toward the opposite side should be avoided to prevent tension on the soft tissues and at the nerve anastomosis site. Additionally, spicy foods should be avoided to prevent excessive secretion from the salivary gland on the operated side.

22.8 Follow-Up

Regular follow-ups at 3, 6, 9, and 12 months post-surgery are essential for accurately assessing the recovery levels of facial nerve function. Electroneurophysiological testing should be conducted, and both static photos and dynamic videos of the patient's face should be retained for evaluation. Additionally, patients should receive rehabilitation guidance during these follow-up visits.

References

1. Peitersen E. Bell's palsy: the spontaneous course of 2,500 peripheral facial nerve palsies of different etiologies. Acta Otolaryngol Suppl. 2002;549:4–30.
2. Samii M, Matthies C. Management of 1000 vestibular schwannomas (acoustic neuromas): the facial nerve—preservation and restitution of function. Neurosurgery. 1997;40(4):684–94; discussion 694–5.
3. Terzis JK, Konofaos P. Nerve transfers in facial palsy. Facial Plast Surg. 2008;24(2):177–93.
4. Ballance SC, Duel AB. The operative treatment of facial palsy by the introduction of nerve grafts into the fallopian canal and by other intratemporal methods. Arch Otolaryngol. 1932;15(1):1–70.
5. Socolovsky M, et al. Treatment of complete facial palsy in adults: comparative study between direct hemihypoglossal-facial neurorrhaphy, hemihipoglossal-facial neurorrhaphy with grafts, and masseter to facial nerve transfer. Acta Neurochir. 2016;158(5):945–57; discussion 957.
6. Campero A, Socolovsky M. Facial reanimation by means of the hypoglossal nerve: anatomic comparison of different techniques. Neurosurgery. 2007;61(3 Suppl):41–9; discussion 49–50.
7. Wilkinson EP, et al. Hypoglossal facial anastomosis. In: Brackmann DE, Shelton C, Arriaga MA, editors. Otologic surgery. Amsterdam: Elsevier; 2016. p. 670–7.
8. Jandali D, Revenaugh PC. Facial reanimation: an update on nerve transfers in facial paralysis. Curr Opin Otolaryngol Head Neck Surg. 2019;27(4):231–6.
9. Ling M, et al. Central functional reorganization and recovery following facial-hypoglossal neurorrhaphy for facial paralysis. Neuroimage Clin. 2021;32:102782.
10. Samii M, et al. Comparison of direct side-to-end and end-to-end hypoglossal-facial anastomosis for facial nerve repair. World Neurosurg. 2015;84(2):368–75.
11. May M, Sobol SM, Mester SJ. Hypoglossal-facial nerve interpositional-jump graft for facial reanimation without tongue atrophy. Otolaryngol Head Neck Surg. 1991;104(6):818–25.

12. Hammerschlag PE. Facial reanimation with jump interpositional graft hypoglossal facial anastomosis and hypoglossal facial anastomosis: evolution in management of facial paralysis. Laryngoscope. 1999;109(2 Pt 2 Suppl 90):1–23.
13. Arai H, Sato K, Yanai A. Hemihypoglossal-facial nerve anastomosis in treating unilateral facial palsy after acoustic neurinoma resection. J Neurosurg. 1995;82(1):51–4.
14. Cusimano MD, Sekhar L. Partial hypoglossal to facial nerve anastomosis for reinnervation of the paralyzed face in patients with lower cranial nerve palsies: technical note. Neurosurgery. 1994;35(3):532–3; discussion 533–4, 532.
15. Rebol J, Milojkovic V, Didanovic V. Side-to-end hypoglossal-facial anastomosis via transposition of the intratemporal facial nerve. Acta Neurochir. 2006;148(6):653–7; discussion 657.
16. Ferraresi S, et al. End-to-side intrapetrous hypoglossal-facial anastomosis for reanimation of the face. Technical note. J Neurosurg. 2006;104(3):457–60.
17. Darrouzet V, Guerin J, Bebear JP. New technique of side-to-end hypoglossal-facial nerve attachment with translocation of the infratemporal facial nerve. J Neurosurg. 1999;90(1):27–34.
18. Asaoka K, et al. Surgical anatomy for direct hypoglossal-facial nerve side-to-end "anastomosis". J Neurosurg. 1999;91(2):268–75.
19. Frazier CH. The treatment of paralysis of the recurrent laryngeal nerve by nerve anastomosis. Ann Surg. 1924;79(2):161–71.
20. Miyauchi A, et al. The role of ansa-to-recurrent-laryngeal nerve anastomosis in operations for thyroid cancer. Eur J Surg. 1998;164(12):927–33.
21. Gao Y, et al. The efficacy of ansa cervicalis anterior root for unilateral recurrent laryngeal nerve injury. Chin J Otorhinolaryngol Head Neck Surg. 2018;53(9):655–60.
22. Ji R, et al. Applied anatomy of anastomosis between the cervical loopor sternocleidomastoid muscular branches of the accessory nerve and the phrenic nerve for treatment of dyspnea after paraplegia. Chin J Clin Anat. 2001;19(4):319–20.
23. Conley J, Baker DC. Hypoglossal-facial nerve anastomosis for reinnervation of the paralyzed face. Plast Reconstr Surg. 1979;63(1):63–72.
24. Steiner HH, et al. The ansa cervicalis hypoglossal-facial nerve coaptation for indirect facial nerve repair. Clin Neurol Neurosurg. 1997;99:S120.
25. Schipper J, et al. Paralyzed face. Ansa-cervicalis-nervi-hypoglossi. Chirurg. 2005;76(1):47–53.
26. Leong SC, Lesser TH. Long-term outcomes of facial nerve function in irradiated and nonirradiated nerve grafts. Ann Otol Rhinol Laryngol. 2013;122(11):695–700.
27. Liang J, et al. Descending hypoglossal branch-facial nerve anastomosis in treating unilateral facial palsy after acoustic neuroma resection. Zhonghua Yi Xue Za Zhi. 2015;95(47):3856–8.
28. Shen L, et al. Clinical analysis of hypoglossal nerve descending branch facial nerve anastomosis for facial paralysis in acoustic neuroma surgery. Chin J Neurotraum Surg. 2017;3(5):294–6.
29. Kessler LA, Moldaver J, Pool JL. Hypoglossal-facial anastomosis for treatment of facial paralysis. Neurology. 1959;9(2):118–25. https://doi.org/10.1212/wnl.9.2.118.
30. Chang CG, Shen AL. Hypoglossofacial anastomosis for facial palsy after resection of acoustic neuroma. Surg Neurol. 1984;21(3):282–6. https://doi.org/10.1016/0090-3019(84)90203-9.
31. Pitty LF, Tator CH. Hypoglossal-facial nerve anastomosis for facial nerve palsy following surgery for cerebellopontine angle tumors. J Neurosurg. 1992;77(5):724–31. https://doi.org/10.3171/jns.1992.77.5.0724.
32. Kukwa A, Marchel A, Pietniczka M, Rakowicz M, Krajewski R. Reanimation of the face after facial nerve palsy resulting from resection of a cerebellopontine angle tumour. Br J Neurosurg. 1994;8(3):327–32.
33. Tang Y, Chen Z, Zhu J, et al. Salvaging the transected hypoglossal nerve using descendens hypoglossi in patients undergoing hypoglossal-facial nerve anastomosis for facial palsy: a randomized clinical trial. J Neurosurg. 2024;141:1578–86. https://doi.org/10.3171/2024.4.JNS232971.
34. Tayebi Meybodi A, et al. Anatomical assessment of the digastric branch of the facial nerve as a landmark to localize the extratemporal facial nerve trunk. Surg Radiol Anat. 2019;41:657.
35. Salame K, et al. Microsurgical anatomy of the facial nerve trunk. Clin Anat. 2002;15(2):93–9.
36. Iaconetta G, et al. The hypoglossal nerve: anatomical study of its entire course, vol. 109. World Neurosurg; 2017. p. e486.
37. Vacher C, Dauge MC. Morphometric study of the cervical course of the hypoglossal nerve and its application to hypoglossal facial anastomosis. Surg Radiol Anat. 2004;26(2):86–90.
38. Banneheka S. Anatomy of the ansa cervicalis: nerve fiber analysis. Anat Sci Int. 2008;83(2):61–7.

23 Extracranial Neurolysis for Sequelae of Spastic Facial Paralysis

Baimiao Wang and Shi-Ting Li

23.1 Introduction

A wide variety of etiologies can be responsible for facial paralysis: e.g., idiopathic (Bell's palsy), traumatic, infectious, neoplastic, and congenital. Those with incomplete recovery often have sequelae of facial paralysis of varying degrees, which can be broadly categorized into spastic and flaccid symptoms. Flaccid symptoms are manifested by preexisting weakness in the face, such as weakness in lifting the eyebrows, incomplete eye closure, and limited movement of the mouth. The sequelae of spastic facial palsy include six major symptoms: synkinesis (meaning that unintentional muscular movement of one portion of the face when another portion of the face moves voluntarily [1]), hemifacial muscle tremble, tension in the affected facial, stiff facial expressions, narrowing orbital fissure, and eye opening difficulty. Different patients may come to the doctor with different symptoms as their main complaint, all of which can seriously affect the patient's quality of life and the patient's desire for treatment is very urgent.

The pathogenesis of sequelae of spastic facial paralysis is very complex and remains inconclusive, and currently consists of the following four main hypotheses.

B. Wang · S.-T. Li (✉)
Department of Neurosurgery, XinHua Hospital, Shanghai JiaoTong University School of Medicine, Shanghai, China

1. The first is that axons undergo aberrant regeneration after injury, resulting in its inability to innervate the original correct target muscle [2]. Sunderland described five possible degrees of facial nerve injury, which, also known as grade I through V, are classified from mild to severe as neurapraxia, axonotmesis, neurotmesis, neurotmesis with disruption of the perineurium, and neurotmesis with total disruption of the entire nerve trunk [3]. In grade I and II injuries, due to the integrity of the endoneurium, the regenerating axon will still innervate the correct target muscle along the original pathway, and there will not be synkinesis. In grade III–V injuries, the integrity of the endoneurium is damaged, and the regenerated fibers are likely to grow into other nerve fiber bundles by mistake or sprout side branches, thus innervating the wrong target muscles and generating synkinesis [4].
2. A second potential pathophysiology is ephaptic transmission. Demyelination of nerve axons occurs after the onset of facial paralysis, and with incomplete formation of myelin sheaths, nerve impulses can be transmitted between neighboring axons by means of an electrical tension mechanism, resulting in a "short-circuit" phenomenon or jumping excitation between neighboring axons [4, 5].
3. The enhanced excitability patterns at the facial nucleus may also play a role in the development of sequelae of spastic facial

S.-T. Li et al. (eds.), *Microvascular Decompression Surgery*,
https://doi.org/10.1007/978-981-96-0767-9_23

paralysis, which has been validated by animal experiments and electrophysiological evidence [6, 7].
4. Finally, cortical reorganization may also participate in the development of sequelae of spastic facial paralysis. Several studies have demonstrated that secondary cortical reorganization occurs in primary sensorimotor and supplementary motor area in patients with sequelae of facial paralysis, manifested by decreased activation in motor cortical area on the affected side and increased activation in supplementary motor areas on the contralateral side [8–10].

Current international treatment options for sequelae of spastic facial paralysis can be divided into three broad categories: botulinum toxin injection therapy, physical rehabilitation therapy, and surgical treatment.

23.1.1 Botulinum Toxin Injection Therapy

This therapy improves the static and dynamic appearance of a patient's face by blocking the presynaptic release of acetylcholine, which produces a functional denervation effect at the motor endplate. This is only a temporary phenomenon and always reverses in a period of 3 to 5 months when collateral axonal sprouting reestablishes the motor synapses [4]. Therefore, once a patient with sequelae of spastic facial paralysis decides to receive botulinum toxin treatment, he or she is destined to need repeated injections. However, the accumulation of injections may result in the increase of antibodies in the body, leading to a gradual decrease in the efficacy of the treatment [11]. At the same time, patients may experience a series of complications such as oral incompetence, ptosis, diplopia, exposure keratopathy, and worsened cosmesis. The higher the dose of botulinum toxin injected, the higher the risk of the above complications [12, 13]. Botulinum toxin treatment is effective in patients with sequelae of spastic facial paralysis, but a significant decline in its efficacy is inevitable after multiple injections.

23.1.2 Physical Rehabilitation Therapy

Balliet proposed neuromuscular retraining (NMR) for facial neuromuscular retraining in 1982 [14]. NMR is a highly patient-centered, individualized physical therapy program designed based on the patient's facial muscle function and psychological state. Its successful implementation requires not only a thorough pretreatment assessment by an NMR specialist but also in-depth learning, good compliance, and active exercise by the patient. Under the guidance of the therapist, the patient should be familiar with which muscles need to be engaged and which ones do not for each type of expressive activity. After the onset of facial paralysis, the lack of facial muscle movement feedback will affect the brain's ability to receive relevant facial movement information. The incorporation of biofeedback mechanisms in physical therapy facilitates immediate facial movement analysis and error correction by the brain, which is beneficial in increasing efficacy. Commonly used biofeedback methods include surface electromyography (sEMG) feedback, mirror vision (mirror) feedback, half-mirror vision feedback, sensory feedback, and proprioceptive feedback [5, 13, 15, 16]. Many studies have suggested that botulinum toxin injections combined with physical therapy may increase the long-term efficacy of targeting synkinesis movements [12].

23.1.3 Surgical Treatment

Surgical treatment includes selective neurectomy, selective myotomy, and masseteric nerve-facial nerve anastomosis.

1. *Selective neurotomy*: Selective neurotomy is a procedure that relieves symptoms by selectively cutting the abnormally conducting nerves in the face. It was first reported in 1950, and four patients with synkinesis achieved satisfactory efficacy after surgery [17]. In 1986, DOBIE and FISCH [18] applied selective neurotomy to treat patients with syn-

kinesis, and the short-term follow-up results showed satisfactory efficacy; however, all the patients had the adverse effect of shrinkage of the eye fissure of the affected side at 2 to 3 years after surgery. Since then, some scholars have improved the procedure [19], and proposed two-step Highly Selective Neurectomy to treat patients with synkinesis, with no obvious postoperative complications. Although the short-term effect of selective peripheral neurotomy was satisfactory, the long-term follow-up results showed that the synkinesis was prone to recurrence [20].

2. *Selective Myotomy*: The symptoms are controlled by direct excision of the target muscle of abnormal movement. It was first reported in 1991, when GUERRISSI [21] obtained satisfactory postoperative results by selectively removing the zygomaticus major muscle in 5 patients and the upper lip lifting muscle in 1 patient. Currently, the most commonly resected target muscle is the platysma muscle, and it has been reported in the literature that platysma muscle resection is effective in relieving the symptoms of cervical synkinesis [22]. However, postoperative complications such as swelling of the operative area, lymphedema, ecchymosis, bleeding, and irreversible postoperative trauma may occur [4].
3. *Masseteric-Zygomatic Nerve Transfer*: The principle of the surgery is to cut the zygomatic branch of the facial nerve and disconnect the abnormal innervation, to relieve the symptoms. It is often used to improve the eye–mouth and mouth–eye synkinesis. Subsequently, the ipsilateral masseteric nerve is anastomosed to the distal end of the dissected zygomatic branch of the facial nerve so that the zygomatic muscle complex is reinnervated. This surgical procedure can be performed as a single procedure for synkinesis or combined with a cross facial nerve graft to improve the synkinesis while decreasing facial muscle tone, resulting in a more symmetrical static appearance of the face and better smile movement. However, this procedure is highly invasive, involves many steps, and requires a high degree of technical skill for end-to-end anastomosis and end-to-side anastomosis (when cross facial nerve grafting is involved), and long-term follow-up of postoperative outcomes is lacking [23–25].

We propose the surgical procedure of extracranial neurolysis for sequelae of spastic facial paralysis for the first time in our center. The results of the previous animal experiments confirmed that there were pathological changes such as membrane structural disorders, abnormal proliferation of nerve fibers, and misdistribution of the extracranial facial nerve trunk in the guinea pig model of spastic facial paralysis. Abnormal proliferation of nerve fibers was also found in the epineurium and perineurium of FNT in patients with sequelae of spastic facial paralysis [26]. Therefore, the abnormal proliferation of facial nerve fibers and the fascicular distribution of regenerated fibers in the epineurium and perineurium of the facial nerve trunk may be an important etiology for the development of the sequelae of spastic facial paralysis such as synkinesis, which is the pathological and histological basis for our proposal of extracranial neurolysis for sequelae of spastic facial paralysis.

23.2 Evaluation

The diagnosis of sequelae of spastic facial paralysis is made in patients with varying degrees of spastic facial palsy sequelae symptoms combined with electrophysiologic abnormal muscular response of the facial nerve (AMR positivity). A detailed preoperative evaluation is essential for each patient. Patients are required to complete a detailed clinical scale assessment and electrophysiologic and imaging assessments upon admission.

23.2.1 Clinical Scale Assessment

1. The House-Brackmann Grading System [27] (HBGS), Facial Nerve Grading System 2.0 (FNGS2.0) [28], Sunnybrook facial grading system [29] are often used to objectively

assess the degree of facial paralysis and sequelae in patients.

   (a) The House-Brackmann Grading System (HBGS) categorizes the degree of facial paralysis into six grades, i.e., grades I to VI, which involves the assessment of static and dynamic facial function and secondary damage, and is convenient for clinical application, but lacks the assessment of the sequelae of spastic facial paralysis.
   (b) FNGS 2.0 also uses a six-level classification, with the first part assessing the static and dynamic conditions of the four regions of the brow, eye, nasolabial fold, and oral; and the second part assessing the severity of the sequelae of facial paralysis (synkinesis and facial contractures).
   (c) The Sunnybrook Facial Nerve Scoring System assesses not only the patient's static facial appearance, including the size of the eye slits, nasolabial folds, and the morphology of the corners of the mouth, but also assesses the patient's dynamic facial function based on five standardized facial expression movements (forehead wrinkle, gentle eye closure, open mouth smile, snarl, and lip Pucker). The scale also provides a detailed assessment of the patient's synkinesis.

2. The severity of synkinesis is also evaluated using the Synkinesis Assessment Questionnaire (SAQ) self-assessment scale [30]. The SAQ scale consists of nine questions that allow patients to rate their own self-perceived degree of eye–mouth, mouth–eye, and other kinds of synkinesis, and often responds to the patient's synkinesis score along with the synkinesis score on the Sunnybrook scale.
3. The FDI [31] (Facial Disability Index) and FaCE [32] scales are used to understand the impairment of patients' somatic and social functioning due to the sequelae of facial paralysis. The FDI is a commonly used self-assessment scale, which consists of two subscales, namely, physical functioning and social functioning, and it responds well to the subjective feelings of the patients.

23.2.2 Electrophysiologic Evaluation

1. *Facial nerve abnormal muscle response (AMR) test*: Abnormal muscle response (AMR), also known as lateral spread response (LSR), AMR refers to the abnormal electromyographic response that can be recorded on the facial muscle innervated by another branch of the facial nerve when one branch of the nerve is stimulated. And a positive AMR is a necessary indicator for the clinical diagnosis of sequelae of spastic facial paralysis. It is worth noting that the AMR waveforms of patients with sequelae of spastic facial paralysis and hemifacial spasm are similar, but the mechanisms of their formation are not the same. The mechanism of AMR waveform formation in spastic facial paralysis sequelae is related to the abnormal vagal distribution of the facial nerve, while the mechanism of AMR waveform formation in patients with hemifacial spasm is related to the contact between the facial nerve and the responsible blood vessels in the cerebellopontine angle, as well as the formation of abnormal neural circuits [33].
2. *Electroneurography (ENoG)*: The ENoG value is expressed as the ratio of the amplitude of the compound muscle action potentials (CMAPs) evoked by facial nerve electrical stimulation on the affected side to that on the normal side. The degree of neurological damage is determined by the amount of degeneration of the facial nerve fibers on the affected side. Combined with the results of electromyography, the damage to the facial nerve can be judged comprehensively. A >90% decrease in ENoG wave amplitude 10–14 days after the onset of facial paralysis is one of the predictive factors for the development of synkinesis after 12 months, which is more likely to occur in these patients [34].
3. *Electromyography (EMG)*: EMG is an examination to record the nerve–muscle electrical

activity under quiet and random muscle contraction, which is the main method to examine the functional status of the peripheral nervous system. Through the characteristics of motor unit potential (MUP) such as morphology, time course, wave amplitude, phase, recruitment, and type of release, the nature and duration of facial neuropathy can be determined.

23.2.3 Imaging Evaluation

We use thin-section CT of the temporal bone and cranial 3D navigation-enhanced MRI to exclude intracranial facial nerve occupying lesions.

23.3 Surgery

Abnormal muscle response (AMR) testing was performed throughout the operation; anesthesia was induced using short-acting muscle relaxants. After satisfactory general anesthesia and tracheal intubation of the patient, the skin was presterilized with anerdian at the electrode insertion point. Subcutaneous needle electrodes were used for the recording electrode, reference electrode, stimulation electrode, and grounding electrode. The grounding electrode was inserted at the chin. The recording and reference electrodes were inserted into the frontal muscle, orbicularis oculi muscle, orbicularis oris muscle, and depressor anguli oris muscle on the affected side from top to bottom, with about 5 mm, and were inserted into the subcutaneous area for about 5 mm. The stimulation electrodes were inserted into the supraorbital lateral and anterior and inferior part of the angle of the mandible, and the temporal and marginal branches of the facial nerve were stimulated and recorded, respectively, after the metabolism of short-acting myorelaxants was complete.

All patients were put in a lateral decubitus position, and their heads were fixed in a frame, positioning the mastoid tip at the highest level. About 5 cm long retroauricular curved incision around the mastoid tip was made (Fig. 23.1a). The skin and subcutaneous tissue were incised sequentially, and the flap was turned anteriorly to expose the underlying sternocleidomastoid muscle. An “L”-shaped incision was made in the sternocleidomastoid muscle (Fig. 23.1b), with a transverse edge used to disengage the sternocleidomastoid muscle from the mastoid process, and a vertical edge located at the most anterior edge of the mastoid tip. Thereby, the sternocleidomastoid muscle was slightly stripped from the mastoid process. The bone of mastoid tip was exposed to the level of the digastric groove, and the posterior belly of digastric muscle was exposed (Fig. 23.1c). Then, blunt dissection was carried out to separate the posterior belly of digastric muscle from the parotid gland, thus enlarging the exposure of the posterior aspect of the parotid gland. The facial nerve trunk (FNT) was then exposed under the microscope. The FNT is often located below the posterior auricular artery, so which is often used as an anatomic marker to find the facial nerve (Fig. 23.1d). Along the anterior margin of the digastric groove, the FNT and the bifurcation of the facial nerve was visualized on the deep side of the parotid gland (Fig. 23.1e). The final exposure length of FNT was about 1 to 1.5 cm. If further exposure was required, the most proximate part of the FNT could be reached at the stylomastoid foramen level by drilling a portion of mastoid tip.

The well-exposed FNT can be manipulated only after an intraoperatively stable AMR waveform has been induced (Fig. 23.2a, b). The FNT was stimulated by a probe from the proximal end, and EMG images of the facial nerve branches (frontal, orbicularis oculi, orbicularis oris, and depressor anguli oris muscles) were obtained (Fig. 23.2c). Along the long axis of the FNT, the epineurium was gently picked with a nerve neurolysis knife (Fig. 23.1f), and then the epineurium was held by microfine forceps and excised by microscopic scissors after careful stripping of the epineurium. Subsequently, the perineurium was continued to be picked with a nerve neurolysis knife, and the perineurium was excised in the same way. Once the dual AMR related to the oral-ocular and oculo-oral synkinesis disappeared, the release surgery was stopped immediately (Fig. 23.2d, e). The nerve probe was placed

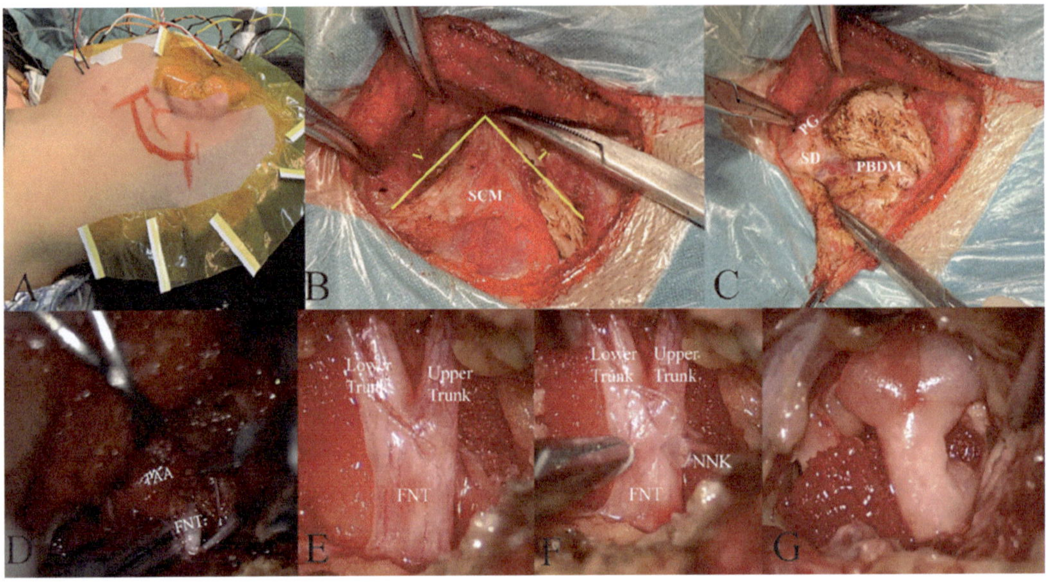

Fig. 23.1 Surgical procedures of extracranial neurolysis for sequelae of spastic facial paralysis. (**a**) 5 cm-long retroauricular curved incision around the mastoid tip (MT). (**b**) The "L" incision of the sternocleidomastoid muscle. *T* transverse side of the "L" incision, *V* vertical side of the "L" incision. (**c**) Flip of the sternocleidomastoid muscle to expose the mastoid tip, styloid diaphragm, and posterior belly of the digastric. (**d**) The posterior auricular artery is located superficial to the main trunk of the facial nerve and can be used as an intraoperative marker to find the facial nerve. (**e**) Under the microscope view, the exposure of the main trunk of the facial nerve as well as the upper and lower trunks. (**f**) The epineurium was gently picked with a nerve neurolysis knife. (**g**) The main trunk and branches of the facial nerve were wrapped with an artificial nerve sheath. *SCM* sternocleidomastoid muscle, *PG* parotid gland, *SD* styloid diaphragm, *PBDM* posterior belly of the digastric muscle, *PAA* posterior auricular artery, *FNT* facial nerve trunk, *NNK* nerve neurolysis knife

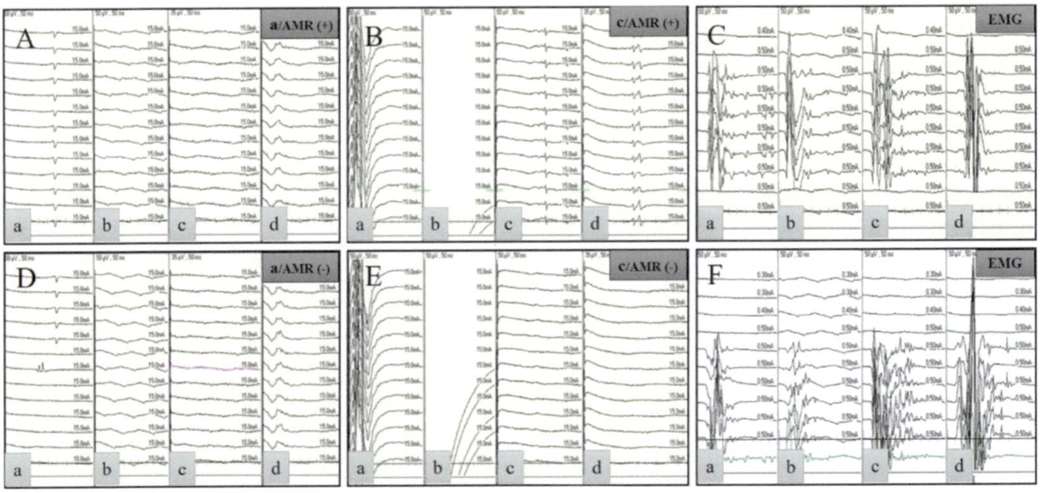

Fig. 23.2 Intraoperative neurophysiological monitoring via synkinesis associated AMR and facial EMG. The dual AMR recordings were achieved from the orbicularis oculi by electrical stimulation of the marginal mandibular branch (**a**) and the orbicularis oris by stimulation of the facial nerve's temporal branch (**b**). Before neurolysis, the FNT was stimulated by a probe from the proximal end, and EMG images of the facial nerve branches were obtained (**c**). The oral-ocular synkinesis associated AMR disappeared when stimulating the marginal mandibular branch during neurolysis (**d**). The stimulation of the temporal branch failed to induce the oculo-oral synkinesis associated AMR during neurolysis (**e**). The proximal end of FNT was stimulated with the probe, and the EMG of the facial nerve branches was re-recorded (**f**). Columns a, b, c, and d in each chart represent frontal muscle, orbicularis oculi muscle, orbicularis oris muscle, and depressor anguli oris muscle, respectively. *AMR* abnormal muscle response, *EMG* electromyography, *FNT* facial nerve trunk

again at the same site proximal to the main trunk of the facial nerve, and the EMG waveforms were collected, and the latency and amplitude were recorded after the relaxation procedure (Fig. 23.2f). The main trunk and branches of the facial nerve were wrapped with an artificial nerve sheath (Fig. 23.1g), and the parotid gland, muscle, and subcutaneous tissue were sutured layer by layer. The wound is sterilized and bandaged.

The patients received identical rehabilitation therapy three times per day for 12 months, administered by physiotherapists who were aware of the treatment assignments. Rehabilitation therapy included identical active exercise, functional training, physical therapy, and massage.

Long-term postoperative follow-up of about 200 patients in our center found that all postoperative spastic facial palsy sequelae symptoms improved significantly, with the most obvious improvement in facial tightness and stiffness, a significant improvement in Sunnybrook score, and no aggravation of worsen facial palsy, parotid leakage, poor wound healing, and other complications in the postoperative period.

23.4 Discussion

Sequelae of spastic facial paralysis can occur when incomplete recovery occurs from different causes of facial palsy. Symptoms of spastic facial palsy sequelae, such as synkinesis, hemifacial muscle tremble, tension in the affected facial, stiff facial expressions, asymmetry in eye opening width, and eye-opening difficulty, often appear 3 to 6 months after the onset of the disease, and the above symptoms worsen with the passage of time [35]. When symptoms appear, we recommend early surgical intervention. Detailed preoperative evaluation of the patient's clinical symptoms and electrophysiologic parameters is essential, and a positive AMR waveform is instructive.

The pathogenesis of facial palsy sequelae is complex, and the vagal distribution of nerve fibers in the extracranial segment may be an important causative factor. Extracranial neurolysis surgery can remove most of the abnormal nerve conduction of the facial nerve, and intraoperative attention should be paid to the following: (1) The scope of facial nerve membrane release includes the main trunk of the facial nerve, the bifurcation of the facial nerve, and the beginning of the upper and lower trunks of the facial nerve in the area far away from the sternomastoid foramen. Combined with the actual intraoperative experience: the disappearance of AMR waveforms mostly occurs when the facial nerve bifurcation is loosened, and the operation for the bifurcation is the key to the operation. (2) The operation should be carried out in layer-by-layer depth, and the separation should be carried out step by step from the inner end to the distal end, avoiding the use of bipolar electrocoagulation as far as possible and minimize the direct pulling on the facial nerve fibers. The whole operation is carried out by microsurgical techniques to remove the proliferated membranous connective tissues around the facial nerve as much as possible. Finally, the artificial nerve sheath was used to wrap the main trunk and branches of the facial nerve to prevent the occurrence of postoperative adhesions in the operated area. (3) The complete disappearance of the AMR waveform is the main basis for determining the surgical process, and the partial disappearance of the AMR or the absence of AMR often suggests that the neurolysis is not complete, and the operation cannot be ended arbitrarily. Combined with the results of long-term clinical follow-up in our center, the safety and effectiveness of this procedure have been fully confirmed and should be fully promoted by our colleagues.

References

1. Crumley RL. Mechanisms of synkinesis. Laryngoscope. 1979;89(11):1847–54.
2. Montserrat L, Benito M. Facial synkinesis and aberrant regeneration of facial nerve. Adv Neurol. 1988;49:211–24.
3. Sunderland S. Nerve and nerve injuries. 2nd ed. London: Churchill Livingstone; 1978.
4. Husseman J, Mehta RP. Management of synkinesis. Facial Plast Surg. 2008;24(2):242–9.
5. Maria CM, Kim J. Individualized management of facial synkinesis based on facial function. Acta Otolaryngol. 2017;137(9):1010–5.

6. Choi D, Raisman G. Somatotopic Organization of the facial nucleus is disrupted after lesioning and regeneration of the facial nerve: the histological representation of synkinesis. Neurosurgery. 2002;50(2):355–63.
7. Oge AE, Yayla V, Demir GA, et al. Excitability of facial nucleus and related brain-stem reflexes in hemifacial spasm, post-facial palsy synkinesis and facial myokymia. Clin Neurophysiol. 2005;116(7):1542–54.
8. Rijntjes M, Tegenthoff M, Liepert J, et al. Cortical reorganization in patients with facial palsy. Ann Neurol. 1997;41(5):621–30.
9. Wang Y, Wang WW, Hua XY, et al. Patterns of cortical reorganization in facial synkinesis: a task functional magnetic resonance imaging study. Neural Regen Res. 2018;13(9):1637–42.
10. Wang Y, Yang L, Wang WW, et al. Decreased distance between representation sites of distinct facial movements in facial synkinesis—a task fMRI study. Neuroscience. 2019;397:12–7.
11. Göschel H, Wohlfarth K, Frevert J, et al. Botulinum a toxin therapy: neutralizing and nonneutralizing antibodies—therapeutic consequences. Exp Neurol. 1997;147(1):96–102.
12. Mehdizadeh OB, Diels J, White WM. Botulinum toxin in the treatment of facial paralysis. Facial Plast Surg Clin North Am. 2016;24(1):11–20.
13. Chuang DCC, Chang TNJ, Lu JCY. Postparalysis facial synkinesis: clinical classification and surgical strategies. Plast Reconstr Surg Glob Open. 2015;3(3):e320.
14. Balliet R, Shinn JB, Bach-Y-Rita P. Facial paralysis rehabilitation: retraining selective muscle control. Int Rehabil Med. 1982;4(2):67–74.
15. Lapidus JB, Lu JCY, Santosa KB, et al. Too much or too little? A systematic review of postparetic synkinesis treatment. J Plast Reconstr Aesthet Surg. 2020;73(3):443–52.
16. Fujiwara K, Furuta Y, Yamamoto N, et al. Factors affecting the effect of physical rehabilitation therapy for synkinesis as a sequela to facial nerve palsy. Auris Nasus Larynx. 2018;45(4):732–9.
17. Marino H, Alurralde A. Spastic facial palsy; peripheral selective neurotomy. Br J Plast Surg. 1950;3(1):56–9.
18. Dobie RA, Fisch U. Primary and revision surgery (selective neurectomy) for facial hyperkinesia. Arch Otolaryngol Head Neck Surg. 1986;112(2):154–63.
19. Hohman MH, Lee LN, Hadlock TA. Two-step highly selective neurectomy for refractory periocular synkinesis. Laryngoscope. 2013;123(6):1385–8.
20. Van Veen MM, Dusseldorp JR, Hadlock TA. Long-term outcome of selective neurectomy for refractory periocular synkinesis. Laryngoscope. 2018;128(10):2291–5.
21. Guerrissi JO. Selective myectomy for postparetic facial synkinesis. Plast Reconstr Surg. 1991;87(3):459–66.
22. Henstrom DK, Malo JS, Cheney ML, et al. Platysmectomy: an effective intervention for facial synkinesis and hypertonicity. Arch Facial Plast Surg. 2011;13(4):239–43.
23. Biglioli F, Kutanovaite O, Rabbiosi D, et al. Surgical treatment of synkinesis between smiling and eyelid closure. J Craniomaxillofac Surg. 2017;45(12):1996–2001.
24. Biglioli F, Soliman M, El-Shazly M, et al. Use of the masseteric nerve to treat segmental midface paresis. Br J Oral Maxillofac Surg. 2018;56(8):719–26.
25. Gray ML, Hu S, Gorbea E, et al. Masseteric-zygomatic nerve transfer for the management of eye closure-smile excursion synkinesis. Am J Otolaryngol. 2020;41(4):102479.
26. Wei X, Chang B, LI S. Epineurectomy of facial nerve trunk for refractory oral-ocular and oculo-oral synkinesis following Bell palsy. J Craniofac Surg. 2021;32(8):e822–6.
27. House JW, Brackmann DE. Facial nerve grading system. Otolaryngol Head Neck Surg. 1985;93(2):146–7.
28. Facial Nerve Disorders Committee, Vrabec JT, Backous DD, et al. Facial nerve grading system 2.0. Otolaryngol Head Neck Surg. 2009;140(4):445–50.
29. Ross BG, Fradet G, Nedzelski JM. Development of a sensitive clinical facial grading system. Otolaryngol Head Neck Surg. 1996;114(3):380–6.
30. Mehta RP, Wernickrobinson M, Hadlock TA. Validation of the Synkinesis assessment questionnaire. Laryngoscope. 2007;117(5):923–6.
31. Vanswearingen JM, Brach JS. The facial disability index: reliability and validity of a disability assessment instrument for disorders of the facial neuromuscular system. Phys Ther. 1996;76(12):1288–98.
32. Kahn JB, Gliklich RE, Boyev KP, et al. Validation of a patient-graded instrument for facial nerve paralysis: the FaCE scale: validation of a patient-graded instrument for facial nerve paralysis: the FaCE scale. Laryngoscope. 2001;111(3):387–98.
33. Zheng X, Hong W, Tang Y, et al. Sympathetic nerves bridge the cross-transmission in hemifacial spasm. Neurosci Lett. 2012;517(1):52–5.
34. Nakano H, Haginomori SI, Wada SI, et al. Electroneurography value as an indicator of high risk for the development of moderate-to-severe synkinesis after Bell's palsy and Ramsay Hunt syndrome. Acta Otolaryngol. 2019;139(9):823–7.
35. Alipour S, Pick C, Jansen S, et al. Long-term therapy with botulinum toxin in facial synkinesis: Retrospective data analysis of data from 1998 to 2018. Clin Otolaryngol. 2021;46(4):758–66.

Intraoperative Monitoring

24

Shi-Ting Li and Ying Ting-Ting

24.1 Introduction

Cranial nerves are susceptible to injury during microvascular decompression (MVD) procedures. Intraoperative Neurophysiological Monitoring (IOM or IONM) allows for a reliable and effective evaluation of patients' neurological conditions while under anesthesia by analyzing alterations in electrophysiological signals associated with motor and sensory conduction pathways, variations in cortical bioelectric activity, and cerebral blood flow. The adoption of IOM is increasingly becoming a standard practice in medicine. It has the potential to identify reversible neurological impairments early in the surgical process. Prompt and appropriate actions informed by these early warnings can avert permanent nerve damage. Furthermore, neurophysiological techniques are being utilized more frequently for preoperative diagnostics, intraoperative assessments, and postoperative evaluations of neurological injuries. In the context of MVD, neurophysiological monitoring enhances both the safety and effectiveness of surgical interventions. Presently, the techniques most commonly employed for neurophysiological monitoring during the perioperative phase of MVD include brainstem auditory evoked potentials (BAEP), electromyography (EMG), and abnormal muscle response, Z-L response.

24.2 Equipment and Electrodes

Selecting the right equipment for intraoperative monitoring is crucial. While not all features are essential for standard clinical recordings, several specific attributes become particularly important for intraoperative applications. For example, the system should support simultaneous multimodal recordings, such as electromyography (EMG) and evoked potentials, to cater to the requirements of different surgical procedures. A standard monitoring system typically comprises one or more programmable devices capable of delivering auditory, visual, and electrical stimuli with varying amplitudes, durations, and rates. It includes a range of electrodes for administering electrical stimuli and capturing electrophysiological signals from the scalp, nerves, and muscles, as well as a head box for connecting different electrode groups to amplifiers. Additional components include amplifiers, a display monitor, a printer, and often a modem or network link for remote monitoring [1]. All components are linked to a computer that controls stimulus delivery,

The original version of the chapter has been revised. A correction to this chapter can be found at https://doi.org/10.1007/978-981-96-0767-9_25

S.-T. Li (✉) · Y. Ting-Ting
Department of Neurosurgery, XinHua Hospital, Shanghai JiaoTong University School of Medicine, Shanghai, China

S.-T. Li et al. (eds.), *Microvascular Decompression Surgery*, https://doi.org/10.1007/978-981-96-0767-9_24

data acquisition, filtering, averaging, visualization, printing, and sometimes remote transmission and permanent data storage [1]. The system should also allow for modifications in recording protocols and display settings as needed, enabling rapid interpretation of results.

Various types of stimulation electrodes can be used for both stimulating and recording, such as adhesive electrodes, metal cup electrodes, subdermal needles, corkscrew electrodes, and metal probes, which can function as monopolar or bipolar. The effectiveness of stimulus delivery and data recording largely depends on the choice of electrode type and its precise placement [2].

Subdermal needles are particularly advantageous in the operating room, as they can be applied quickly after the patient is anesthetized, without requiring skin preparation. They are generally easy to secure, ensuring stable and low electrode-skin impedances. If feasible, incorporating additional "redundant" electrodes at both the recording and grounding sites can be beneficial, providing a safeguard against dislodgment during surgical procedures.

24.3 Effects of Anesthetics on Intraoperative Neurophysiology Studies

Different anesthetic agents have been shown to influence neurophysiology studies conducted during intraoperative monitoring due to their impact on cerebral blood flow, tissue perfusion, and metabolic rates. General anesthesia encompasses multiple components, including analgesia (the reduction of pain response), sedation (the induction of sleep), amnesia (the prevention of memory formation regarding the surgical experience), and muscle relaxation (the inhibition of muscle activity). Additionally, it may lead to hypotension (a decrease in blood pressure) and hypothermia (a drop in body temperature), both of which can also modify neurophysiological signals [1]. Consequently, when interpreting neurophysiological recordings, it is essential to consider the effects of any alterations in the anesthesia protocol, as these changes can closely resemble those induced by surgical interventions. Routine monitoring of vital signs such as pulse oximetry, electrocardiograms (ECG), arterial blood pressure, capnography, body temperature, and muscle twitch responses is crucial during surgical procedures. Effective communication with the anesthesiology team is vital for the success of neurophysiologic intraoperative monitoring. A collaborative approach involving the anesthesiology, surgical, and neurophysiological monitoring teams is essential [3]. A comprehensive discussion regarding the different types of anesthetics and their specific effects on neurophysiological monitoring will be provided at the conclusion of each monitoring method.

24.4 Monitoring Techniques

24.4.1 Brainstem Auditory Evoked Potentials

Brainstem auditory evoked potentials monitoring (BAEPs), also named auditory brainstem responses (ABRs), is a widely utilized, classical, and noninvasive method aimed at minimizing the risk of hearing loss during surgeries in the cerebellopontine angle (CPA), such as microvascular decompression (MVD) [4]. Normal BAEPs are characterized by the presence of 5 to 7 vertex-negative peaks, which appear between 2 ms and 10 ms following the presentation of a high-intensity transient sound, like a click or a brief, loud tone burst (Fig. 24.1). Specific anatomical locations have been identified as the primary sources for the generation of these waveforms: Wave I originates from the distal auditory nerve; Wave II from the cochlear nucleus and proximal auditory nerve; Wave III from the superior olivary nucleus (located in the lower pons); Wave IV from the lateral lemniscus; Wave V from the inferior colliculus; Wave VI from the medial geniculate body; and Wave VII from the auditory radiations. Besides indicating the conduction pathways in the auditory system, BAEPs also offer significant insights into the overall functionality of the brainstem.

The cochlear nerve may sustain damage during surgery for several reasons: (1) stretching of the cochlear nerve while retracting the cerebel-

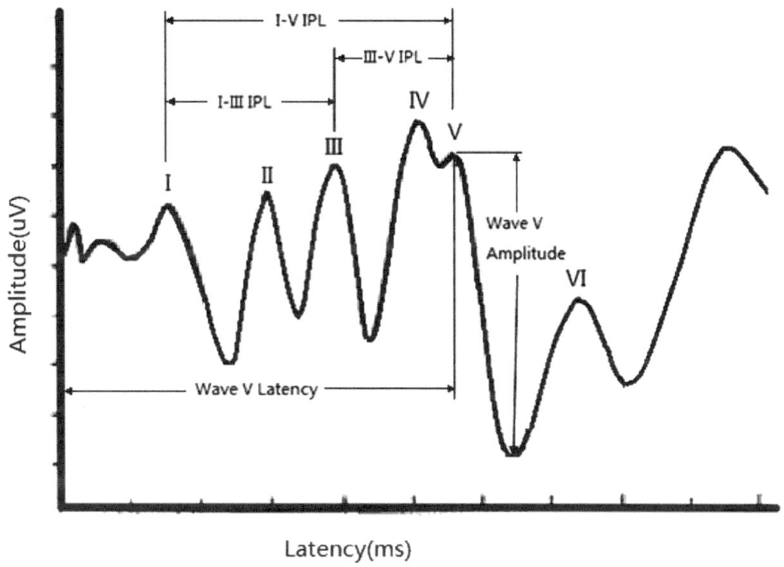

Fig. 24.1 Typical recording of brainstem auditory evoked potentials

lum; (2) manipulation of the labyrinthine artery and/or the antero-inferior cerebellar artery; (3) direct trauma from surgical instruments or nearby coagulation; and (4) newly introduced compression of the cochlear nerve at the end of the procedure due to interposed Teflon between the compressive vessel and the VIIth-cochlear nerve complex [5, 6]. During the monitoring of BAEPs, it is crucial to closely evaluate any changes in the BAEP patterns and analyze how these alterations correlate with the surgical maneuvers performed. This evaluation will help determine whether the observed changes indicate damage or potentially reversible dysfunction in the auditory pathways of the ear, the auditory nerve, or the brainstem. Consequently, this testing method is applicable in surgical interventions such as microvascular decompression of the facial or trigeminal nerve, as well as tumor resections in the CPA region.

24.4.1.1 Stimulation and Recording

Stimulation The sound stimulus is delivered through miniature electromagnetic earphones that are placed into the ear canals and secured with sponge (molded foam) ear inserts, which are connected to a transducer via plastic tubing. Any dislodgment or kinking of this tubing can result in the complete absence of all BAEP components, or may lead to reduced amplitudes and delayed latencies.

Sound Intensity For intraoperative monitoring, clicks of alternating polarity are typically employed to minimize stimulus artifacts. The required stimulus intensity is generally set at or above 70 dB nHL, although higher intensities may be necessary if the patient has preexisting hearing loss.

Stimulus Rate To avoid contamination from electrical artifacts, it is essential to steer clear of stimulus rates at exactly 10 Hz or its multiples. Instead, a frequency between 20 and 40 Hz (e.g., 33.1 Hz) is commonly utilized, and this rate should be maintained consistently throughout the surgical procedure. Achieving reliable signals often necessitates several hundred averaged trials to effectively reduce electrical noise in the operating room.

Recording Electrodes and Band Pass Electrode placement adheres to the EEG 10–20 International System. The standard configuration for recording electrodes is as follows: Channel 1 connects the vertex to the ipsilateral earlobe/mastoid (Cz–Ai/Mi); Channel 2 connects the vertex to the contralateral earlobe/mastoid (Cz–Ac/Mc). Two additional channels can be included:

Channel 3 connects the ipsilateral earlobe/mastoid to the contralateral earlobe/mastoid (Ai–Ac or Mi–Mc); Channel 4 connects the vertex to a non-cephalic reference (Cz–Nc), such as from the vertex to the cervical area (Cz–Cv2). Typical filter settings include a low-frequency filter at 100 Hz and a high-frequency filter at 3 kHz. Given that BAEPs exhibit very short latencies and small amplitudes, a time base of 1 ms (with a sweep of 10 ms) and sensitivity settings of 0.1–0.2 μV/division are employed [2].

24.4.1.2 Intraoperative Interpretation

Baseline data should be established following the induction of anesthesia and the positioning of the patient. These baseline responses must exhibit clear and reliable components, and they should be compared throughout the surgery using consistent acquisition and stimulus parameters. Waves I, III, and V consistently show stability and serve as the primary basis for interpreting BAEP results. Waves IV and V frequently merge into a morphologically varied IV-V complex. In certain individuals, the V wave may manifest at the inflection point of the descending segment of the IV wave, or it may seamlessly blend into a broader complex [4, 7].

According to the standards set by the American Clinical Neurophysiology Society for recording BAEPs, the analysis typically focuses on the detection of waves I, III, and V. Key measurements include: (1) peak latency of wave I; (2) peak latency of wave III; (3) peak latency of wave V; (4) interpeak interval between waves I and III; (5) interpeak interval between waves III and V; (6) interpeak interval between waves I and V; (7) amplitude of wave I; (8) amplitude of wave V; and (9) the amplitude ratio of waves IV-V to I [8]. The criteria for identifying significant intraoperative changes in BAEPs are not uniformly accepted across hospitals, which often implement varying protocols for monitoring hearing loss, alert criteria, and definitions of hearing loss [2]. Traditionally, the most critical indicators include the latency and amplitude of peak V, with a commonly accepted criterion being a 1 ms increase in wave V latency or a 50% decrease in wave V amplitude, both of which are sensitive predictors of potential postoperative hearing loss [9].

A significant limitation of this technique is the poor signal-to-noise ratio associated with BAEPs, which necessitates extended data acquisition times to achieve adequate quality. There is a notable incidence of unsatisfactory recordings due to substantial artifacts, which diminishes the effectiveness of intraoperative ABR monitoring and prevents real-time results [10]. As a far-field recording potential, BAEPs are vulnerable to various artifacts, including those arising from body temperature fluctuations, changes in intracranial pressure due to cerebrospinal fluid release, saline perfusion in the surgical area, and interference from surgical tools such as microscopes, drills, and ultrasonic aspirators [11]. Despite these limitations, the noninvasive nature of BAEPs and their fundamental neurological principles render this technique the most widely adopted monitoring method in the operating room.

24.4.1.3 Anesthesia Requirements

BAEPs are generally not significantly influenced by anesthetic agents; however, they can be affected by temperature changes. A reduction in the temperature of the proximal section of the VIIIth cranial nerve leads to a slowdown in its conduction velocity, resulting in delays in the latencies of waves III and V. Fortunately, these effects are reversible once normal body temperature is restored.

24.4.2 Cochlear Nerve Compound Action Potential

The cochlear nerve compound action potential (CNAP) is a monitoring technique in surgeries where there is a risk of injury to the cochlear nerve or distal VIIIth cranial nerve. Compared to other monitoring techniques such as BAEP, CNAP allows for real-time cochlear nerve assessment because it is a near-field recording technique. Furthermore, CNAP wave amplitudes are typically much larger and less affected by electrical artefacts than far-field BAEP recorded from the scalp, so that the time to superimpose the signals can be less (Fig. 24.2). This increases the frequency of assessment of the cochlear nerve

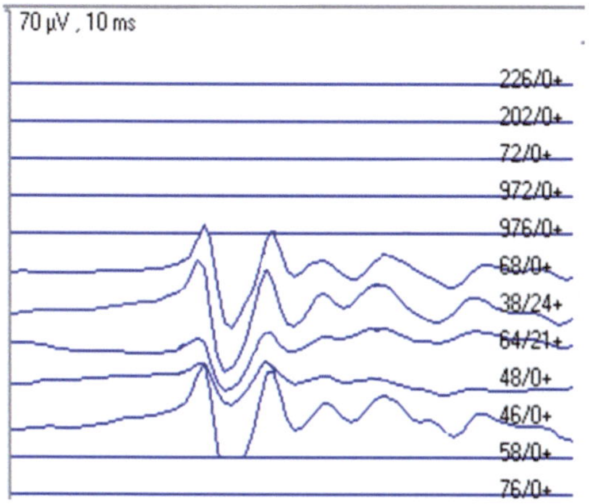

Fig. 24.2 CNAP recorded from the cisternal portion of the cochlear nerve during operation

and distal auditory nerve, and can provide nearly real-time cochlear neurophysiological feedback [12]. CNAP is more advantageous for use in noisy environments or in patients where preoperative ABR waves are absent, and is currently used primarily for the monitoring of cochlear nerve function during tumor resection of the CPA [7, 13].

24.4.2.1 Stimulation and Recording

Stimulation The CNAP was recorded using the same acoustic stimulus as the BAEP: broadband alternating clicks at a stimulus intensity of 100–110 dB. The other ear canal received white noise 30–40 dB lower than the stimulus intensity to eliminate bone conduction cross-reactivity.

Recording Electrodes and Band Pass Another electrode was placed proximal to the VIIIth nerve to record complex action potentials from the auditory nerve, with a filter range of 100/150–15,000 Hz and a signal analysis time of 10 ms, averaging 10–100 events.

24.4.2.2 Intraoperative Interpretation

Reduced amplitude and prolonged latency of CNAP potentials usually indicate a reduction in the number of neurons and nerve fibers, as well as disruption of stimulation and response of spiral ganglion neurons [10]. However, the main disadvantage of this technique is that it requires the electrodes to be placed directly on the auditory nerve. This requires the surgeon to place the electrodes carefully and keep them stable during the procedure while avoiding damage to the nerve fibers. There is currently no standard alarm threshold for CNAP, and the literature has classified monitoring results into three categories based on amplitude: no change, attenuation (amplitude attenuation of more than 80%), and disappearance (not possible to obtain a waveform with good reproducibility) [14]. In some studies, CNAP predicts postoperative hearing loss with up to 83% sensitivity and 100% specificity [15].

24.4.3 Brainstem Trigeminal Evoked Potentials

The trigeminal somatosensory system, responsible for sensation in the face and the anterior two-thirds of the tongue, can be effectively monitored using standard somatosensory evoked potentials (SSEPs). Research has demonstrated that SSEP monitoring is beneficial during intraoperative assessments of the medulla oblongata and is particularly useful in trigeminal rhizotomy procedures for patients with trigeminal neuralgia, where monitoring neural conduction in the trigeminal nerve is valuable [16]. Electrodes placed on the scalp can record activity related to the ascending trigeminal sensory pathways, stimulated by electrical impulses delivered to the peripheral trigeminal nerve.

24.4.3.1 Stimulation and Recording

Stimulation Sites The trigeminal nerve is stimulated using needle electrodes that are inserted subcutaneously into the upper (anode) and lower (cathode) lips [17].

Stimulation Intensity and Rate For each set of trigeminal evoked potentials (BTEP), stimulation is conducted over 300 trials to ensure the repeatability of the recorded cortical response. The stimulation frequency is set at 4.7 Hz, with each stimulus lasting 0.2 ms. An alternating polarity is employed to minimize significant baseline shifts.

The intensity of stimulation varies between 7 and 16 mA during these trials [17].

Recording Electrodes and Band Pass Cortical responses are recorded using electrodes positioned on the scalp. The recordings are conducted with needle electrodes placed at locations C5 or C6 on the contralateral side of the scalp, with Fpz serving as the reference point, following the International 10/20 system [17]. The waveform pattern remains consistent regardless of whether the reference site is Fpz or Cv7. The signals are filtered using a bandpass filter with a range of 0.1 to 1000 Hz, and the sampling rate is set at 5000 Hz.

24.4.3.2 Intraoperative Interpretation

Sensation in the head and face is innervated by the trigeminal nerve and can be assessed by stimulating the trigeminal branches while recording somatosensory evoked potentials (SEPs). This is technically difficult in practice, and large electrical stimulation artefacts often appear in the SEP waveform due to the short distance between the stimulating electrode of the BTEP and the scalp recording site. Because of the short latency period, large stimulation artefacts often overlap and blur with trigeminal SEPs, making them technically difficult to record.

Negative components generated by electrical stimulation of the trigeminal nerve branches have been recorded with latencies of 0.9, 1.6, and 2.6 ms at the point where the trigeminal nerve enters the brainstem [16]. These potentials specifically reflect neural activity within the trigeminal nerve, excluding other rostral structures, which means such recordings are solely applicable for monitoring the trigeminal (sensory) nerve [18]. Additionally, long-latency components are also monitored, with the latencies and amplitudes of the N13 and P19 peaks being recorded [17] (Fig. 24.3).

24.4.4 Somatosensory Evoked Potentials of Upper Extremity

Somatosensory evoked potentials (SSEPs) can be generated through electrical stimulation of peripheral nerves, such as the median or ulnar nerve at the wrist or the posterior tibial nerve at the ankle. This technique is utilized intraoperatively to monitor cortical or spinal cord blood perfusion, as well as to assess the structural and functional integrity of peripheral nerves and spinal nerve roots [19].

Injury to the brachial plexus due to improper patient positioning during surgery poses a significant perioperative risk and is a common complication following microvascular decompression (MVD). Typically, monitoring the SSEPs produced in this area through stimulation of the ulnar and median nerves can help prevent such nerve damage [20].

24.4.4.1 Stimulation and Recording

Stimulation Sites For upper extremity assessments, stimulation is applied to the median or ulnar nerve at the wrist, while for lower extremity evaluations, the posterior tibial nerve is stimulated at the ankle.

Stimulus Intensity and Rate The standard intensity for arm stimulation is approximately

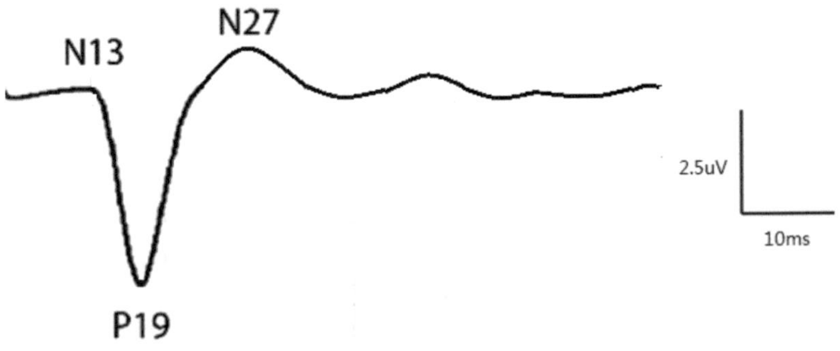

Fig. 24.3 Characteristic wave of trigeminal SSEP under general anesthesia

25 mA, and for leg stimulation, it is about 50 mA. The duration of each stimulus is set to 0.3 ms. A non-integer stimulation rate, such as 4.7 or 5.1 Hz, is employed to prevent synchronization with power line interference.

Recording Electrodes and Band Pass Electrodes are positioned on the scalp according to the 10–20 International System commonly used in clinical settings. For upper extremity stimulation, recordings are captured from the shoulder, cervical spine, and scalp. The setup requires three cortical channels (C′3-Fpz, C′4-Fpz, C′3-C′4), one cervical channel (Cs2-Fpz/Cs5-Fpz), and one peripheral channel (Erb's ipsilateral-contralateral) for monitoring median/ulnar nerve activity. Reference electrodes may be placed on the forehead or mastoid sites. Optimal low filter settings are typically around 30 Hz, while high filter settings range from 1500 to 3000 Hz. Notch filters at 60 Hz and 50 Hz should be disabled. Approximately 300 to 500 stimuli are necessary to produce a clear SSEP response.

24.4.4.2 Intraoperative Interpretation

The recording channel Erbi-Erbc captures the initial recorded potential known as Erb's point or N9, characterized by a negative upward deflection occurring approximately 9 ms after stimulating the median or ulnar nerve at the wrist. This deflection reflects the electronegativity resulting from the electrical impulse reaching the region of the evoked potential.

The channel Cs2-Fz/Cs5-Fz records the second potential, the cervicomedullary junction potential, represented by the P/N13 complex. This potential appears as a negative upward deflection around 13 ms after median nerve stimulation at the wrist.

The most significant component recorded from the scalp displays a negative peak at approximately 20 ms, followed by a positive peak at around 25 ms, forming the N20–P25 complex. The N20 component is thought to originate from the cortical area contralateral to the side of stimulation (C′3-Fpz/C′4-Fpz) (Fig. 24.4).

SSEPs have become a crucial component in a variety of surgical procedures. They are utilized to monitor the function of the large fiber sensory system during operations that pose a risk of damage to this system. A decrease in SSEP amplitude of 50% or more, or an increase in latency of 20% or greater, is considered a significant change that may indicate a potential postoperative neurological deficit. It is noteworthy that the amplitudes of the various components of evoked potentials are more prone to random fluctuations compared to the latencies of specific components.

During microvascular decompression (MVD) surgery, patients are positioned in a park bench configuration, which involves lateral positioning with the neck flexed and the head rotated downward. To enhance exposure and access, the upper shoulder and arm are depressed and secured using tape. However, the pronation and flexion of the lower arm can lead to compression of the ulnar nerve between the operating table and the cubital tunnel. Continuous intraoperative SSEP monitoring of ulnar and median nerve function serves as an effective indicator of brachial plexus

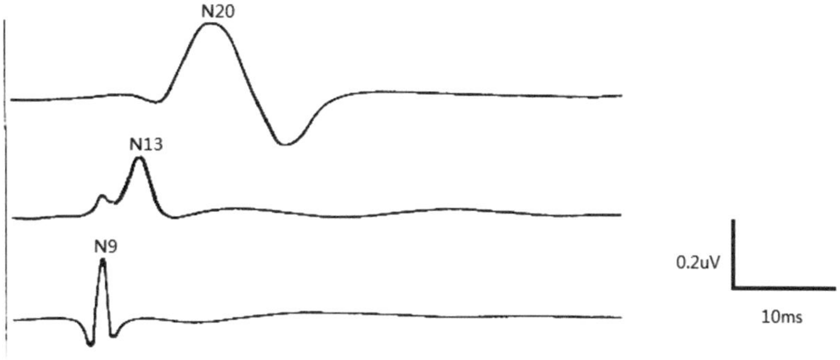

Fig. 24.4 Somatosensory evoked potentials from median nerve stimulation are shown. Typical peaks are shown in each of three recording channels

function, helping to minimize intraoperative neurological injuries during MVD surgeries [20].

24.4.4.3 Anesthesia Requirements

Inhalational anesthetics, including isoflurane, halothane, and enflurane, are known to reduce the amplitude and increase the latency of cortical components, with these effects directly correlating to the concentration of the agents administered in a dose-dependent manner [21]. Various intravenous agents such as propofol, benzodiazepines, barbiturates, etomidate, ketamine, and opiates also impact the amplitude and latency of SSEPs. Hypothermia can lead to increased latency and a slight decrease in the amplitude of SSEPs, whereas hyperthermia tends to decrease latency and further reduce amplitude. Additionally, severe hypotension may result in a significant decrease or even a complete loss of cervical and cortical responses.

24.4.5 Electromyography

Most cranial nerves are monitored by assessing their motor components to evaluate motor nerve function integrity. This process includes the recording of spontaneous electromyographic (EMG) activity as well as EMG activity triggered by electrical stimulation of the patient, the latter referred to as "triggered EMG." Free-run EMG (fEMG) involves capturing spontaneous muscle activity, which is valuable in intraoperative neurophysiology for identifying motor nerve depolarization caused by surgical irritation, ideally before any irreversible damage occurs to these structures. Triggered electromyographic (tEMG) activity can be recorded from the corresponding muscle following direct electrical stimulation of the motor nerve or nerve root. These recordings are often referred to as compound muscle action potentials (CMAPs). This technique is particularly useful for identifying specific cranial nerves or nerve roots that may be challenging to differentiate from surrounding tumoral, fibrous, or fatty tissues, thereby helping to preserve the structural and functional integrity of cranial nerves and spinal roots [22].

24.4.5.1 Stimulation and Recording

Stimulation Sites No stimulation is needed for fEMG recording, as this method relies solely on capturing spontaneous muscle activity and detecting irritation-induced muscle responses. In contrast, triggered EMG requires an electrical stimulus applied directly to the nerve structures. The EMG response is typically elicited by the surgeon using a probe to deliver electrical stimulation within the operative field. Both unipolar and bipolar stimulation techniques can be employed. A bipolar stimulator generates a current that flows more closely around the probe's tip compared to unipolar stimulation. As a result, unipolar stimulation may be more effective for determining whether the target nerve is in proximity to the probe, while bipolar stimulation offers enhanced precision in localization [23].

Stimulus Intensity and Rate The stimulation technique involves delivering constant current through repetitive square wave pulses lasting 0.1 to 0.2 ms at a frequency of 1 Hz, averaging 4 to 8 trials. The intensity of the stimulus for direct nerve or nerve root stimulation is gradually increased from 0 mA until an EMG response is observed, with a maximum limit of approximately 2 mA.

Recording Electrodes and Band Pass For both methods, electrodes are positioned in the target muscles that correspond to the nerve of interest. Given the relatively superficial nature of the muscles located in the head, face, neck, and tongue, paired unipolar needle electrodes are commonly used during surgery. This approach allows for quick placement and secure attachment of the electrodes without causing displacement. The specific muscles typically monitored for cranial nerve activity are detailed in Table 24.1 [22]. In monitoring the motor function of the glossopharyngeal nerve, recordings can be obtained not only by placing needle or hook wire electrodes in the laryngeal muscles but also from an endotracheal tube equipped with built-in recording wire electrodes [24]. Relatively broad filter settings are employed, with low-frequency filters set between 20 and 30 Hz and high-frequency filters between 5 and 10 kHz. The sweep speed is

Table 24.1 Cranial nerves and the corresponding muscles used in IOM

Cranial nerve	Nerve name	Muscles
III	Oculomotor	Inferior rectus, inferior oblique
IV	Trochlear	Superior oblique
V	Trigeminal	Masseter, temporalis
VI	Abducens	Lateral rectus
VII	Facial	Frontalis, orbicularis oculi, nasalis, orbicularis oris, mentalis
IX	Glossopharyngeal	Lateral soft palate
X	Vagus	Vocal cords, cricothyroid
XI	Accessory	Trapezius/stemocleidomastoid
XII	Hypoglossal	Tongue/genioglossus

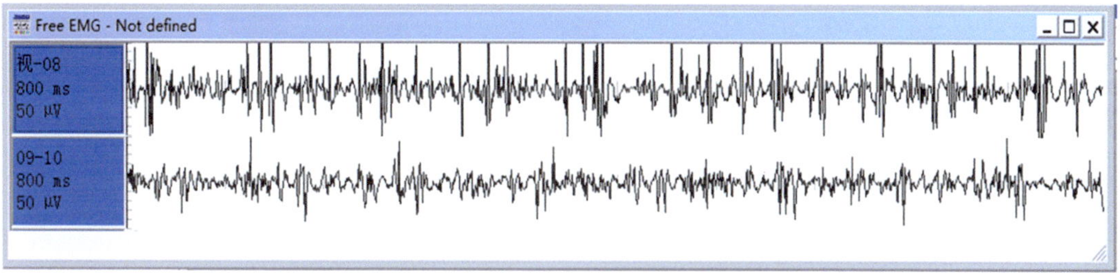

Fig. 24.5 An example of high-frequency "A-train" EMG activity refers to rapid, repetitive motor unit discharges, typically indicating nerve irritation during surgery

generally adjusted to 70–200 ms per division for continuous EMG recordings and 2–5 ms per division for recording electrically evoked EMG potentials. Sensitivity is typically calibrated to 50–200 μV per division.

24.4.5.2 Intraoperative Interpretation

Monitoring both spontaneous and triggered electromyography (EMG) is highly recommended during MVD procedures. Continuous recording of spontaneous EMG provides early warnings of nerve irritation.

Free-Run EMG Activity

During free-run EMG monitoring, muscle activity is continuously evaluated during parts of the surgery where motor nerves are at risk. Manipulation of these nerves can trigger depolarization of motor axons, leading to activation of motor units in the monitored muscle. The motor unit potentials (MUPs) generated can present a variety of patterns that need to be interpreted to understand and predict the consequences of surgical maneuvers that might provoke this activity. Making the EMG signal audible significantly enhances the monitoring process, allowing both the neurophysiologist and the surgeon to hear it. Surgeons may then correlate specific surgical actions with the onset or increase of EMG activity. Although observed EMG activity does not always indicate nerve damage, it at least signals depolarization of the corresponding nerve [22, 25].

Romstöck classified EMG patterns into three types of train-like waves: type A, type B, and type C. A-trains, similar to neuronal tonic discharges, consist of rapid, repetitive discharges (Fig. 24.5). These waves typically show some frequency variation, which suggests significant neural provocation or potential injury. Three key indicators that may signal nerve injury include: (1) sustained high-frequency firing lasting several seconds, (2) multiple large bursts of activity with complex morphology, and (3) abrupt bursts of high-amplitude spikes followed by complete silence [26, 27]. As a general rule, higher numbers and rates of recurrent MUPs are associated with increased nerve irritation. Mechanical compression can cause significant EMG activity, though in extreme cases, nerve injury could occur without any EMG activity being recorded, espe-

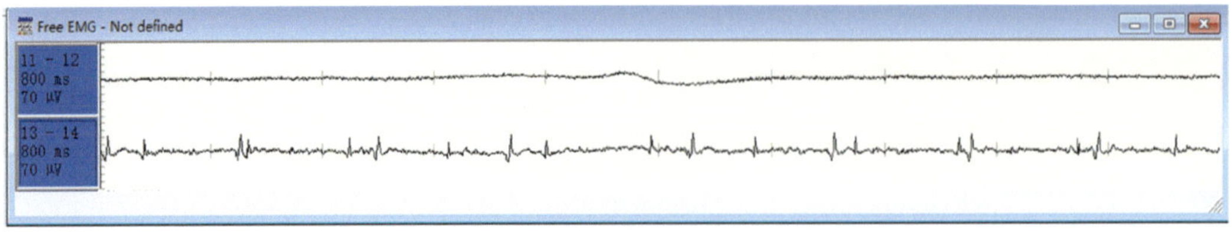

Fig. 24.6 A slowly repetitive B-train recorded from the orbicularis oris muscle during surgery for a right side vestibular schwannoma

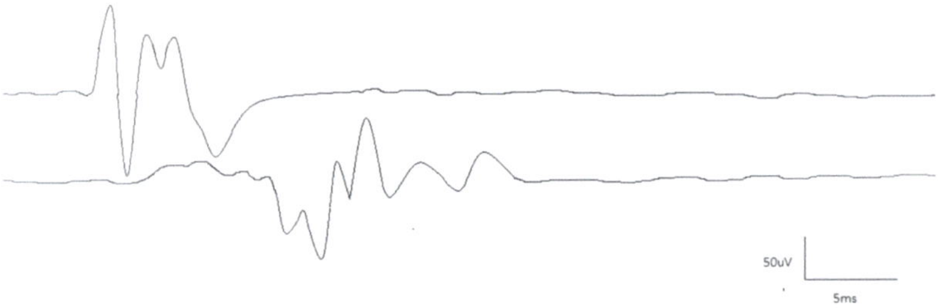

Fig. 24.7 Upper curve: EMG potentials recorded from electrodes placed in the Masseter muscles. Lower curve: EMG potentials recorded from electrodes placed in the orbicularis oculi muscles

cially in cases of complete nerve transaction [27, 28]. There are other factors that can produce EMG patterns resembling A-trains. For example, flushing the surgical site with cold water can induce EMG discharges. Although this response is benign, it is indistinguishable from neuronal discharges caused by mechanical nerve stimulation. Additionally, electrocoagulation can create artifacts that resemble neuronal discharges. It's important to recognize that spontaneous EMG activity may not reliably detect motor cranial nerve stimulation or damage during electrocoagulation due to the electrical artifacts it generates. B-trains (Fig. B-trains) are slower, repetitive discharges that are generally benign and do not predict postoperative neurological dysfunction (Fig. 24.6). Sporadic single EMG discharges are also frequently encountered and are usually considered harmless. C-trains consist of irregular EMG discharges that resemble interference patterns, which can be seen during shallow anesthesia [2].

Triggered EMG Activity

Triggered EMG recordings are utilized to locate or identify cranial nerves or their nuclei that cannot be visually distinguished in the surgical field. Monitoring EMG activity in muscles innervated by cranial nerves VII, IX, and X during surgery helps prevent complications such as facial palsy, dysphonia, and dysphagia [2, 29, 30]. While these cranial nerve palsies are usually temporary, they are often caused by cauterization, pulling, retraction, or sectioning of these nerves during the procedure [31]. The identity of the cranial nerve can be determined by observing which muscle responds to stimulation. If the same electrode detects activity from muscles innervated by two different nerves, the latency of the response can be used to differentiate them. For instance, stimulation of the trigeminal nerve elicits a CMAP with an onset latency of 3.5 to 5 ms [32], while stimulation of the facial nerve results in a CMAP with an onset latency of 6 to 8 ms (Fig. 24.7).

Spontaneous EMG activity may also be recorded from the target muscle during triggered EMG if it occurs simultaneously. The key difference between spontaneous and triggered EMG activity is that triggered EMG produces a consistent latency after the stimulus, while spontaneous EMG appears randomly, without a fixed relationship to the stimulus.

It's important to note that during bipolar stimulation, the presence of fluid in the surgical area may cause the stimulating current to pass through the fluid rather than reaching the nearby nerves. Therefore, the area should be aspirated before stimulation. Additionally, pharmacological neuromuscular blockade (NMB) may result in false-negative findings, so it is essential to confirm the absence of NMB before performing triggered EMG recordings.

24.4.5.3 Anesthesia Requirements

The level of muscle relaxation or pharmacologically induced paralysis is the most critical factor influencing EMG monitoring. It is advisable for the patient to be free from the effects of muscle relaxants during the EMG monitoring period. While literature confirms that EMG monitoring can be performed adequately with controlled partial neuromuscular blockade (NMB), we prefer to avoid using any neuromuscular blocking agents (NMBAs) during critical phases of the procedure to prevent potential confounding variables. In general, both inhalational and intravenous anesthetics have minimal or no impact on EMG monitoring. However, certain inhalational anesthetics, such as isoflurane, can lead to muscle relaxation [21].

The degree of muscle relaxation can be assessed using the train of four (TOF) method, which involves delivering a series of four electrical stimuli, typically at an intensity of about 25 mA, to the median or facial nerve, and measuring the resultant muscle contractions. The absence of twitches indicates complete paralysis, while the presence of at least three twitches signifies that the patient remains only minimally relaxed or practically not paralyzed [1].

24.4.6 Abnormal Muscle Response

In 1985, Moller and Jannetta first demonstrated that in patients with hemifacial spasm, stimulating one branch of the facial nerve could activate facial muscles innervated by other branches, due to the hyperexcitability of the facial nerve. This phenomenon, known as the abnormal muscle response (AMR) or lateral spreading response (LSR), is believed to be associated with synaptic transmission, although the exact mechanism of the lateral spread remains unclear. Notably, the AMR typically disappears immediately in most patients when the offending vessel is moved away from the facial nerve; this disappearance may help predict both short- and long-term success of microvascular decompression (MVD) for hemifacial spasm [33].

24.4.6.1 Stimulation and Recording

Stimulation Sites Stimulation needle electrodes are primarily placed over either the temporal branch or the marginal mandibular branch of the facial nerve.

Stimulation Intensity and Rate A single constant current stimulus lasting 0.1 to 0.2 ms, delivered at a rate of 1 Hz, is used to elicit lateral spread. Typically, a stable AMR is recorded at a stimulation intensity level between 5 and 15 mA.

Recording Electrodes and Band Pass Recording needles are inserted subcutaneously, spaced 0.5 to 1 cm apart, into the mentalis muscle if the temporal branch of the facial nerve is stimulated, or into the orbicularis oculi muscles if the marginal mandibular branch is stimulated.

24.4.6.2 Intraoperative Interpretation

During intraoperative monitoring, an AMR wave with a latency of approximately 10 ms after stimulation is recorded. The baseline threshold for eliciting the AMR is established, and stimulation may proceed close to this level. When the offending vessel is repositioned away from the facial nerve, the AMR is known to either disappear or become significantly attenuated [34] (Fig. 24.8). The intensity is then increased for a few seconds to confirm the permanent disappearance of the AMR.

However, it is possible for the AMR to dissipate prior to performing MVD, such as when the dura is opened. In these cases, it is advisable to increase the stimulation intensity to reestablish the presence of the AMR [35]. Changes in the AMR should be closely monitored throughout the MVD until complete decompression is achieved and the dura is sutured.

Clinical studies have shown that the disappearance of the AMR or a decrease in wave

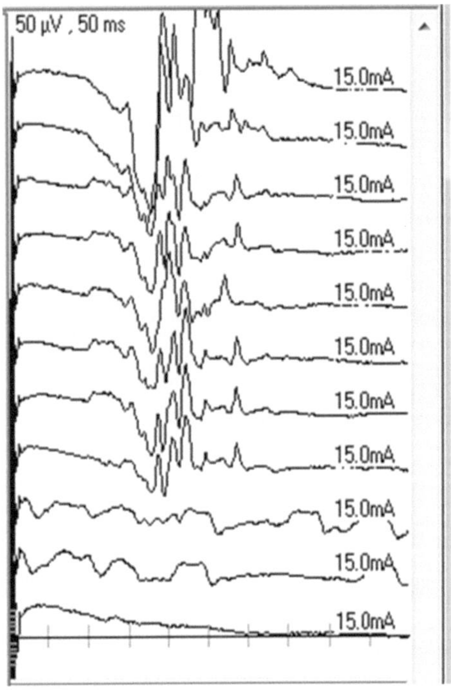

Fig. 24.8 Typical changes of AMR during MVD for HFS

amplitude is a good predictor of clinical response to MVD [36–39]. However, others have questioned the reliability of LSR in predicting postoperative clinical outcomes [40]. The practical value of AMR disappearance as a method to evaluate MVD efficacy is still controversial. Sekula conducted a meta-analysis on this issue. The pooled probability was 4.2 (95% CI 2.7–6.7)—if the abnormal muscle response (AMR) disappeared during surgery, the chances of cure were 4.2 times greater than if lateral spread persisted. They concluded, "Routine AMR monitoring should be performed in the operating theater, and surgical decisions in the operating theater should be enhanced by AMR" [35].

The criteria for determining the disappearance of the AMR are not uniform. Some studies consider the AMR to be resolved if its amplitude decreases by more than 50%, whereas others consider it to be resolved only if the AMR disappears completely. Overall, the majority of the clinical literature supports the disappearance of the AMR as a valid marker of adequate nerve decompression and predictive of clinical cure; if the AMR persists intraoperatively after decompression, the probability of postoperative symptomatic relief in such patients is low, but this does not exclude the possibility of postoperative benefit [25].

It is worth noting that in patients with post-paralytic facial dyskinesia (PFS), AMR may also be recorded in the orbicularis oculi or orbicularis oculi muscles, respectively. AMR is present in all patients with HFS and in most patients with PFS. However, the latency of the AMR in patients with HFS is more stable (approximately 10 ms), whereas in patients with PFS, the latency of the AMR is likely to be longer, and the waveforms more discrete.

24.4.6.3 Anesthesia Requirements

Since the abnormal muscle response (AMR) is a type of triggered electromyography, the level of muscle relaxation is crucial for effective monitoring. No muscle relaxants are administered following the induction of anesthesia.

24.4.7 Z-L Response

The Z-L Response (ZLR) was first introduced by Zheng et al. [41] for intraoperative monitoring of HFS. This response is particularly useful when AMR is absent before decompression or persists even after all vascular compressions have been addressed. The ZLR can assist neurosurgeons in identifying the true source of compression when multiple offending vessels are present.

24.4.7.1 Stimulation and Recording

Stimulation Sites The stimulating electrode is placed on the wall of the offending artery, near the site of compression (within 5 mm), during MVD for HFS [41].

Stimulation Intensity and Rate A single constant current stimulus lasting 0.1 to 0.2 ms, delivered at a rate of 1 Hz, is used to elicit the ZLR. The intensity of stimulation ranges from 0.5 to 2 mA.

Recording Electrodes and Band Pass ZLR is recorded from the orbicularis oculi, orbicularis oris, and mentalis muscles using needle electrodes. The filter settings for ZLR are identical to those used for AMR.

24.4.7.2 Intraoperative Interpretation

The morphology of the ZLR is similar to that of the AMR. The latency of the ZLR is approximately 7.3 ± 0.8 ms, which is significantly shorter than the latency of the AMR (Fig. 24.9). In most patients, where a single offending vessel compresses the facial nerve at a specific site, both the ZLR and AMR provide similar information during surgery: both responses disappear immediately when the offending artery is removed from the facial nerve. However, if the AMR is absent initially or persists after the offending vessel has been repositioned with Teflon sponges, the ZLR becomes critical for assessing whether sufficient decompression has been achieved [41, 42]. In cases where multiple arteries compress the facial nerve, the ZLR can only be recorded from the facial muscles when the true offending vessel is stimulated. Therefore, the ZLR may be valuable for identifying the actual source of compression [43].

Overall, the combined intraoperative monitoring of AMR and ZLR offers valuable neurosurgical guidance during MVD for HFS, particularly when AMR waves are not detected. The integration of AMR and ZLR can help reduce both the false-positive and false-negative rates associated with AMR [44].

24.4.7.3 Anesthesia Requirements

The anesthesia requirements for ZLR monitoring are identical to those for AMR. No muscle relaxants should be administered following the induction of anesthesia.

24.4.8 Blink Reflexes

In 1952, Kugelberg was the first to identify two electrically induced blink reflex (BR) components, R1 and R2 [45]. Typically, an electrical stimulus applied to the supraorbital nerve (V1) produces two measurable responses in the orbicularis oculi muscles: an early response known as R1, which is ipsilateral to the stimulated side, and a later response, R2, which is expressed bilaterally. The ipsilateral R2 is often referred to as R2i, while the contralateral response is denoted as R2c, also known as the "consensual response," similar to the photomotor pupillary reflex [46]. The latency of the R1 component of the BR is relatively stable at approximately 10 ms. In contrast, R2 typically exhibits more variable latencies and larger magnitudes compared to R1, with a lower threshold [24].

The blink response is a valuable technique for investigating trigeminal and facial nerve pathways and is commonly employed for the preoperative assessment of nerve and brainstem function. Deletis demonstrated a method for recording the R1 component of the BR under

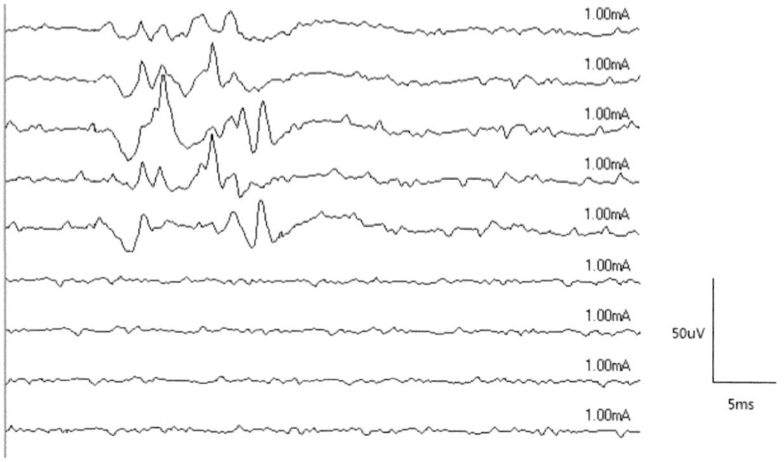

Fig. 24.9 ZLR is recorded from the facial muscles while stimulating the offending artery

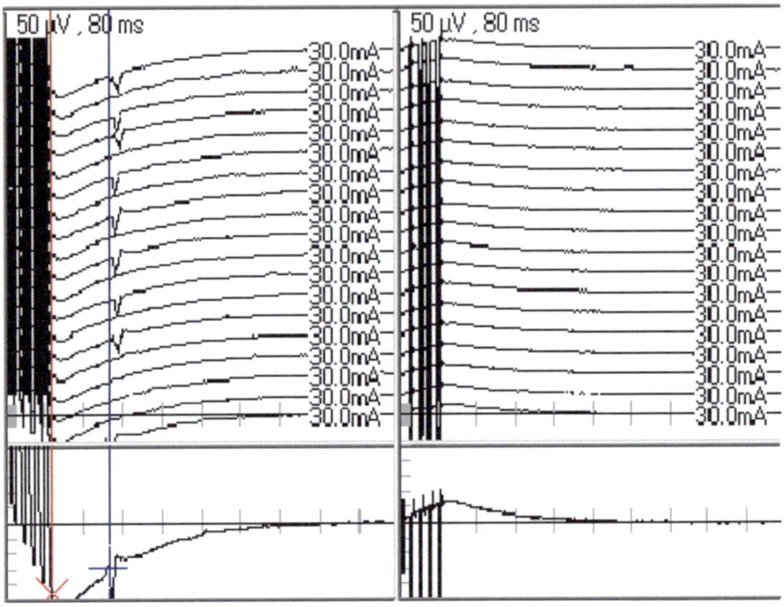

Fig. 24.10 The R1 component can be recorded ipsilaterally by stimulating the supraorbital nerve with a short train of electrical stimuli intraoperatively

intraoperative general anesthesia [47]. They stimulated the supraorbital nerve with a short train of electrical impulses, successfully eliciting the R1 component of the BR after delivering four stimulus sequences (Fig. 24.10). Therefore, employing this test for intraoperative neuromonitoring appears to be feasible. The following section will focus on the methods and applications of the blink reflex in intraoperative monitoring.

24.4.8.1 Stimulation and Recording

Stimulation Sites Stimulation of the supraorbital nerve was conducted using a pair of electroencephalographic needle electrodes inserted subcutaneously over the nerve.

Stimulus Intensity and Rate Four to seven rectangular constant-current stimuli were applied, with an interstimulus interval (ISI) of 2 ms, an intensity ranging from 20 to 40 mA, and a train repetition rate of 0.4 Hz.

Recording Electrodes and Band Pass Recording was performed using needle electrodes similar to those employed for stimulation. These electrodes were placed in the lower lateral region of the orbicularis oculi muscle, both ipsilateral and contralateral to the stimulated side. Recordings utilized a 50-ms epoch with bandpass digital filters set between 70 and 1219 Hz. Attempts to record the blink reflex (BR) were made after intubation, during the surgery, and after the initiation of skin closure [47].

24.4.8.2 Intraoperative Interpretation

The supraorbital nerve was stimulated with a short train of electrical stimuli, and the R1 component of the BR was elicited when there were four stimulus strings in the sequence. No patient elicited R2, probably due to the effect of anesthetics on the R2 polysynaptic pathway.

Although the blink reflex is usually normal in patients with idiopathic trigeminal neuralgia. The possibility to achieve continuous monitoring of the sensory part of the trigeminal nerve, brainstem, and facial nerve is a further important development. It has also been recently reported that the use of concurrent BR and LSR monitoring during MVD maximizes the ability to predict patient prognosis and determine the extent of facial nerve decompression [48]. Although the potential value of BR monitoring has yet to be fully elucidated, it is an ideal candidate for novel ION methods. In addition, this reflex-based approach could facilitate additional simultaneous monitoring of the trigeminal afferents and brainstem connections that make up the reflex arc [48]. BR may be a useful intraoperative monitoring technique for monitoring the sensory portion of the trigeminal nerve when brainstem and facial nerve function are normal. When intraoperative trigeminal nerve injury occurs, the R1 latency on the affected side may be delayed or absent. When brainstem and trigeminal function are normal, BR provides insight into facial nerve function throughout [49, 50].

Currently, the number of studies utilizing the blink reflex (BR) remains relatively limited. Therefore, additional prospective studies with larger sample sizes and extended follow-up periods are necessary to validate the effectiveness of these reflex monitoring techniques.

24.4.8.3 Anesthesia Requirements

Recording the BR in patients under general anesthesia is feasible when using low doses of desflurane or sevoflurane during surgery. If total intravenous anesthesia is employed, boluses of propofol should be avoided, as they inhibit the elicitation of the BR. Additionally, the use of muscle relaxants should also be avoided.

24.4.9 Facial F-Wave

The F-wave is an antidromic pulse that travels to an alpha motoneuron in the anterior horn of the spinal cord and then returns orthodromically down the same axon. It is a standard electrophysiological technique used to identify lesions in the proximal segments of peripheral nerves. Recent findings regarding facial F-waves in various conditions affecting the intracranial and intracanalicular portions of the nerve have demonstrated the diagnostic value of this method [51, 52].

24.4.9.1 Stimulation and Recording

Stimulation Sites The stimulating electrodes are positioned proximally over the zygomatic branch of the facial nerve.

Stimulus Intensity and Rate The facial nerve is stimulated using constant current rectangular monophasic pulses (duration of 0.1 to 0.2 ms) delivered transcutaneously (for extraoperative studies) or via subdermal needle electrodes (for intraoperative measurements). The stimulation frequency is set at 1 Hz [53]. The stimulation strength is adjusted to supramaximal levels to achieve stable M-waves with minimal stimulus intensity, typically between 3 and 10 mA.

Recording Electrodes and Band Pass Recording electrodes are placed on both sides of the nose to capture the compound action potentials of the paranasal muscles [54, 55]. The F-wave varies with each stimulus, and the F/M amplitude ratio (the percentage of the peak F-wave amplitude relative to the peak M-wave amplitude) and latency are analyzed. Recordings are processed through preamplifiers and amplifiers (set to 100 μV/div) and then bandpass filtered between 20 and 3000 Hz without averaging.

24.4.9.2 Intraoperative Interpretation

The implementation of intraoperative facial F-wave monitoring provides continuous and accurate real-time insights into the functional status of the nerve. Additionally, it offers a reliable prognostic evaluation of postoperative facial nerve function. An advantage of F-wave recordings is their utility in detecting facial nerve function during the perioperative period. F-waves have been reported as useful indicators of lower motor neuron excitability. In the ipsilateral mentalis muscles, the F wave, elicited by stimulating the marginal mandibular branch of the facial nerve, is also an antidromic pulse that propagates to the facial motonucleus and returns orthodromically down the same axon. Consequently, the F wave in facial muscles may reflect the excitability of the facial motonucleus (Fig. 24.11).

Electrophysiological studies have shown that F waves are more persistent in patients with HFS. There is evidence that as soon as the AMR disappears, so do the F waves [56].

Facial nerve F-wave monitoring is now employed for intraoperative assessment of facial nerve function. It delivers continuous, validated, real-time information regarding the nerve's functional state during surgical manipulation. Changes in intraoperative F-waves are closely

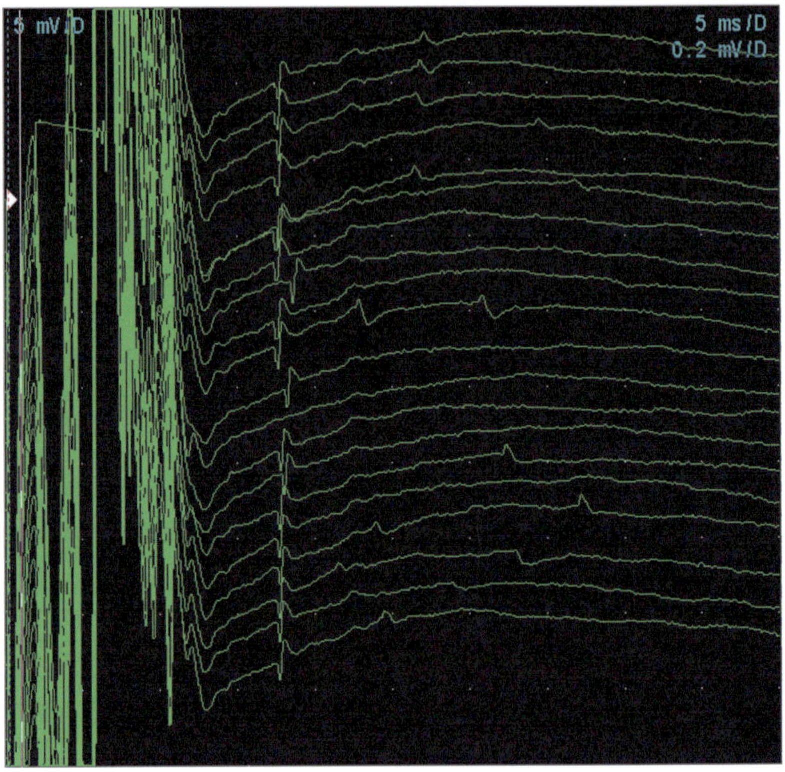

Fig. 24.11 Typical facial F-waves recorded from the Scalenus depressor muscle when stimulating the mandibular marginal branch of the facial nerve

associated with the actual handling of the nerve. Additionally, intraoperative F-wave monitoring can detect a transient disappearance of the F-wave, which indicates an imminent risk of significant facial dysfunction. Wedekind and Klug [57] reported that the permanent absence of the F-wave has a sensitivity of 91% and a specificity of 100% in predicting poor outcomes for facial nerve function.

24.4.9.3 Anesthesia Requirements

The effectiveness of facial nerve F-wave monitoring during surgery is limited by its sensitivity to anesthesia and may be absent in some healthy adults [53, 55].

24.4.10 Motor-Evoked Potentials

Transcranial electrical stimulation was first introduced to the human brain by Merton and Morton [58]. This technique can be performed through electrical stimulation of the cortex or the spinal cord. It involves applying an electrical current to depolarize the corticospinal system proximal to the surgical level, surpassing its threshold. This method evaluates the integrity of motor pathways from the cortex to the muscles. It has been demonstrated to be practical and effective during surgery, and is now widely regarded as essential in the neurosurgical field [59, 60]. For neurophysiological intraoperative monitoring of motor pathways, the use of motor-evoked potentials (MEPs) triggered by electrical cortical stimulation is successfully performed under anesthesia (Fig. 24.12).

24.4.10.1 Stimulation and Recording

Stimulation Sites The standard 10–20 EEG electrode placement system is employed. Scalp electrodes are often positioned more laterally than in the standard montage for spinal surgeries [56]. C3-Cz is used for stimulation of the left hemisphere, while C4-Cz is utilized for the right hemisphere [61]. Using a Cz cathode may reduce the likelihood of extracranial activation of the facial nerve.

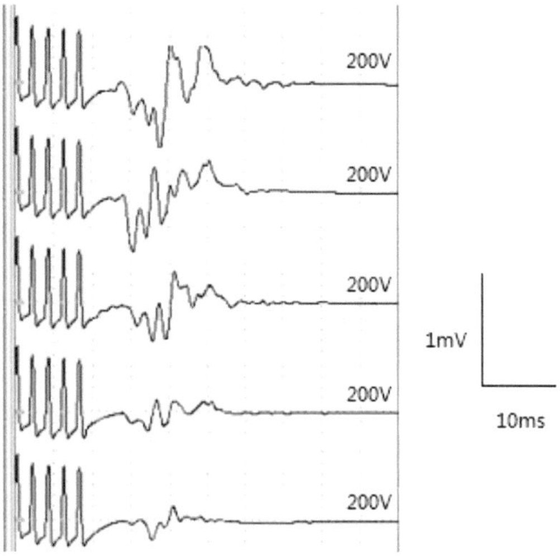

Fig. 24.12 It takes a short train stimuli of 200 V to eliciting MEP before decompression. After MVD completed, the amplitude of MEP decreased significantly

Stimulus Intensity and Rate Transcranial stimulation may utilize constant voltage (ranging from 180 to 600 V) or constant current (ranging from 50 to 220 mA) with durations varying from 0.5 to 3 ms and interstimulus intervals of 1 to 5 ms. Typically, three or more pulses are delivered at a train repetition rate of 2 Hz.

Recording Electrodes and Band Pass Electrodes are placed in the target muscles corresponding to the nerve of interest. Pairs of monopolar needle electrodes are most commonly employed. Filter settings typically range between 5 and 10 kHz [62, 63].

24.4.10.2 Intraoperative Interpretation

Preserving postoperative facial nerve function is a key objective of microvascular decompression (MVD). Monitoring motor-evoked potentials (MEPs) has been reported to be valuable for assessing postoperative cranial nerve function [62, 64]. MEP monitoring can significantly impact the prevention of paraplegia and paralysis during surgeries where the motor pathways may be at risk. It enables observation of the functionality of both the first and second motor neurons and aids in predicting postoperative nerve function. However, continuous intraoperative monitoring of MEPs is challenging due to artifacts caused by body movements. Consequently, surgical manipulation must be paused during MEP recordings [59, 60].

The criteria for alarming MEP changes remain a topic of debate. Some experts advocate for an “all or nothing” approach, suggesting that the complete absence of MEPs should indicate impaired neurological function. Others argue that an intraoperative increase in stimulation threshold and a decrease in amplitude are closely linked to postoperative nerve dysfunction [63, 65].

MEPs are also employed during MVD to identify and avoid lesions to the facial nerve while manipulating the vessels compressing it. Facial compound muscle action potentials (CMAPs) in transcranial MEPs appear with a short latency of approximately 15 ms [62]. Fernandez [56] reported that MEP monitoring in patients with hemifacial spasm (HFS) shows distinctive characteristics due to the hyperexcitability of the facial nerve and facial motor nucleus. Facial cortical motor evoked potentials (FCoMEPs) are continuously recorded before, during, and after MVD, alongside lateral spreading responses (LSRs). The major excitability changes in FCoMEPs are indicated by an increased number of stimuli required to elicit responses or by an increase in the intensity of current compared to baseline measurements. Therefore, transcranial MEPs have also been explored as an adjunct to monitoring during MVD for hemifacial spasm (Fig. 24.11). Although FCoMEPs have been increasingly utilized in MVD surgery for patients with HFS, further well-designed controlled studies are necessary to determine the clinical utility of FCoMEP monitoring as a predictor of postoperative outcomes [66].

It is important to note that when recording from the facial muscles, the current may have directly stimulated the extracranial segment of the facial nerve without assessing the intracranial portion. This can be verified by comparing responses to strings of stimuli versus single stimuli. Pulse trains of stimuli are often required during MEP monitoring to reach the threshold and excite neurons, while a single stimulus is typically sufficient to activate peripheral nerves. Thus, a response observed in a train stimulus but absent in a single stimulus may indicate involvement of the intracranial segment of the facial nerve, whereas a response in both may suggest stimulation of the extracranial segment.

24.4.10.3 Anesthesia Requirements

In general anesthetic techniques should be used with minimized inhalational agents, such as nitrous oxide and Isoflurane and minimized neuromuscular blockade. Anesthesia techniques using a combination of less than 50% nitrous oxide and narcotics, Etomidate, or Ketamine allow the recording of reliable MEPs [21].

24.5 Summary

In recent years, intraoperative neuromonitoring techniques have been used not only to assess the integrity of cranial nerve, sensory, and motor pathways but also to improve outcomes and reduce postoperative complications in MVD. Some of the newer advances in ION for MVD have provided clinicians with a deeper understanding of the pathophysiology of these disorders. Although the neurological prognostic benefits of current IONM modalities have been questioned: they may lead to increased costs, false-positive or false-negative results, or prolonged operative times. However, many experts continue to advocate for the use of IONM because its potential benefits to neurological prognosis greatly outweigh the associated costs and risks. Many studies have found that a multimodal IONM approach is often more advantageous than a single modality using the IONM modality. The knowledge and experience of clinical neurophysiologists in basic electrophysiology and operating room electrophysiology, comprehensive training of monitoring technicians, active communication between IOM team members, and a customized approach suited to the purpose of IOM in a particular procedure will greatly contribute to the accuracy of the IOM. Future research should focus on improving and developing new IONM techniques with high sensitivity and specificity in improving clinical outcomes and predicting neurological damage after all types of MVD treatment.

References

1. George Zouridakis ACP. A concise guide to intraoperative monitoring. Boca Raton, FL: CRC; 2000.
2. López JR, Legatt AD. Monitoring surgery around the cranial nerves. Handb Clin Neurol. 2022;186:319–51.
3. Gloria M, Galloway MRN, Lopez JR, Zamel KM. Intraoperative neurophysiologic monitoring. New York, NY: Cambridge University Press; 2010.
4. Thirumala PD, Carnovale G, Loke Y, Habeych ME, Crammond DJ, Balzer JR, et al. Brainstem auditory evoked potentials' diagnostic accuracy for hearing loss: systematic review and meta-analysis. J Neurol Surg B Skull Base. 2017;78(1):43–51.
5. Lee MH, Lee S, Park SK, Lee JA, Park K. Delayed hearing loss after microvascular decompression for hemifacial spasm. Acta Neurochir. 2019;161(3):503–8.
6. Li N, Zhao WG, Pu CH, Yang WL. Correlation between cerebellar retraction and hearing loss after microvascular decompression for hemifacial spasm: a prospective study. World Neurosurg. 2017;102:97–101.
7. Ariano M, Franchella S, Tealdo G, Zanoletti E. Intraoperative Cochlear nerve function monitoring in hearing preservation surgery: a systematic review of the literature. Audiol Res. 2022;12(6):696–708.
8. Society ACN. Guideline 9C: guidelines on short-latency auditory evoked potentials. Am J Electroneurodiagnostic Technol. 2006;46(3):275–86.
9. Sprenghers L, Lemmens R, Loon JV. Usefulness of intraoperative monitoring in microvascular decompression for hemifacial spasm: a systematic review and meta-analysis. Br J Neurosurg. 2022;36(3):346–57.
10. Pobożny I, Lachowska M, Bartoszewicz R, Niemczyk K. Detailed insight into transtympanic electrocochleography (TT-ECochG) and direct cochlear nerve action potential (CNAP) for intraoperative hearing monitoring in patients with vestibular schwannoma—methodology of measurements and interpretation of results. Otolaryngol Pol. 2020;74(6):1–8.
11. Yamakami I, Yoshinori H, Saeki N, Wada M, Oka N. Hearing preservation and intraoperative auditory brainstem response and cochlear nerve compound action potential monitoring in the removal of small acoustic neurinoma via the retrosigmoid approach. J Neurol Neurosurg Psychiatry. 2009;80(2):218–27.
12. Miyazaki H, Caye-Thomasen P. Intraoperative auditory system monitoring. Adv Otorhinolaryngol. 2018;81:123–32.
13. Watanabe N, Ishii T, Fujitsu K, Kaku S, Ichikawa T, Miyahara K, et al. Intraoperative cochlear nerve mapping with the mobile cochlear nerve compound action

potential tracer in vestibular schwannoma surgery. J Neurosurg. 2018;1:1–8.
14. Li X, Liang J, Song G, Jiao H. Using a facial nerve stimulator to record the auditory nerve compound action potential to locate the auditory nerve during vestibular schwannoma resection. World Neurosurg. 2023;175:e582–e92.
15. Sun DQ, Sullivan CB, Kung RW, Asklof M, Hansen MR, Gantz BJ. How well does intraoperative audiologic monitoring predict hearing outcome during middle fossa vestibular schwannoma resection? Otol Neurotol. 2018;39(7):908–15.
16. Stechison MT, Kralick FJ. The trigeminal evoked potential: part I. Long-latency responses in awake or anesthetized subjects. Neurosurgery. 1993;33(4):633–8.
17. Malcharek MJ, Landgraf J, Hennig G, Sorge O, Aschermann J, Sablotzki A. Recordings of long-latency trigeminal somatosensory-evoked potentials in patients under general anaesthesia. Clin Neurophysiol. 2011;122(5):1048–54.
18. Oikawa T, Matsumoto M, Sasaki T, Kodama N. Experimental study of medullary trigeminal evoked potentials: development of a new method of intraoperative monitoring of the medulla oblongata. J Neurosurg. 2000;93(1):68–76.
19. Ghatol D, Widrich J. Intraoperative neurophysiological monitoring. In: StatPearls [Internet]. Treasure Island, FL: StatPearls; 2023.
20. Ying T, Wang X, Sun H, Tang Y, Yuan Y, Li S. Clinical usefulness of somatosensory evoked potentials for detection of peripheral nerve and brachial plexus injury secondary to malpositioning in microvascular decompression. J Clin Neurophysiol. 2015;32(6):512–5.
21. Gruenbaum BF, Gruenbaum SE. Neurophysiological monitoring during neurosurgery: anesthetic considerations based on outcome evidence. Curr Opin Anaesthesiol. 2019;32(5):580–4.
22. Holland NR. Intraoperative electromyography. J Clin Neurophysiol. 2002;19(5):444–53.
23. Kennelly KD. Electrodiagnostic approach to cranial neuropathies. Neurol Clin. 2012;30(2):661–84.
24. Singh R, Husain AM. Neurophysiologic intraoperative monitoring of the glossopharyngeal and vagus nerves. J Clin Neurophysiol. 2011;28(6):582–6.
25. Kennelly KD. Clinical neurophysiology of cranial nerve disorders. Handb Clin Neurol. 2019;161:327–42.
26. Moller AR. Intraoperative neurophysiologic monitoring. Am J Otol. 1995;16(1):115–7.
27. Romstöck J, Strauss C, Fahlbusch R. Continuous electromyography monitoring of motor cranial nerves during cerebellopontine angle surgery. J Neurosurg. 2000;93(4):586–93.
28. Nelson KR, Vasconez HC. Nerve transection without neurotonic discharges during intraoperative electromyographic monitoring. Muscle Nerve. 1995;18(2):236–8.
29. Harper CM. Intraoperative cranial nerve monitoring. Muscle Nerve. 2004;29(3):339–51.
30. Minahan RE, Mandir AS. Neurophysiologic intraoperative monitoring of trigeminal and facial nerves. J Clin Neurophysiol. 2011;28(6):551–65.
31. Habeych MECD, Gardner P, Thirumala PD, Horowitz MB, Balzer JR. Intraoperative neurophysiological monitoring of microvascular decompression for glossopharyngeal neuralgia. J Clin Neurophysiol. 2014;31(4):337–43.
32. Moller AR. Intraoperative neurophysiological monitoring. 3rd ed. New York: Springer-Verlag; 2011.
33. Moller AR, Jannetta PJ. Monitoring facial EMG responses during microvascular decompression operations for hemifacial spasm. J Neurosurg. 1987;66(5):681–5.
34. Thirumala PD, Shah AC, Nikonow TN, Habeych ME, Balzer JR, Crammond DJ, et al. Microvascular decompression for hemifacial spasm: evaluating outcome prognosticators including the value of intraoperative lateral spread response monitoring and clinical characteristics in 293 patients. J Clin Neurophysiol. 2011;28(1):56–66.
35. Sekula RF Jr, Bhatia S, Frederickson AM, Jannetta PJ, Quigley MR, Small GA, Breisinger R. Utility of intraoperative electromyography in microvascular decompression for hemifacial spasm: a meta-analysis. Neurosurg Focus. 2009;27(4):E10.
36. Sun C, Xu J, Zhu W, Zhang X, Zhao P, Zhang Y. Beyond the observation of all or nothing: the clinical significance of the pre-decompression instability of abnormal muscle response in microvascular decompression for hemifacial spasm. J Clin Neurosci. 2022;104:64–8.
37. Yang W, Kuroi Y, Yokosako S, Ohbuchi H, Tani S, Kasuya H. Hemifacial spasm caused by veins confirmed by intraoperative monitoring of abnormal muscle response. World Neurosurg X. 2018;1:100002.
38. Ying T-T, Li S-T, Zhong J, Li X-Y, Wang X-H, Zhu J. The value of abnormal muscle response monitoring during microvascular decompression surgery for hemifacial spasm. Int J Surg. 2011;9(4):347–51.
39. Zhang X, Zhao H, Zhu J, Tang Y-D, Ying T-T, Yuan Y, et al. Electromyographically guided nerve combing makes microvascular decompression more successful in hemifacial spasm with persistent abnormal muscle response. World Neurosurg. 2017b;102:85–90.
40. Joo WI, Lee KJ, Park HK, Chough CK, Rha HK. Prognostic value of intra-operative lateral spread response monitoring during microvascular decompression in patients with hemifacial spasm. J Clin Neurosci. 2008;15(12):1335–9.
41. Zheng X, Hong W, Tang Y, Ying T, Wu Z, Shang M, et al. Discovery of a new waveform for intraoperative monitoring of hemifacial spasms. Acta Neurochir. 2012;154(5):799–805.
42. Yang M, Zheng X, Ying T, Zhu J, Zhang W, Yang X, et al. Combined intraoperative monitoring of abnormal muscle response and Z-L response for hemifacial spasm with tandem compression type. Acta Neurochir. 2014;156(6):1161–6; discussion 6.

43. Zhang X, Zhao H, Tang Y-D, Zhu J, Zhou P, Yuan Y, et al. The effects of combined intraoperative monitoring of abnormal muscle response and Z-L response for Hemifacial spasm. World Neurosurg. 2017a;108:367–73.
44. Son B-C, Ko H-C, Choi J-G. Intraoperative monitoring of Z-L response (ZLR) and abnormal muscle response (AMR) during microvascular decompression for hemifacial spasm. Interpreting the role of ZLR. Acta Neurochir. 2018;160(5):963–70.
45. Kugelberg E. Facial reflexes. Brain. 1952;75(3):385–96.
46. Esteban A. A neurophysiological approach to brainstem reflexes. Blink reflex. Neurophysiol Clin. 1999;29(1):7–38.
47. Deletis V, Urriza J, Ulkatan S, Fernandez-Conejero I, Lesser J, Misita D. The feasibility of recording blink reflexes under general anesthesia. Muscle Nerve. 2009;39(5):642–6.
48. Hsu P-C, Yang T-F, Hsu SPC, Yen Y-S, Lin C-F, Tsai Y-Y, et al. Blink synkinesis monitoring during microvascular decompression for hemifacial spasm. J Chin Med Assoc. 2019;82(6):519–23.
49. Simioni V, Capone JG, Sette E, Granieri E, Farneti M, Cavallo MA, et al. Intraoperative monitoring of sensory part of the trigeminal nerve using blink reflex during microvascular decompression for trigeminal neuralgia. Acta Neurochir. 2018;160(1):165–9.
50. Ying T, Bao B, Yuan Y, Zhong W, Zhu J, Tang Y, et al. Blink reflex monitoring in microvascular decompression for trigeminal neuralgia. Neurol Res. 2021;43(7):591–4.
51. Jerath N, Kimura J. F wave, a wave, H reflex, and blink reflex. Handb Clin Neurol. 2019;160:225–39.
52. Wedekind C, Klug N. Nasal muscle F-wave for peri- and intraoperative diagnosis of facial nerve function. Electromyogr Clin Neurophysiol. 1998;38(8):481–90.
53. Wedekind C, Klug N. Facial F wave recording: a novel and effective technique for extra- and intraoperative diagnosis of facial nerve function in acoustic tumor disease. Otolaryngol Head Neck Surg. 2003;129(1):114–20.
54. Wedekind C, Klug N. Assessment of facial nerve function in acoustic tumor disease by nasal muscle F waves and transcranial magnetic stimulation. Muscle Nerve. 2000;23(1):58–62.
55. Wedekind C, Stauten W, Klug N. A normative study on human facial F waves. Muscle Nerve. 2001;24(7):900–4.
56. Fernandez-Conejero I, Ulkatan S, Sen C, Deletis V. Intra-operative neurophysiology during microvascular decompression for hemifacial spasm. Clin Neurophysiol. 2012;123(1):78–83.
57. Wedekind C, Klug N. Recording nasal muscle F waves and electromyographic activity of the facial muscles: a comparison of two methods used for intraoperative monitoring of facial nerve function. J Neurosurg. 2001;95(6):974–8.
58. Merton PAMH. Stimulation of the cerebral cortex in the intact human subject. Nature. 1980;285(5762):227.
59. MacDonald DB. Safety of intraoperative transcranial electrical stimulation motor evoked potential monitoring. J Clin Neurophysiol. 2002;19(5):416–29.
60. Motoyama YKM, Yamada S, Nakagawa I, Nishimura F, Hironaka Y, Park YS, Hayashi H, Abe R, Nakase H. Evaluation of combined use of transcranial and direct cortical motor evoked potential monitoring during unruptured aneurysm surgery. Neurol Med Chir (Tokyo). 2011;51(1):15–22.
61. Dong CCMD, Akagami R, Westerberg B, Alkhani A, Kanaan I, Hassounah M. Intraoperative facial motor evoked potential monitoring with transcranial electrical stimulation during skull base surgery. Clin Neurophysiol. 2005;116(3):588–96.
62. Fukuda M, Oishi M, Takao T, Saito A, Fujii Y. Facial nerve motor-evoked potential monitoring during skull base surgery predicts facial nerve outcome. J Neurol Neurosurg Psychiatry. 2008;79(9):1066–70.
63. MacDonald DB, Dong CC, Uribe A. Intraoperative evoked potential techniques. Handb Clin Neurol. 2022;186:39–65.
64. Matthies C, Raslan F, Schweitzer T, Hagen R, Roosen K, Reiners K. Facial motor evoked potentials in cerebellopontine angle surgery: technique, pitfalls and predictive value. Clin Neurol Neurosurg. 2011;113(10):872–9.
65. Pepa GMD, Stifano V, D'Alessandris QG, Menna G, Burattini B, Domenico MD, et al. Intraoperative corticobulbar motor evoked potential in cerebellopontine angle surgery: a clinically meaningful tool to predict early and late facial nerve recovery. Neurosurgery. 2022;91(3):406–13.
66. Joo B-E, Kim J-S, Deletis V, Park KS. Advances in intraoperative neurophysiology during microvascular decompression surgery for hemifacial spasm. J Clin Neurol. 2022;18(4):410–20.

Correction to: Intraoperative Monitoring

Shi-Ting Li and Ying Ting-Ting

Correction to:
Chapter 24 in: S.-T. Li et al. (eds.), *Microvascular Decompression Surgery*, https://doi.org/10.1007/978-981-96-0767-9_24

The author has included Dr. Ting-Ting Ying as co-author for this chapter. The chapter has now been updated.

The updated version of this chapter can be found at
https://doi.org/10.1007/978-981-96-0767-9_24

S.-T. Li et al. (eds.), *Microvascular Decompression Surgery*,
https://doi.org/10.1007/978-981-96-0767-9_25

MIX
Papier aus verantwortungsvollen Quellen
Paper from responsible sources
FSC® C105338

If you have any concerns about our products,
you can contact us on
ProductSafety@springernature.com

In case Publisher is established outside the EU,
the EU authorized representative is:
Springer Nature Customer Service Center GmbH
Europaplatz 3, 69115 Heidelberg, Germany

Printed by Libri Plureos GmbH
in Hamburg, Germany